Practical
Cookery level 3

for VRQ and NVQ courses

John Campbell • David Foskett • Neil Rippington • Patricia Paskins

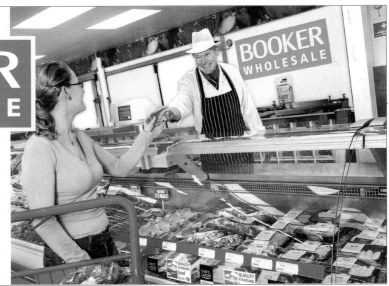

DYNAMIC LEARNING

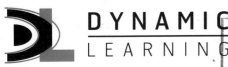

HODDER EDUCATION
AN HACHETTE UK COMPANY

Orders: please contact Bookpoint Ltd, 130 Milton Park, Abingdon, Oxon
OX14 4SB. Telephone: (44) 01235 827720. Fax: (44) 01235 400454. Lines are
open from 9.00–5.00, Monday to Saturday, with a 24-hour message answering
service. You can also order through our website www.hoddereducation.co.uk

If you have any comments to make about this, or any of our other titles, please
send them to educationenquiries@hodder.co.uk

British Library Cataloguing in Publication Data
A catalogue record for this title is available from the British Library

ISBN: 978 1444 122770

Previous editions published as *Advanced Practical Cookery*
First edition published 1995
Second edition published 1997
Third edition published 2002
Fourth edition published 2006
This edition published 2011

Impression number   10 9 8 7 6 5 4 3 2 1
Year   2013 2012 2011

Copyright © 2011 John Campbell, David Foskett, Neil Rippington and Patricia
Paskins

Hachette UK's policy is to use papers that are natural, renewable and recyclable
products and made from wood grown in sustainable forests. The logging and
manufacturing processes are expected to conform to the environmental regulations
of the country of origin.

Cover photo by Andrew Callaghan
Typeset by Fakenham Prepress Solutions, Fakenham, Norfolk NR21 8NN
Printed in Italy for Hodder Education, An Hachette UK Company, 338 Euston Road,
London NW1 3BH

Contents

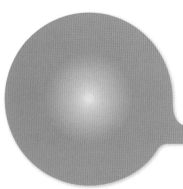

Introduction

This book will build on the practical skills you developed at Level 2, introducing you to the new techniques and theoretical knowledge you need to become a competent chef in the global hospitality industry.

Hospitality and the cooking and serving of food are an important part of our lives and can be traced back to the ancient Greeks and Romans. Hospitality and food have always been about entertaining, nourishment, friendship, celebration and the creation of satisfaction and happiness.

Good chefs are educators and communicators; their creativity inspires people. John Campbell is one of the UK's most respected chefs. He was classically trained and he has achieved a high standard of excellence, developing his professional skills into a modern classical cuisine. Many of his recipes are featured in this book, and you will learn a great deal from them, and from his demonstrations, available on Dynamic Learning.

We wish you well in your learning and future careers. Hopefully, studying and using this book will give you the competitive edge so that you can become a great chef, communicator and educator.

About the Level 3 qualifications

The Level 3 diploma (VRQ) focuses on advanced culinary skills, with a sound theoretical foundation. The techniques can be applied across a range of recipes and products. To achieve the diploma, you will complete practical tasks and theoretical assessments. Each chapter of this book relates to one unit of the diploma.

The diploma is highly regarded by the industry across a range of disciplines.

This book also fully supports the Level 3 NVQs in Professional Cookery and Professional Cookery (Patisserie and Confectionery). The mapping grid on page ix shows where each NVQ unit is covered in the book.

Remember that learning is for life; the journey continues.

Nutritional evaluation of the recipes in this book

The healthy eating and nutrition information in this book has been provided by Dr Jenny Poulter and Jane Cliff. Both are public health nutritionists with a proven track record in chef education, catering training, research and evaluation. It is because of national concern with the alarming increase in cases of obesity, particularly in the young, that we invited Jenny and Jane to develop the nutritional analysis for the recipes and provide healthy eating tips where appropriate.

Vegetable oil was used as the first choice of oil for the nutritional analysis, unless specified otherwise, and butter was used as the first choice over margarine. Semi-skimmed milk was used as the first choice unless otherwise stated.

We are most grateful to Jenny and Jane for their contribution and our special thanks go to Pat Bacon SRD, who undertook the recipe analysis with efficiency and patience.

Some of the recipes in this book have been analysed using a specialised computer software program (CompEat Pro, Version 5.8.0, released in 2002). This program converts foods into nutrients by drawing on a massive compositional database derived from the laboratory analysis of representative foods. The most recent version of this database, from the Food Standards Agency, has been used, alongside additional compositional data from manufacturers and approved texts.

Every effort has been made to ensure that the figures are as accurate as possible — however they must be treated as estimates only, for a number of reasons:

- the nutrient composition of individual foods can vary and an average value has been used (based on McCance and Widdowson (2002) *The Composition of Foods* (6th edn), Cambridge: Royal Society of Chemistry/Food Standards Agency)
- where it is more appropriate, analysis is based on the cooked weights (assumed edible portions) of a recipe item
- estimates of average weights have been made for ingredients where no weight was given (e.g. 3 eggs, 12 king-sized prawns)
- where compositional data is not available for a specific 'less common' ingredient (e.g. capers, foie gras, wild mushrooms) then the nearest best equivalent food has been used to provide the nutritional data.

In order to help you interpret this nutritional information, a system has been developed that bands recipes by virtue of their saturated fat content (see the diagram below). In terms of health these are perhaps two of the most important parameters to look at, because:

- saturated fat content gives some indication of heart health value

- calories give an indication of fat content (usually the higher the fat content the higher the calorie content) and portion size; this is where people need to exert more control in order to tackle obesity in the UK.

The bands are:
- Below 4 g saturated fat/portion:

- 4–6.9 g saturated fat/portion:

- Above 7 g saturated fat/portion:

Lots of the recipes in this book are high in saturated fat (red banding), total fat and calories. This is illustrated well in the fish section, where many recipes are 'red' (i.e. contain more than 7 g saturated fat/portion) and have high calorie values even though white fish is inherently low in fat (both saturated and unsaturated). The main reasons for this are that many of these recipes:
- rely on butter and cream to add flavour and texture
- often add large quantities of oil — to fry, seal or as a dressing
- provide very large portion sizes.

Creative chefs can use their expertise to modify these dishes sensitively, to make healthier changes in a way that does not compromise flavour, texture or appearance. This is the challenge for the next decade.

Acknowledgements

We are most grateful to Booker PLC, in particular Ron Hickey and Niall Brannigan, for their support in the development of the book, including the provision of the food shown in the photographs.

We are also very grateful to the following for their assistance in preparing this book:

- Steve Thorpe, Iain Middleton, Tony Taylor, Martin Houghton and Alan Baxter for their advice
- Atul Kochhar, Marc Sanders, René Pauvert, Gary Thompson and Neil Yule, who contributed recipes
- The staff at Coworth Park, part of the Dorchester Collection
- Alexia Chan, Deborah Edwards Noble and Melissa Brunelli at Hodder Education, and Rick Jackman, Sylvia Worth and Jane Jackson.

Photography

Most of the photos in this book are by Andrew Callaghan of Callaghan Studios. The photography work could not have been done without the help of the authors and their colleagues and students at Thames Valley University (TVU) and Colchester Institute. The publishers would particularly like to acknowledge the following people for their work.

John Campbell and Olly Rouse organised the photography at TVU. They were assisted in the kitchen by:

- Ryan Anthony
- Jovita Dmello
- Michael Greenham
- Lim Hyeonsik
- James Knowles
- Tarkan Nevzat
- Yulee Shin.

Neil Rippington, Chris Barker, Stephanie Conway and Paula Summerell organised the photography at Colchester Institute. They were assisted in the kitchen by:

- Nicholas Henn
- Chris Hopkins
- Georgie Lund
- Alice Wright.

The authors and publishers are grateful to everyone involved for their hard work.

About the contributors

Chris Barker completed his apprenticeship with Trust House Forte before working at The Intercontinental Hotel, London in the pastry section under Michael Nadell. He then moved to The Ritz Hotel as Chef Patissier. As well as teaching patisserie at Colchester Institute, Chris is currently Curriculum Manager with responsibility for part-time and Level 3 full-time chefs' programmes.

Stephanie Conway has worked in some of the finest country house hotels including Rhinefield House Hotel under Richard Bertinet. After a stint at the White Barn Inn in Maine, USA, Stephanie worked at London's Royal Garden Hotel under Nick Hollands, later becoming Chef Patissier at the London Marriott County Hall. Stephanie is currently employed as a chef lecturer at Colchester Institute, teaching patisserie.

Peter Eaton is Head Chef of Coworth Park, part of the Dorchester Collection. Peter followed John Campbell to Coworth Park in 2009, after being part of his kitchen team at the Vineyard at Stockcross since September 2004 as Head Chef, helping to earn the two Michelin stars. Peter previously spent seven and a half years at the two Michelin star *Le Manoir aux Quat'Saisons* in Oxford, working under Gary Jones and Raymond Blanc. Before that Peter spent four and a half years at Homewood Park Hotel where, during this time, the restaurant gained a Michelin star and received 8 out of 10 in the *Good Food Guide*.

Olly Rouse is Head Chef of Restaurant John Campbell at The Dorchester Collection's Coworth Park, Surrey. Formerly sous chef at the two Michelin starred restaurant The Vineyard at Stockcross, Olly consults internationally on the modern use of cooking techniques including sous vide.

Paula Summerell started her career with Michael Nadell in the pastry section of The Intercontinental Hotel, London. After a summer season working in Luzern, Switzerland, she returned to London to work in the Pastry section at the Dorchester Hotel under Anton Mossimann. Paula then spent time working with Mark Hix at the Candlewick Room in the City of London and for Shell UK at their London headquarters. Paul is currently employed at Colchester Institute as a chef lecturer, teaching patisserie, food hygiene and nutrition.

Zamzani Abdul Wahab is a celebrity chef who has presented television programmes around the world and has published two books. He is Head of Special Projects at the School of Hospitality, Tourism and Culinary Arts, KDV College, Malaysia.

Wong Song Shing is Head of Culinary Arts at Silver Spoon International College, Malaysia. Previously he held the same role at Genting Inti International College. He has worked at the Wigmore Hall restaurant and Westminster City Inn Hotel, both in London, and at restaurants in the USA, Australia and Malaysia.

Picture credits

Every effort has been made to trace the copyright holders of material reproduced here. The authors and publishers would like to thank the following for permission to reproduce copyright illustrations:

pp.2, 3 © Bananastock/Photolibrary Group Ltd; p.5 © boumenjapet – Fotolia.com; p.6 © TA Craft Photography – Fotolia; p.10 © Bananastock/Photolibrary Group Ltd; p.13 © sylvie peruzzi – Fotolia.com; p.15 © Ken Ng – Fotolia.com; p.20 © Stockbyte/Getty Images; p.23 © Blend Images/Getty Images; p.24 © Steve Nagy/Design Pics Inc./Rex Features; pp.25, 26 © erwinova – Fotolia.com; p.32 © Bananastock/Photolibrary Group Ltd; p.38 © Ingor Normann – Fotolia; p.41 © Bananastock/Photolibrary Group Ltd; p.42 © Suhendri Utet – Fotolia.com; p.45 (left) © Bogdan Dumitru – Fotolia.com, (right) © Ayupov Evgeniy – Fotolia.com; p.50 © A.B. Dowsett/Science Photo Library; p.52 © quayside – Fotolia.com; p.55 © Eye Of Science/Science Photo Library; p.56 © Sozaijiten/Getty Images; p.61 © Bananastock/ Photolibrary Group Ltd; p.70 ©Olaf Doering/Alamy; p.73 © Bananastock/Photolibrary Group Ltd; p.75 © Ingram Publishing Ltd; p.77 (top) © Photolibrary.com, (bottom) © CuboImages srl/Alamy; p.84 © Ingram Publishing Ltd; p.85 © Awe Inspiring Images – Fotolia.com; pp.99 (top), 104 (top), 106 (top), 108 (top), 119, 134, 158 (top) Sam Bailey/Hodder Education; p.166 Zamzani Abdul Wahab; p.174 Sam Bailey/Hodder Education; p.179 Zamzani Abdul Wahab; pp.181, 186, 195 Sam Bailey/Hodder Education; pp.203, 204 Zamzani Abdul Wahab; p.215 Sam Bailey/Hodder Education; p.216 Zamzani Abdul Wahab; pp.225, 227, 229, 236–8, 240, 253, 256, 263, 274, 278 (bottom), 373 (bottom) Sam Bailey/Hodder Education; p.389 reproduced under the terms of the click-use licence.

Except where stated above, photographs are by Andrew Callaghan, and illustrations by Barking Dog Art.

Reasons to come to Booker the UK's biggest wholesaler

To find your nearest branch visit www.booker.co.uk

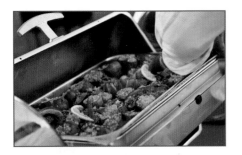

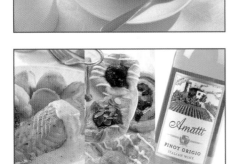

choice up

Huge range
The average branch carries over 10,000 lines in stock the whole time, with even more available to order.

New Lines
Our expert buyers are constantly sourcing great new lines for you. Look for the 'New Line shelf' cards in branch, every week.

prices down

Catering Price check
Our catering price check service allows you to enter your current Brakes or 3663 prices and, with one click, instantly see if you can buy cheaper from Booker. Why not compare our prices for yourself by visiting www.booker.co.uk today!

Essentials - every day low price
We have lock down prices on a range of products that are essential to your business. From bread, milk, eggs and potatoes through to sugar, tuna, chips and peas we will give you a low price, every day to help you plan your menu and your budget.

better service

Internet ordering
The easiest way to place your order with your branch is via our website. Simply log on to www.booker.co.uk, and register for online ordering. Its so simple - start today!

Free, 7 days a week, delivery service*
All your fresh produce, frozen, wet and dry goods delivered to your door on the one vehicle - 7 days a week.

*Terms and conditions apply - see in branch for details.

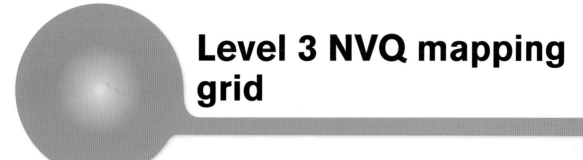

Level 3 NVQ mapping grid

This grid will help you find the information you need for every unit of your Level 3 NVQ.

For NVQ Professional Cookery (Patisserie and Confectionery), only the highlighted units apply.

NVQ Professional Cookery Level 3

NVQ unit	Sections of the book
CU1063 Maintain Food Safety when Storing, Preparing and Cooking Food	Chapter 2
CU339 Maintain the Health, Hygiene, Safety and Security of the Working Environment	Chapter 1
CBU26 Develop Productive Working Relationships with Colleagues	Chapter 1
CU944 Produce Healthier Dishes	Chapter 13 pages 388–93
CU1015 Cook and Finish Complex Fish Dishes	Chapter 7
CU1016 Cook and Finish Complex Shellfish Dishes	Chapter 7
CU1017 Cook and Finish Complex Meat Dishes	Chapter 5
CU1018 Cook and Finish Complex Poultry Dishes	Chapter 6
CU1020 Cook and Finish Complex Vegetable Dishes	Chapter 4
CU1021 Prepare Fish for Complex Dishes	Chapter 7
CU1022 Prepare Shellfish for Complex Dishes	Chapter 7
CU1023 Prepare Meat for Complex Dishes	Chapter 5
CU1024 Prepare Poultry for Complex Dishes	Chapter 6
CU1025 Prepare Game for Complex Dishes	Chapter 6
CU1026 Prepare, Cook and Finish Complex Hot Sauces	Chapters 4 to 7 and 11
CU1027 Prepare, Cook and Present Canapés and Cocktail Products	Chapters 4 to 7
CU1028 Prepare, Cook and Finish Dressings and Cold Sauces	Chapter 4, particularly pages 96–7 and 122–6
CU1029 Prepare, Cook and Finish Complex Hot Desserts	Chapter 9
CU1030 Prepare, Cook and Finish Complex Cold Desserts	Chapter 9

NVQ unit	Sections of the book
CU1031 Produce Sauces, Fillings and Coatings for Complex Desserts	Chapters 9 and 11
CU1032 Prepare, Cook and Finish Complex Soups	Pages 116–21, 258–60, 274 and 277
CU1033 Prepare, Cook and Finish Fresh Pasta Dishes	Pages 140, 141, 171, 185, 255, 267 and 275
CU1034 Prepare, Cook and Finish Complex Bread and Dough Products	Chapter 8
CU1035 Prepare, Cook and Finish Complex Cakes, Sponges, Biscuits and Scones	Chapter 12
CU1036 Prepare, Cook and Finish Complex Pastry Products	Chapter 10
CU1037 Prepare, Process and Finish Complex Chocolate Products	Chapters 9 and 12
CU1038 Prepare, Process and Finish Marzipan, Pastillage and Sugar Products	Chapters 9 and 12
CU1039 Prepare, Cook and Present Complex Cold Products	Chapters 4 and 7
CU920 Employment Rights and Responsibilities in the Hospitality, Leisure, Travel and Tourism Sector	Chapter 1
CU338 Contribute to the Control of Resources	Chapter 1
CU364 Ensure Food Safety Practices are Followed in the Preparation and Serving of Food and Drink	Chapter 2
CU350 Contribute to the Development of Recipes and Menus	Chapter 3

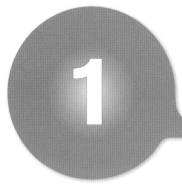

Supervisory skills

This chapter covers Unit 301: Supervisory Skills in the Hospitality Industry. In this chapter you will learn how to:

1. Apply and monitor good health and safety practices
2. Apply and monitor good health and safety training
3. Apply staff supervisory skills within a small team.

1.1   Apply and monitor good health and safety practices and training

Supervising health and safety in the workplace

Chefs de partie, sous chefs and head chefs are all responsible for supervising health and safety. It is important that such people in the kitchen supervise the day-to-day work, train employees in good practice and ensure that they achieve high standards in maintaining health and safety. As part of their roles they also advise management on health and safety issues. The management of health and safety at work involves:

- Organising managers, supervisors and employees in ways so that they can implement the health and safety policy of the establishment
- Measuring health and safety performance and reviewing that performance
- Auditing of the whole health and safety system
- Planning for health and safety, setting standards and implementing the health and safety policy
- Reviewing and developing the health and safety policy.

The chef as a supervisor

Many chefs have the role of supervisor built into their job specification and job responsibilities. As a supervisor you have a key role to play in maintaining health and safety and will need to put into practice the health and safety systems and controls designed by the management team with the involvement of the supervisor.

As a chef acting as a supervisor, you need to be involved in planning health and safety initiatives, training employees and monitoring health and safety performance standards. In order to identify hazards you must carry out safety inspections. This means observing how people carry out their daily work. If you have any concerns you must discuss them with the employees and the manager.

As a working chef you will need to identify the training needs of the establishment. You need to review each individual training need and assess how safe people are when doing their jobs. Often the chef as a supervisor will be part of a committee on health and safety which establishments are required to have to ensure safety inspections are carried out and so that accidents are investigated.

Supervising work tasks

Chefs are responsible for overseeing and carrying out work tasks. These tasks and procedures must adhere to the establishment's health and safety policy. The employee must carry out all procedures and tasks that he or she needs to complete safely and to a high standard.

The supervisor must, at all times, give guidance, demonstrate good practice and ensure that all work activities are carried out in a disciplined manner. Different employees will need varying levels of supervision. Competent people also need supervising to check that they do not fall into bad habits or take dangerous short cuts.

Particular attention must be paid to people who are vulnerable to a higher risk of injury.

Jobs in the kitchen Name three jobs in the kitchen that you consider present a higher risk of injury than others.

Develop effective working relationships

In the hospitality industry it is essential that as a supervisor you develop effective working relationships with other supervisors. It is important to discuss health and safety and monitoring issues at team meetings as well as any major issues relating to health and safety. When new equipment has been installed, for example, there will be a need for written safety procedures and for staff to be trained in how to use the equipment.

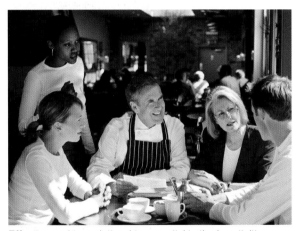
Effective working relationships are vital in the hospitality industry

Supervisors are an important link between employees and managers. You must communicate effectively about health and safety issues. Good communication can maintain employee motivation; this, in turn, helps to build the team and creates a health and safety culture that engages and supports staff so that they are able to eliminate risks and control them. Always welcome staff comments and encourage staff to report problems. Treat those who report problems openly and fairly. Give them confidence in you and your ability. Make sure that you deal promptly with any conflicts on health and safety amongst staff and reach solutions quickly. You may, on occasions, be involved in disciplining an employee for a breach of health and safety rules.

What is a good supervisor?
A good supervisor is someone who:
- Is open
- Is fair
- Is well informed
- Is well organised
- Is a good communicator
- Shows respect for others
- Gives support to others to establish policies and procedures.

Health and safety is about protecting people from harm, injuries and illness. It is important that you and other employees always act within the procedures laid down in the health and safety policy.

Supervisors must have completed a recognised training programme and attend regular updates.

Maintaining security and health and safety procedures
As a supervisor it is essential that you maintain security and health and safety procedures in own areas of responsibility. To ensure that legislation regarding safety and security is implemented, it is necessary:
1. For the legislation to be known
2. That the requirements are carried out
3. That a system of checks makes certain that the legislation is complied with.

First, all people involved in an establishment must be made aware of the need for safety and security and their legal responsibilities towards themselves, their colleagues, their employers and members of the public.

A system of checks, both spot-checks and regular inspections at frequent intervals, needs to be set up and the observations and recommendations resulting from these inspections should be recorded and passed to superiors for action. The details would include time and date of inspection, exact site and a clear description of the breach of security or fault of safety equipment. This information would be acted upon promptly according to the policy of the organisation.

It is the responsibility of everyone at the workplace to be conscious of safety and security and to pass on to the appropriate people recommendations for improving the procedures for maintaining safety and security. The types of equipment that need to be inspected to make certain that they are available and ready for use include security equipment, in addition to first-aid and fire-fighting equipment. The supervisor or person responsible for these items needs to regularly check and record that they are in working condition and that, if they have been used, they are restored ready for further use. Security systems and fire-fighting equipment are usually checked by the makers. It is the responsibility of the management of the establishment to ensure that this equipment is maintained correctly. First-aid equipment is usually the responsibility of the designated first aider, whose functions include replenishing first-aid boxes. However, a chef de partie or supervisor will be aware that if fire extinguishers and first-aid equipment are used, he or she has a responsibility to take action to maintain the equipment by reporting to the appropriate person. It is advisable that all staff are trained in the use of fire extinguishers.

Routine checks or inspections need to be carried out in any establishment to see that standards of hygiene, health and safety are maintained for the benefit of workers, customers and other members of the public. Visitors, suppliers and contractors are also entitled to expect the premises to be safe when they enter. Particular attention needs to be paid to exits and entrances, passageways and the provision of adequate lighting. Floors need to be sound, uncluttered and well lit. Disposal of rubbish and bin areas need particular care regarding cleanliness, health and safety. Toilets, staff rooms and changing rooms need to be checked regularly. All staff must adopt hygienic and safe work practices. They should be conscious at all times and in all places of work of the health and safety of the premises. Failure to do so may result in accidents and the spread of infections. Any discrepancies and damage should be reported, as should any unsafe or unhealthy features.

Checks or inspections would usually be carried out by a person responsible for health and safety within the organisation, with authority to take action to remedy faults and discrepancies, and to implement improvements.

Monitoring inspections and recording evidence is an important aspect of the supervisor's role. Even more important is that any shortcomings are remedied at once. Inspections should be regular and particular attention should be paid to hazards, security, safety equipment and cleanliness.

Records, which should be accurate and legible, should include the date and time of inspection, by whom the entry was made and details of what has

been checked. Any hazards, faults, lack of cleanliness, damage or discrepancies should be recorded.

If you observe any unhygienic and unsafe practices they can best be remedied by training the individuals involved and giving constructive explanations as to why their practices are unhygienic and unsafe. Persons with infections or notifiable diseases must be made aware of their responsibility to inform their employer.

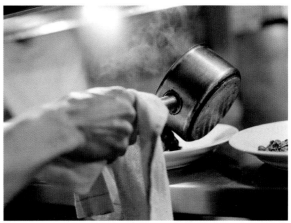

An example of safe practice: using a cloth when holding a hot pan handle

Maintain a healthy and safe working environment

It is necessary to be aware of the policy and procedures of the organisation in relation to health and safety legislation. Every individual at work anywhere on the premises needs to develop an attitude towards possible hazardous situations in order to prevent accidents to themselves and others. Training is also essential to develop good practice and should include information on what hazards to look for, hygienic methods of working and the procedures to follow in the event of an incident. You should keep records of staff training in these areas.

It is essential that checks are made to maintain high standards of health and safety at work and to comply with the law, so that employees, employers and members of the public remain safe and healthy.

Every organisation will have procedures to follow in the event of a fire, accident, flood or bomb alert; every employee needs to have knowledge of these procedures.

Every establishment must have a book to record accidents. It is also desirable to have a book to record items that are in need of maintenance due to wear and tear or damage, so that these faults can be remedied. Details of incidents, such as power failure, flooding, infestation, contamination, and so on, which do not result in an accident, should be recorded in an incident book.

Records should be kept of items lost, damaged or discarded, giving details of why and how it happened and what subsequent steps have been taken.

It is the responsibility of chefs, supervisors and others concerned with health and safety to ensure that training and instruction are given so as to prevent accidents and to help staff work efficiently and safely. Problems that may occur as a result of any staff failing to comply with health and safety standards should be identified and appropriate action taken.

Lapse in security Write down what could happen if security lapses or breaks down in a hotel's kitchen and restaurant.

Health and safety at work

What is health?

Health is normally defined as the soundness of body. The World Health Organisation defines it as 'The state of complete physical, mental and social well-being and not merely the absence of disease or infirmity'.

When we consider health, we associate it with adequate ventilation, lighting and overall cleanliness, correct temperature levels and no overcrowding; with everyday practices in particular workplaces such as handling chemicals; and with procedures to deal with hazards like exposure to dust, fumes and biological agents.

Lack of control in the workplace over work procedures involving health risks can lead to ill health or lead to conditions that will result in ill health.

What does it mean to be safe?

It means that the individual is free from danger or risk of danger from:

- The contracting and use of machinery in the workplace
- Handling dangerous substances
- The lifting of heavy equipment
- Slippery floors, passageways and stairs
- Personal injury because personal protection clothing is used.

Work under the Health and Safety at Work Act 1974 means work as an employee or as a self-employed person. An employee is a person who works under a contract of employment. A self-employed person can be described as someone who works for reward or gain for his or herself rather than under a contract of employment. A self-employed person may or may not employ others.

The Health and Safety at Work Act makes it clear that employees are at work when carrying out tasks that are in their job description, for which they are paid by their employer; so employees are not 'at work' when they are engaged in activities that are not within the course of their specific employment. Employees cannot be asked to carry out a work task that is not in their job description or that they are not qualified to do.

Voluntary workers and those on work experience are also regarded as being employees as far as health and safety at work is concerned.

i Terms associated with health and safety at work:

Workplace This is a place or places where employees are likely to work or which they have to frequent in the course of their employment.

Welfare May be referred to as looking after people's well-being at work, providing good changing facilities, staff feeding and washing facilities, sanitary conveniences and ensuring that the facilities are comfortable and safe.

Occupational health This covers the overall state of the person's mental and social well-being at work as a consequence of their work. A wide range of workplace conditions and practices is usually associated with occupational health. These include air quality, manual handling, the use of and exposure to chemicals and biological agents, exposure to fumes and dust, and work stress.

Assessment and reduction of risk

The prevention of both accidents and food poisoning in catering establishments is essential. It is necessary to assess each situation and decide what action should be taken.

In most professionally operated catering establishments the hazards are few and easy to check and much of what is called for is a matter of common sense.

Accidents do occur in kitchens but rarely lead to serious injury. However, all accident situations are undesirable and minimising their numbers depends on the development and maintenance of a safety culture. The first step in accident control is identifying potential hazards.

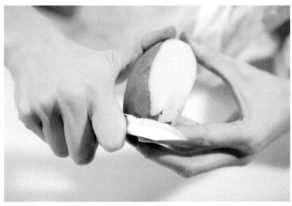

Everyday kitchen tasks have the potential to cause injuries

Injuries can result from slips, trips, falls and knife cuts, and people may suffer scalds and burns as a result of being in contact with hot liquids, hot surfaces and steam. Despite the existence of these hazards, experienced and knowledgeable chefs tend to foresee and avoid them.

An awareness of how to work in a kitchen and avoid these hazards develops through experience but can be facilitated through induction and training.

It is important to understand the meaning of the following three terms, which are in regular use:

1. **Hazard:** the potential to cause harm
2. **Risk:** the likelihood that harm will result from a particular hazard (the catering environment may have many hazards but the aim is to have few risks)
3. **Accident:** an unplanned or uncontrolled event that leads to or could have led to an injury, damage to plant or other loss.

Carrying out a risk assessment

A risk assessment can be divided into four areas:

1. Minimal risk: safe conditions with safety measures in place

2. Some risk: acceptable risk; however, attention must be paid to ensure that safety measures operate
3. Significant risk: where safety measures are not fully in operation (also includes food most likely to cause food poisoning); requires immediate action
4. Dangerous risk: where processes and operation of equipment should stop immediately; the system or equipment should be completely checked and operation recommenced after clearance.

In carrying out a risk assessment ensure that you:

- Assess the risks
- Determine preventative measures
- Decide who carries out safety inspections
- Decide frequency of inspection
- Determine methods of reporting back and to whom
- Detail how to ensure inspections are effective
- Carry out safety training related to the job.

The purpose of the exercise of assessing the possibility of risks and hazards is to prevent accidents.

Under the Control of Substances Hazardous to Health Regulations (COSHH) 1999, it is necessary for employers to carry out risk assessments of all hazardous chemicals and substances that employees may be exposed to at work and to survey all areas, in order to ascertain the chemicals and substances in use.

Some examples of chemical substances found in kitchens are:

- Cleaning chemicals, alkalis and acids
- Detergents, sanitisers, descalers
- Chemicals associated with burnishing
- Pest control chemicals, insecticides and rodenticides

Chefs and kitchen workers must also be aware of the correct handling methods required.

Kitchen equipment: risk Consider a kitchen in which you have worked and list the equipment that you considered to be (a) low risk and (b) high risk.

Accidents

What is an accident?

An accident is an unlooked-for mishap, an untoward event which is not expected or designed and is unintended and an unexpected loss or hurt. What is clear is that an accident is an:

- Unplanned and uncontrolled event
- Event that causes injury, damage or loss
- Event that could lead to a near-miss accident or could result in no loss or damage at all.

Accidents do not just happen. They arise from uncontrolled events, usually from a chain of uncontrolled events.

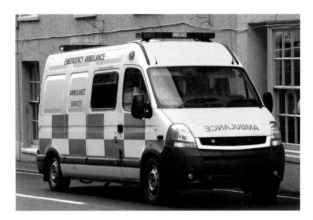

The outcome of an accident may be:
- Death
- Personal injury
- Long-term health problems
- Damage to property or premises
- Damage to the environment
- No injury or damage at all.

Why do accidents occur?

Human, occupational, environmental and organisational factors may all contribute to accidents that occur in the workplace (see Table 1.1).

The causes of accidents

Accidents happen in many ways. The three main causes are:

1. Unsafe actions
2. Unsafe conditions
3. A combination of unsafe actions and unsafe conditions.

Unsafe acts in the kitchen may include:
- Using unsafe equipment such as sharp or mechanical equipment without guards
- Walking on slippery floors
- Carrying saucepans of boiling water
- Carrying sharp knives
- Using damaged equipment
- Lifting heavy loads in an unsafe manner
- Not wearing protective clothing
- Using unsafe chemicals or cleaning chemicals without following the manufacturers' instructions
- Inadequate maintenance of work equipment
- Poor environmental conditions, such as poor lighting, extreme temperatures, high humidity, poorly designed buildings
- Dirty environment
- Broken machine guards
- Poor work system in place
- Wearing loose clothing that can get trapped in machines.

Accidents will occur in the workplace if health and safety is not taken seriously and there is no culture of safety. There is a low risk of accidents in an organisation that has an effective health and safety policy and a strong safety culture and a real commitment from management.

Table 1.1 Factors that may contribute to accidents

Human factors	These include the inability to recognise hazards and risks; lack of skills; general attitude to safety (e.g. taking short cuts, insufficient care); tiredness; effects of alcohol and drugs.
Occupational factors	These involve being exposed to risk in the workplace due to your occupation. For example, a chef may risk cuts, a computer operator risks eye strain.
Environmental factors	These refer to the working environment such as poor lighting, poor air quality and excessively high temperatures in the kitchen. The time available to carry out certain jobs and the pressure of the work environment are also significant.
Organisational factors	The organisation or establishment could affect the safety of staff; for example, the safety standards of the organisation, safety precautions that are enforced and encouraged by the employer. The effectiveness of communication between work colleagues and the employer. The amount of training individuals have received; advice and supervision.

The cost of accidents

The results of accidents may mean that:

- Lives can be lost
- People are injured
- Money is wasted
- Machinery is damaged
- Products are damaged
- Reputation is lost.

Employees, their friends and close relatives, as well as the general public, may all incur costs following an accident. See Table 1.2.

For the employers there are direct and indirect costs associated with accidents. See Table 1.3.

Personal negligence Think of an accident that could occur through personal negligence at your workplace. What effect would that have on the individual employee and the employer?

Management of occupational health

Occupational health is usually associated with illness and disease caused by work and the workplace. In some cases, the cause of disease is not known for several years.

The management of occupational health is about controlling hazards that affect the body over a long period such as, for example, breathing in asbestos fibres, or a back injury from frequent lifting. In a kitchen you will find chemicals for cleaning which may cause skin problems. It is important to understand how such substances are able to enter the body and cause health problems so that preventative measures can be implemented.

Substances such as chemicals enter the body by:

- Breathing in (inhalation)
- Absorption (through the skin or eyes)
- Ingestion (eating or drinking)
- Infection (puncturing the skin).

Harmful substances include:

- Aerosols
- Fumes
- Dust
- Fibres
- Liquids

Table 1.2 Cost of accidents to employees, their friends and family and the general public

Cost of accidents to:		
Employees	**Close friends and family of employees**	**General public**
• Personal injury or death • Pain and suffering • Loss of earnings • Loss of quality of life	• Distress and grief • Anxiety • Loss of earnings while looking after sick or injured person • Loss of quality of life	• Personal injury or death • Pain and suffering • Loss of earnings • Loss of quality of life • Medical costs

Table 1.3 Costs of accidents to employers

Costs of accidents to employers	
Direct costs	**Indirect costs**
• Damage and repairs to buildings, vehicles, machinery or stock • Legal costs • Fines (criminal court case) • Compensation (civil court case or agreed compensation) • Loss of product • Overtime payments • Employee medical costs • Employer's liability and public liability claims • Increased insurance premiums	• Loss of output to business • Product liability payments • Time and money spent on investigating an accident • Loss of good will between employees and management • Loss of consumer confidence • Damage to corporate reputation • Hiring and training of replacement staff • Loss of expertise

- Vapours
- Gases.

> **Occupational health and a healthy lifestyle** Explain why companies should take occupational health seriously. How can managers and companies assist in promoting a healthy lifestyle?

The symptoms or effects of harmful substances are grouped together as:

- Irritations: can develop into a rash or dermatitis
- Sensitisation: skin rashes, allergies, asthma, coughing and sneezing
- Carcinogenic: that is, causing cancer, usually over a long period.

Occupational health hazards which may occur through work include:

- Noise and vibration
- Ionising radiation
- Biological hazards
- Work-related upper limb disorders
- Back problems
- Stress
- Passive smoking
- Repetitive strain injury.

> **Promoting good health** Design a poster to promote occupational health and a healthy lifestyle. Think of a celebrity sports person you could use in your promotional material.

Reducing accidents and illness

By law workplaces must take steps to prevent and control accidents, incidents, personal injury and ill health.

The stages involved in reducing the risk from accidents and illness in the workplace are as follows:

- Find out what causes harm in the workplace
- Decide who in the workplace can be harmed
- Determine what preventative measures are needed to reduce the risk of harm
- Plan the actions to introduce the measures
- Implement the measures
- Record the outcomes of the work, procedures and actions introduced to reduce risk.

Monitoring system

To help reduce accidents, set up a monitoring system. This is a system of regular daily checks on what is going on in the workplace that helps to identify the safety practices that the business needs to adopt in order to reduce the risk to employees and others.

Employ a system of control

In order to reduce or eliminate any risk you should use a system of control. Ensure that you:

- Eliminate or avoid the hazard in the workplace
- Substitute a less hazardous piece of work equipment or substance
- Control the risk at source by separating the people from the hazard to reduce risk
- Implement safe working procedures. Decide a safe system of work to control the hazards and risk
- Provide training: always provide training information and instruction for employees and supervise them
- Use personal protective equipment (PPE). Always use personal protective equipment to reduce the risk of harm.

Intervention programmes

These are actions which aim to change the way health and safety is dealt with in an organisation. The actions are interwoven into the policies and procedures of an organisation and they introduce new ways of working that aim to reduce the number of hazards and the number and severity of risks to health and safety.

When designing and implementing intervention programmes it is important to:

- Get the commitment of service managers to sign up to high standards of health and safety
- Analyse the causes of accidents
- Carry out an audit of safety plans
- Raise awareness in the workplace about the risks
- Identify all preventative measures
- Design systems to protect the employee by reviewing the method of work and ensuring the environment is suitable for the work being carried out
- Set up education, training and instruction programmes for employees.

It is important to get all employees involved in designing the intervention programmes. Work as a team and listen to what people have to say. Everyone has an interest in making the workplace safe.

Management systems

Management systems are designed to reduce accidents and illness. The management system should include:

- The health and safety policy
- An organisational structure to implement the policy
- A commitment to health and safety from the employer
- Full integration of health and safety
- Measures and procedures to protect the health and safety of people affected by the operation
- Good communication arrangements
- A commitment from the management team and the workforce to continue to improve and monitor health and safety
- Good monitoring procedures
- A review process.

Health and safety in a production kitchen Design a health and safety policy for a production kitchen.

Legislation and enforcement

Many of the health and safety regulations in the UK are a result of directions from the European Union.

Health and Safety at Work Act

The main piece of legislation dealing with workplace health and safety in England, Wales and Scotland is the Health and Safety at Work Act 1974. Largely similar provision is covered in Northern Ireland under the Health and Safety at Work (Northern Ireland) Order 1978.

The aims of the legislation are:

- To secure the health, safety and welfare of people at work
- To protect people other than those at work against the risks of health and safety that arise out of or in connection with the activities of people at work
- To control the keeping and use of explosive, highly flammable or otherwise dangerous substances at work.

The legislation is about:

- Control
- Providing regulations and approved codes of practice which set the standards of health, safety and welfare.

The Health and Safety Commission

The organisation appointed to regulate health and safety at work is the Health and Safety Commission (HSC).

The HSC is appointed by the Secretary of State. The commission is responsible for proposing health and safety law and standards. It consults professional bodies with an interest in health and safety such as trade unions and industry.

The HSC:

- Appoints the **Health and Safety Executive** (HSE) which regulates health and safety law in industry and public areas
- Gives **local authorities** delegated power to regulate health and safety law in premises such as retail shops, offices, catering services, restaurants, hotels, and so on.

Authorised officers

Health and safety law is enforced by:

- Health and safety inspectors from the HSE
- Environmental health officers (EHOs) and technical officers from local authorities
- Fire officers from the fire service
- For factories, farms and hospitals, a health and safety inspector from the HSE
- For shops, restaurants and leisure centres, the local EHO. Fire officers can visit all these premises for the purposes of enforcing the law on fire safety and fire precautions.

Legal responsibilities

Everyone in the workplace has a responsibility for health and safety. The Act makes it clear that everyone at work – employers, managers and workers – has a responsibility for health and safety. Employers and managers, for example, have the obligation to identify hazards, assess the risks that are present in the workplace and introduce precautions and preventative measures to reduce risks.

Employers' responsibilities to their employees

Every employer has a duty to ensure health and safety and welfare at work of all employees in so far as is reasonably practicable. In hospitality this means:

- Providing and maintaining kitchens, restaurants, accommodation and systems of work that are safe and without risk to health
- Making sure that storage areas and transporting articles such as food, and so on, are safe and there is an absence of risk to health

- There is information and instruction on training and supervision that is necessary to ensure the health and safety of employees at work
- Maintaining the premises and building to make sure they are safe and pose no risk to health
- Maintaining entrances and exits to the workplace and access to work areas that are safe and without risk to health
- Providing a clean and safe environment with good welfare facilities
- Where necessary, providing health surveillance of employees.

Employers must provide a written statement about:

- The general policy towards employees' health and safety at work
- The organisation and arrangements for carrying out that policy.

An organisation with a board of directors/governors must formally and publicly accept its collective role in providing health and safety leadership in the organisation.

Welfare facilities for chefs State what you would consider to be good welfare facilities for chefs.

Duties of employees

Every employee has a duty to take reasonable care of his or her own health and safety and that of other people who may be affected by what he or she does or does not do in the course of carrying out work. Employees must cooperate with the employer to enable the employer to comply with the relevant employer's duties.

Regulations

The main current health and safety regulations were originally made in 1992. Since 1992 some of the regulations have been updated:

- Management of Health and Safety at Work Regulations 1999
- Personal Protective Equipment Regulations 1992
- Provision and Use of Work Equipment Regulations 1998 (PUWER)
- Manual Handling Operations Regulations 1992
- Workplace (Health, Safety and Welfare) Regulations 1992
- Health and Safety (Display Screen Equipment) Regulations 1992.

Other regulations which also apply to the workplace include:

- Lifting Operations and Lifting Equipment Regulations 1998 (LOLER)
- Control of Substances Hazardous to Health Regulations 2002 (COSHH)
- Noise at Work Regulations 1989
- The Health and Safety (First Aid) Regulations 1981
- Reporting Injuries, Diseases and Dangerous Occurrences Regulations 1995 (RIDDOR).

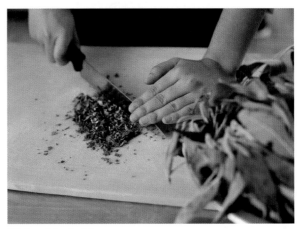

Work safely at all times

Approved codes of practice

The Health and Safety Commission can provide practical guidance for employers and employees to help them to comply with the regulations and duties which apply to them. The advice is issued as a code of practice. If the Health and Safety Commission approves these standards, they can bear the title approved codes of practice. They include a standard, a specification and any other form of practical advice.

Approved codes of practice have a special place in legislation. They are not law, but a failure to observe any part of an approved code of practice may be admissible in criminal court proceedings as evidence about a related alleged contravention of health and safety legislation. If the advice in the approved code of practice has not been followed, then it is up to the defendants to prove that they have satisfactorily complied with the requirement in some other way.

Examples of approved codes of practice are:

- Management of Health and Safety at Work
- Workplace Health, Safety and Welfare

- Control of Substances Hazardous to Health
- Safe Use of Work Equipment
- Safe Use of Lighting Equipment
- First Aid at Work.

Guidance

The Health and Safety Commission also produces guidance on many other technical health and safety subjects. Guidance does not have the same standing in law as approved codes of practice, but it can be used by employers, if followed, to show that they have complied with a recognised standard.

Examples of guidance include:
- Manual Handling
- Reducing Noise at Work
- Guide to COSHH Assessment.

Enforcement

Inspectors are appointed by the enforcing authorities by being issued with a warrant. The warrant specifies the inspector's powers.

The powers of inspectors

Inspectors have a number of powers including the right of entry to workplaces, to serve legal notices requiring improvement work to be done and prohibiting work procedures, processes and the use of work equipment.

Inspectors may:
- Enter premises
- Take a police officer with them
- Take an authorised person or equipment to help with the investigation
- Make necessary examinations and inspections
- Take measurements, photographs or recordings
- Take samples of articles or substances
- Dismantle or test any article or substance
- Take possession of and detain any article or substance for examination or to ensure that no-one tampers with it
- Require any person to give information to assist with any examination or investigation
- Require documents to be produced, inspected or copied
- Require that assistance and facilities be made available to allow the inspector's powers to be exercised
- Seize and render harmless any article or substance which the inspector believes to be a cause of imminent danger or serious personal injury.

Improvement notices

If the inspector thinks there is a contravention of health and safety legislation, he or she can serve an improvement notice on the person responsible stating the details of the contravention. The notice also requires the person responsible to remedy the contravention. The person responsible is the director, manager or supervisor in charge of the premises at the time of the inspection.

The notice must state:
- That a contravention exists
- The details of the law contravened
- The inspector's reasons for his or her opinion
- That the person responsible must remedy the contravention
- The time given for the remedy to be carried out. This must not be less than 21 days.

If a person fails to comply with an improvement notice, he or she commits a criminal offence.

Prohibition notices

If an inspector believes that work activities involve a serious risk of 'personal injury', a prohibition notice may be served on the person in charge of the work activity. The notice must:
- State that, in the inspector's opinion, there is a risk of serious personal injury
- Identify the matters which create the risk
- Give reasons why the inspector believes there to have been a contravention of health and safety law
- Direct that the activities stated in the notice must not be carried on, by or under the control of the person served with the notice, unless the matters which are associated with the risk have been rectified.

Appeals

The person who is served with an improvement on a prohibition notice can appeal against the notice to an employment tribunal. The grounds of the appeal could be based on the following:
- That the inspector interpreted the law incorrectly or exceeded their powers
- A contravention might be admitted but the appeal would be that the remedy was not practicable or not reasonably practicable

- A contravention might be admitted. The appeal would be based on the fact that the incident was so insignificant that the notice should be cancelled.

If an appeal is made against an improvement notice then the notice is suspended until the appeal is heard. If an appeal is made against a prohibition notice the notice is suspended only if the employment tribunal suspends it. If there is no compliance with the notice, the person served with the notice can be prosecuted.

Offences

A contravention of the Health and Safety at Work Act 1974 or any of the regulations made under the Act is a criminal offence. Both an individual and a corporate body can commit an offence and be tried for it in court. It is an offence to:

- Fail to carry out a duty placed on employers, self-employed employees, owners of premises, designers, manufacturers, importers and suppliers
- Intentionally or recklessly interfere with anything provided for safety purposes
- Require payment for anything that an employer must by law provide in the interests of health and safety
- Contravene any requirement of any health and safety regulations
- Contravene any requirement imposed by an inspector
- Prevent or attempt to prevent a person from appearing before an inspector or from answering his/her questions
- Contravene an improvement or prohibition notice
- Intentionally obstruct an inspector in the exercise of his/her powers or duties
- Intentionally make a false entry in a register, book, notice or other document that is required to be kept
- Intentionally or recklessly make false statements
- Pretend to be a health and safety inspector
- Fail to comply with a court order.

Penalties

If a person is found guilty of a health and safety offence, a substantial fine will be imposed.

Manual handling

The incorrect handling of heavy and awkward loads causes accidents and injuries, which can result in staff being off work for some time. It is important to lift heavy items in the correct way. The safest way to lift items is to bend at the knees rather than bending your back. Strain and damage can be reduced if two people do the lifting rather than one.

Design a poster Design a poster to describe correct manual handling.

Manual handling checklist

- When goods are moved on trolleys, trucks or any wheeled vehicles, they should be loaded carefully (not overloaded) and in a manner that enables the handler to see where they are going
- In stores, it is essential that heavy items are stacked at the bottom and that steps are used with care
- Particular care is needed when large pots are moved containing liquid, especially hot liquid. They should not be filled to the brim
- A warning sign that equipment handles, lids, and so on can be hot should be given; this can be indicated by a small sprinkle of flour or something similar
- Extra care is needed when taking a tray from the oven or salamander so that the tray does not burn someone else.

Work equipment

Under the Provision and Use of Work Equipment Regulations (PUWER) 1998, 'work equipment' covers work machinery such as food processors, slicers, ovens, knives and so on. These regulations place duties on employers to ensure that:

- Work equipment is suitable for its intended use and is maintained in efficient working order and in good repair, and
- Adequate information, instruction and training on the use and maintenance of the equipment and any associated hazards are given to employees.

Work equipment that possesses a specific risk must be used only by designated persons who have received relevant training. The regulations' 'specific' requirements cover dangerous machinery parts, protection against certain hazards (falling objects, ejected components, overheating), the provision of

Table 1.4 Significant health and safety factors in the hospitality industry

Cause of accident	Importance	Significant factor
Slips, trips	30% (but they account for 75% of all major injuries)	88% of slips and trips due to slippery floors (spillage not cleared up; wet floors and buckets, etc. in passageways) and uneven floors
Handling	29%	33.3% of handling accidents due to lifting pans, trays, etc. 33.3% due to handling sharp objects, e.g. knives 33.3% are due to awkward lifts from low ovens or high positions
Exposure to hazardous substances, hot surfaces, steam	16%	61% of accidents result from splashes; 13% from hot objects. Causes are poor maintenance in 28% of cases; steam from ovens/steamers 23%; carrying hot liquids 16%; misuse of cleaning materials 14%; cleaning fat fryers 14%; equipment failure 12%; horseplay 4%; hot surfaces 1%
Struck by moving articles including hand tools	10%	33.3% of injuries are from knives; 25% from falling articles; 10% from assault
Walking into objects	4%	75% of injuries the result of walking into a fixed, as opposed to a moveable, object
Machinery	3%	Slicers 30%; mixers 16%; vegetable cutting machines 9%; vegetable slicing, mincing and grating attachments 10%; pie and tart machines 4%; dough mixer, dough moulder, mincing machine, dishwasher 2%
Falls	1.8%	75% of accidents due to persons falling from low height but half of the major injuries occurred on stairs
Fire and explosion	1.6%	80% during manually igniting gas fire appliances, mainly ovens
Electric shock	0.5%	25% due to poor maintenance; 25% of incidents a trolley was involved; 25% unsafe switching and unplugging (75% of these in wet conditions); 25% poor maintenance
Transporter	3%	50% involved lift trucks

Source: Health and Safety Executive

certain stop and emergency stop controls, isolation from energy sources, stability and lighting and markings and warnings. PUWER 1998 replaces the list of prescribed dangerous machines as contained in the Prescribed Dangerous Machines Order 1964.

Fire precautions

Fire safety

Every employer has an explicit duty for the safety of his or her employees in the event of a fire. The Regulatory Reform Fire Safety Order 2005 places a greater focus on fire prevention. It places responsibility for the fire safety of the occupants of premises and people who might be affected by fire on a defined responsible person, usually the employer. The responsible person must:

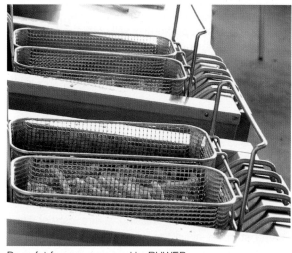

Deep fat fryers are covered by PUWER

- Make sure that the fire precautions, where reasonably practicable, ensure the safety of all employees and others in the building
- Make an assessment of the risk of and from fire in the establishment; special consideration must be given to dangerous chemicals or substances, and the risks that these pose if a fire occurs
- Review the preventative and protective measures.

Fire safety requires constant vigilance to reduce the risk of a fire, using the provision of detection and alarm systems and well-practised emergency and evacuation procedures in the event of a fire. A fire requires heat, fuel and oxygen. Without any one of these elements there is no fire. Methods of extinguishing fires concentrate on cooling or depriving the fire of oxygen (as in an extinguisher that uses foam or powder to smother it).

The following fire precautions must be taken:
- Identified hazards must be removed or reduced so far as is reasonable. All persons must be protected from the risk of fire and the likelihood of a fire spreading
- All escape routes must be safe and used effectively
- Means for fighting fires must be available on the premises
- Means of detecting a fire on the premises and giving warning in case of fire on the premises must be available
- Arrangements must be in place for action to be taken in the event of a fire on the premises, including the instruction and training of employees
- All precautions provided must be installed and maintained by a competent person.

Although businesses no longer need a fire certificate, the fire and rescue authorities will continue to inspect premises and ensure adequate fire precautions are in place. They will also wish to be satisfied that the risk assessment is comprehensive, relevant and up to date.

The fire triangle

For a fire to start, three things are needed:
1. A source of ignition (heat)
2. Fuel
3. Oxygen.

If any one of these is missing, a fire cannot start. Taking steps to avoid the three coming together will therefore reduce the chances of a fire occurring.

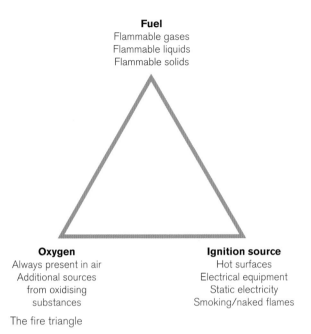

Fuel
Flammable gases
Flammable liquids
Flammable solids

Oxygen
Always present in air
Additional sources
from oxidising
substances

Ignition source
Hot surfaces
Electrical equipment
Static electricity
Smoking/naked flames

The fire triangle

Once a fire starts it can grow very quickly and spread from one source of fuel to another. As it grows, the amount of heat it gives off will increase and this can cause other fuels to self-ignite.

Fire detection and fire warning

You need to have an effective means of detecting any outbreak of fire and for warning people in your workplace quickly enough so that they can escape to a safe place before the fire is likely to make escape routes unusable.

In small workplaces where a fire is unlikely to cut off the means of escape, it is likely that any fire will quickly be detected by the people present and a shout of 'Fire' may be all that is needed. Examples of such workplaces include open-air areas and single-storey buildings where all exits are visible and the distances people need to travel to reach exits are small.

In larger workplaces, particularly multi-storey premises, an electrical fire warning system with manually operated call points is likely to be the minimum needed. In unoccupied areas, where a fire could start and develop to the extent that escape routes may become affected before it is discovered, it is likely that a form of automatic fire detection will also be necessary.

Means of fighting fire

You need to have enough fire-fighting equipment in place for your employees to use, without exposing themselves to danger, to extinguish a fire in its early

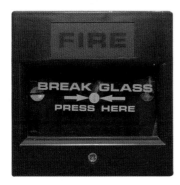

stage. The equipment must be suitable to the risks and appropriate staff will need training and instruction in its proper use.

In small premises, the availability of one or two portable extinguishers in an obvious location may be all that is required. In larger or more complex premises, it is likely that the minimum requirement will be a greater number of portable extinguishers, strategically sited throughout the premises. Means of fighting fire may need to be considered.

Lighting of escape routes

All escape routes, including external ones, must have sufficient lighting for people to see their way out safely. Emergency escape lighting may be needed if areas of the workplace are without natural daylight or are used at night.

Fire-fighting equipment

Portable fire extinguishers

Portable fire extinguishers enable suitably trained people to tackle a fire in its early stage, if they can do so without putting themselves in danger. When you are deciding on the types of extinguisher to provide, you should consider the nature of the materials likely to be found in your workplace. Fires are classified in accordance with British Standard EN2, as shown in Table 1.5.

Table 1.5 British Standard fire classifications

Class A	Fires involving solid materials where combustion normally takes place with the formation of glowing embers
Class B	Fires involving liquids or liquefiable solids
Class C	Fires involving gases
Class D	Fires involving metals
Class F	Fires involving cooking oils or fats

Class A fires involve solid materials, usually of organic matter such as wood, paper and so on. Such fires can be dealt with using water, foam or multi-purpose powder extinguishers, with water and foam considered the most suitable.

Class B fires involve liquids or liquefiable solids such as paints, oils or fats. It would be appropriate to provide extinguishers of foam (including multi-purpose aqueous film-forming foam (AFFF), carbon dioxide, halon or dry powder types). Carbon dioxide extinguishers are also suitable for use on a fire involving electrical equipment.

The fire extinguishers currently available for dealing with Class A or Class B fires should not be used on fires involving cooking oil or fat.

Class C fires involve gases. Dry powder extinguishers may be used on Class C fires. However, you really need to consider what type of portable fire extinguisher to use.

The fire-fighting extinguishing medium in portable extinguishers is expelled by internal pressure, either permanently stored or by means of a gas cartridge. Generally, portable fire extinguishers can be divided into five categories according to the extinguishing medium they contain:

1. Water
2. Foam
3. Powder
4. Carbon dioxide
5. Vaporising liquids, including halons.

Some fire extinguishers can be used on more than one type of fire. For instance, AFFF extinguishers can be used on both Class A and Class B fires. Your fire equipment supplier will be able to advise you.

Hazards in the workplace and risk reduction

The following aspects of the kitchen environment have the potential to give rise to hazards:

- Equipment: liquidisers, food processors, mixers, mincers
- Substances: cleaning chemicals, detergents, sanitisers
- Work methods: carrying knives and equipment incorrectly and not following a logical sequence
- Work areas: spillages not cleaned up, overcrowded work areas, insufficient work space,

uncomfortable work conditions due to extreme heat or cold.

Managing risk

Employers have a duty under the Management of Health and Safety at Work Regulations 1999 to carry out risk assessments and COSHH assessments.

Managing risk is not a complicated procedure. To start with, a health and safety policy must be in place for the business.

Involve employees

Employees are most at risk of having accidents, or experiencing ill health, and they also know the most about the jobs they do so are in the best position to help managers develop safe systems of work that are effective in practice. An actively engaged workforce is one of the foundations that support good health and safety. It ensures that all those involved with a work activity, both managers and workers, are participating in assessing risks.

Assessing risk

Assessing risk is the key to effective health and safety in the workplace. This means nothing more than a careful examination of what, in your work, could cause harm to people, so that you weigh up whether you have taken enough precautions or should do more to prevent harm. See Table 1.6.

Table 1.6 Five steps to assessing risk

1. Look for hazards – the things that could cause harm
2. Decide who might be harmed and how
3. Evaluate the risk and decide whether the existing precautions are adequate, or whether more should be done
4. Write down your findings so you have a record that you can check against
5. Regularly review your assessment and revise it if necessary.

The prevention of accidents and food poisoning in catering establishments is essential; therefore it is necessary to assess the situation and decide what action is to be taken. For more information about carrying out a risk assessment see page 5.

The purpose of the exercise of assessing the possibility of risks and hazards is to prevent accidents. First, it is necessary to monitor the situation, to have regular and spasmodic checks to see that the standards set are being complied with. However, should an incident occur, it is essential that an investigation is made as to the cause or causes and any defects in the system remedied at once. Immediate action is required to prevent further accidents. All personnel need to be trained to be actively aware of the possible hazards and risks and to take positive action to prevent accidents occurring.

Accidents in the workplace

The highest numbers of accidents occurring in catering premises are due to persons falling, slipping or tripping. Therefore, floor surfaces must be of a suitable construction to reduce this risk. A major reason for the high incidence of this kind of accident is that it is likely that water and grease will be spilt and the combination of these substances is treacherous and makes the floor surface slippery. For this reason, any spillage must be cleaned immediately and warning notices put in place, where appropriate, highlighting the danger of the slippery surface. Ideally a member of staff should stand guard until the hazard is cleared.

Placing articles on the floor in corridors, passageways or between stoves and tables may also cause individuals to fall. Persons carrying trays and containers have their vision obstructed and items on the floor may not be visible; the fall may occur onto a hot stove and the item being carried may be hot. These falls can have severe consequences. The solution is to ensure that nothing is left on the floor that may cause a hazard. If it is necessary to have articles temporarily on the floor then it is desirable that they are guarded so as to prevent accidents. Kitchen personnel should be trained to think and act in a safe manner in order to avoid this kind of accident.

Procedures for fire evacuation Design a poster to explain fire evacuation procedures.

Managing health and safety

Employers must have appropriate arrangements in place (recorded where there are five or more employees) for maintaining a safe workplace. These should cover the usual management functions of:

- Planning
- Organisation
- Control.

Reporting hazards

If you see a hazard in your work area that could cause an accident you should do one of two things:

1. Make the hazard safe, as long as you can do so without risking your own safety. Report the hazard to your chef or manager as soon as you can, making sure no one enters the area without being aware of the danger

2. If there is a hazard that you cannot make safe, warn others. Block the route past the hazard. Use a sign (signs are an effective way of informing people).

Safety and hazard signage

These generally take the following forms:

- Prohibition signs are red (for example, a red circle with a line through it tells you something you must not do in the area, for example 'no entry')
- Fire-fighting signs are red with white symbols or writing (for example, fire hose reel)
- Warning signs are yellow (for example, caution – hot surface)
- Mandatory signs are blue (for example, protective gloves must be worn; a solid blue circle with a white picture or writing gives a reminder of something you must do, such as 'shut the door')
- Hazard warning signs are yellow (for example, corrosive). A black and yellow sign is used with a triangular symbol where there is a risk of danger, for example, 'mind your head'
- Emergency/escape and first-aid signs are green with a white picture or writing (for example, emergency sign for escape or first aid).

When using chemicals that could harm you, signs that highlight the following information may be displayed on the container:

- 'Corrosive': could burn your skin
- 'Poison': may kill you if swallowed
- 'Irritant': may cause itching or a rash if in contact with skin.

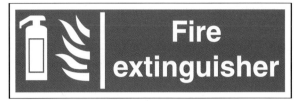

A fire-fighting sign

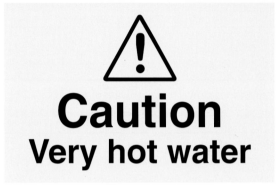

A warning sign

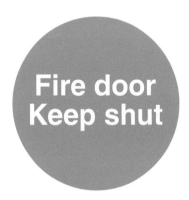

A mandatory sign

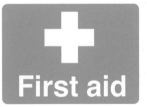 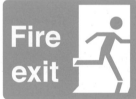

An emergency and escape sign

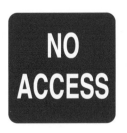 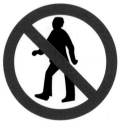

A prohibition sign

Accident recording

All accidents should be reported to your line manager, chef or a supervisor. Each accident is recorded in an accident report form, which must be provided in every business. An example of an incident report form, showing all the detail required, is shown below.

Emergencies in the workplace

Emergencies that might happen in the workplace include:

- Serious accidents
- Outbreak of fire

Full name of injured person:			
Occupation:		Supervisor:	
Time of accident:	Date of accident:	Time of report:	Date of report:
Nature of injury or condition:			
Details of hospitalisation:			
Extent of injury (after medical attention):			
Place of accident or dangerous occurrence:			
Injured person's evidence of what happened (include equipment/items and/or other persons):			
Witness evidence (1):		Witness evidence (2):	
Supervisor's recommendations:			
Date:		Supervisor's signature:	

Incident report form

- Bomb scare
- Failure of a major system, for example water or electricity.

An organisation will have systems in place to deal with emergencies. Key staff are usually trained to tackle emergencies. There will be fire marshals and first aiders. These people will attend regular update meetings. Evacuation procedures will also be held so that employees can practise drill and fire alarms will be tested regularly. Ensure that you know the evacuation procedures in your establishment. If you have to leave the premises, ensure that the following procedures are adhered to:

- Turn off the power supplies: gas and electricity. Usually this means hitting the red button in the kitchen or turning off all appliances individually
- Close all windows and doors
- Leave the building by the nearest emergency exit. DO NOT USE THE LIFTS
- Assemble in the designated area, away from the building
- Check the roll-call of names to establish whether all personnel have left the building safely.

First aid

When people at work suffer injuries or fall ill, it is important that they receive immediate attention and that, in serious cases, an ambulance is called. The arrangements for providing first aid in the workplace are set out in the Health and Safety (First Aid) Regulations 1981. First aiders and facilities should be available to give immediate assistance to casualties with common injuries or illness.

As the term implies, first aid is the immediate treatment given on the spot to a person who has been injured or is ill. Since 1982 it has been a legal requirement that adequate first-aid equipment, facilities and personnel to give first aid are provided at work. If the injury is serious, the injured person should be treated by a doctor or nurse as soon as possible.

First-aid boxes must be easily identifiable and accessible in the work area. They should be in the charge of a responsible person, checked regularly and refilled when necessary.

All establishments must have first-aid equipment and employees qualified in first aid. Large establishments usually have medical staff such as a nurse and a first-aid room. The room should include a bed or couch, blankets, chairs, table, sink with hot and

First-aid equipment

A first-aid box, as a minimum, should contain:

- A card giving general first-aid guidance
- Twenty individually wrapped, sterile, adhesive, waterproof dressings of various sizes
- 25 g cotton wool packs
- A dozen safety pins
- Two triangular bandages
- Two sterile eye pads, with attachment
- Four medium-sized sterile unmedicated dressings
- Two large sterile unmedicated dressings
- Two extra large sterile unmedicated dressings
- Tweezers
- Scissors
- Report book to record all injuries

cold water, towels, tissues and first-aid box. Hooks for clothing and a mirror should be provided. Small establishments should have members of staff trained in first aid and in possession of a certificate. After a period of three years trained first-aid staff must update their training to remain certificated. All catering workers and students are recommended to attend a first-aid course run by St John Ambulance, St Andrew's Ambulance Association or the British Red Cross Society.

First-aid treatment

Shock

The signs of shock are faintness, sickness, clammy skin and a pale face. Shock should be treated by keeping the person comfortable, lying down and warm. Cover the person with a blanket or clothing, but do not apply hot water bottles.

Fainting

Fainting may occur after a long period of standing in a hot, badly ventilated kitchen. The signs of an impending faint are whiteness, giddiness and sweating. A faint should be treated by raising the sick person's legs slightly above the level of their head and, when the person recovers consciousness, putting them in the fresh air for a while and making sure that they have not incurred any injury in fainting.

Cuts

All cuts should be covered immediately with a waterproof dressing, after the skin around the cut has been washed. When there is considerable bleeding it should be stopped as soon as possible. Bleeding may be controlled by direct pressure, by bandaging firmly on the cut. It may be possible to stop bleeding from a cut artery by pressing the artery with the thumb against the underlying bone; such pressure may be applied while a dressing or bandage is being prepared for application, but not for more than 15 minutes.

Nose bleeds

Sit the person down with their head forward and then loosen their clothing around the neck and chest. Ask them to breathe through their mouth and to pinch the soft part of their nose. After ten minutes release the pressure. Warn the person not to blow their nose for several hours. If the bleeding has not stopped, continue for a further ten minutes. If the bleeding has not stopped then, or recurs in 30 minutes, obtain medical assistance.

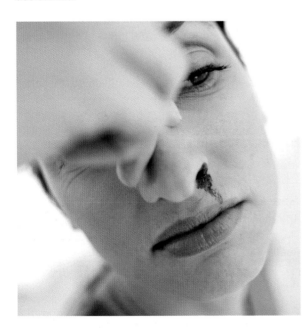

Fractures

A person suffering from broken bones should not be moved until the injured part has been secured so that it cannot move. Medical assistance should be obtained.

Burns and scalds

Place the injured part gently under slowly running water or immerse in cool water, keeping it there for at least ten minutes or until the pain ceases. If serious, the burn or scald should then be covered with a clean cloth or dressing (preferably sterile) and the person sent immediately to hospital. Do not use adhesive dressings, apply lotions or ointments, or break blisters.

Electric shock

Switch off the current. If this is not possible, free the person by using a dry insulating material such as cloth, wood or rubber, taking care not to use bare hands otherwise the electric shock may be transmitted. If breathing has stopped, give artificial respiration and send for a doctor. Treat any burns as above.

Kitchen environment

Kitchens must have a good working environment. This includes:

- **Good clear/clean ventilation systems.** Poor ventilation results in poor quality air. Harmful gases, fumes, vapours and dust can accumulate in the air if there is poor air movement.
- **Comfortable working temperature.** Good ventilation and cooling systems are used to create comfortable working temperatures.
- **Good lighting.** Too little light, either natural or artificial, can lead to eye strain, headaches, fatigue and stress. Poor lighting can create hazards that would otherwise not occur, such as, for example, difficulty in walking down steps and corridors.
- **Cleanliness.** Kitchens must be kept clean and hygienic at all times. Cleanliness is important to prevent slips, trips and falls.
- **Good changing room facilities.** These and good welfare facilities must be provided for staff to enable them to change in a comfortable and hygienic environment.

Supervising health and safety in the kitchen

In order to be a supervisor of health and safety, a chef must have knowledge and understanding of the hazards at work in the kitchen to enable him or her to carry out and organise a risk assessment and to understand how the effective operation of controls can reduce risks. The supervisor must monitor work activities to make sure that health and safety procedures are being followed.

Chefs/supervisors have a central role in dealing with both employees and management. A typical role involves supervising employees' work, mentoring, and so on.

Supervisors must be able to carry out or organise a risk assessment and understand how the effective operation of controls can reduce risks. Always make sure that health and safety principles are being followed. If something goes wrong in the kitchen or restaurant and an accident happens you will be required to investigate and make recommendations to managers on how improvements can be made to prevent future accidents.

A key role is to motivate your staff to follow good health and safety practices, giving them support, advice and guidance in creating a health and safety culture.

Making your work more effective

Make sure you understand the health and safety management system and its procedures. Documents contained within a health and safety management system are:

- The organisation's health and safety policy
- Risk assessments and their findings
- COSHH assessments
- Company rules and procedures
- Systems of safe working

- Monitoring records
- Accident records
- Health and safety training records
- Health surveillance records
- List of staff who are competent in health and safety procedures
- First-aid records
- List of first aiders
- A fire certificate
- Fire and emergency procedures
- Fire inspection records
- Examination and test certificates for work equipment
- Maintenance and repair records for equipment
- Health and safety law poster
- Health and safety committee minutes
- Details of visit by enforcement officers
- Health and Safety at Work Act 1974
- Approval codes of practice.

Having a system of documentation is evidence of a strong commitment to health and safety.

Always record key facts and all record keeping must be accurate.

Table 1.7 Key health and safety terms

Safety	Freedom from danger.
Health	A state of complete physical, mental and social well-being, not merely the absence of disease or infirmity.
Carcinogen	A substance that can cause cancer.
Carcinogenic	Something that could cause cancer.
Fume	Microscopic air-borne particles produced when, for example, metals are heated during welding or as a result of certain chemical processes. A fume may smell foul and may be irritating or toxic.
Vapour	A gaseous form of a substance that is normally solid or liquid.
Accident	Any unplanned event that results or could have resulted in personal injury or ill health; damage to or loss of property, plant or materials; damage to the environment; loss of business opportunity.
Incident	An accident (unplanned event) or a near miss that does not result in personal injury, death or damage but has the potential to do so.
Health and Safety – HSE Executive	The body appointed by the Health and Safety Commission to enforce health and safety law.
Environmental health officer – EHO	An officer employed by local authorities to enforce health and safety law.

Health and Safety Commission – HSC	The body appointed by the government to regulate health and safety law.
Reasonably practicable	What is practicable in the light of whether the time, trouble and expense of the precautions suggested are proportionate or not to the risks involved.
RIDDOR	The Reporting of Injuries, Diseases and Dangerous Occurrences Regulations 1995.
Flammable substances	Any natural or artificial substance in the form of a solid, liquid, gas or vapour that is liable to catch fire.
Danger zone	In relation to work equipment, an area where employees are exposed to dangerous machine parts.
Inspection	An assessment of the health and safety performance of the workplace against pre-set standards so that remedial measures can be taken before equipment becomes dangerous to use.
First aid	The immediate medical treatment given to a person to prevent medical conditions deteriorating or to minimise the consequences of injury or illness.
First aider	A person who has been trained in first aid and holds a current first-aid certificate issued by an organisation approved by the Health and Safety Executive.
Health and safety culture	The integration of health and safety awareness and controls into day-to-day workplace practices.
Risk assessment	A system of identifying workplace hazards and assessing the risks posed by these hazards.
Health surveillance	The systematic monitoring of the health of any worker who may be exposed to harmful substances or harmful work activities.
Reportable accident	An accident that must, by law, be reported to the enforcing authorities. Such accidents are those resulting in death, major injury, injuries as a consequence of which an employee has to take more than three days off work, a dangerous occurrence or certain diseases that occur as a result of work activities specified in RIDDOR.
Safety committee	A committee to deal with health and safety matters in the workplace.

Training and instruction in health and safety

Training is an important and essential part of health and safety management and control. It prepares individuals with information, instruction and practice in order to develop a skill, knowledge, capability and competence.

Advantages of health and safety training

The advantages of giving health and safety training to employees include factors such as it results in their making fewer mistakes; they become aware of hazards, risks and controls; and training reduces risks and the likelihood of injury.

It is important that employers provide good-quality training. The advantages of good training are:

- A reduction in accidents and ill health in the workplace
- A reduction in sickness time, cost of accidents and insurance
- An increase in work productivity
- An increase in hazards being identified by employees
- An improvement in acknowledging the importance of fire drills and alarms
- An improvement in the reputation of an employer who takes health and safety seriously.

Supervisors are often responsible for training and advising managers about the training that is required for employees. It is important to always provide training to new employees; and when people are exposed to new and increased risks in the workplace; and always when new equipment is purchased and installed.

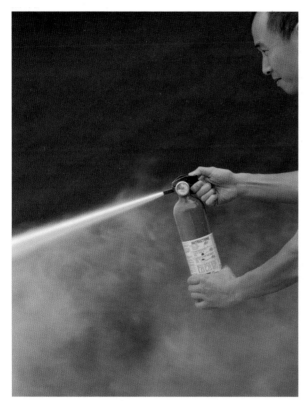

At least some staff need to be trained to use the fire extinguishers

Methods of training include:

- Group training sessions
- Individual training
- Formal training
- Case studies
- Role play: acting out health and safety practice
- Discussion groups
- Interactive computer-based courses.

Health and safety induction course

The following topics could be included on a health and safety induction course:

- Fire safety: emergency evacuation procedures
- Leaflets on health and safety and where to find further information
- Accident and hazard reporting procedures
- The organisation of health and safety policy
- First-aid facilities
- Communication systems of health and safety
- Who the enforcing authority is.

Planning a health and safety induction programme Plan a one-day health and safety induction programme for a new commis chef who will be starting work in your kitchen.

1.2   Applying staff supervisory skills within a small team

Kitchen supervision and management

Organisation of staff and job roles within different industries varies according to their specific requirements and the names given to people doing similar jobs may also vary. Some companies or organisations will require operatives, technicians and technologists; others need crafts people, supervisors and managers. The supervisory function of the technician, chef de partie or supervisor may be similar.

The hospitality and catering industry is made up of people with craft skills. The crafts person is involved with food production; the chef de partie may be the supervisor, supervising a section or sections of the food production system. The head chef will have both managerial and supervisory skills and will determine kitchen policies.

Supervisors are involved with the successful deployment of money, material and people. The primary role of the supervisor is to ensure that a group of people work together to achieve the goals set by the business. Managing physical and human resources to achieve customer service goals requires planning, organising, staffing, directing and controlling.

Supervisors and head chefs need to motivate people, to persuade them to act in certain ways. In the kitchen/restaurant, as in any other department, staff must first be motivated to follow procedures. This can be done in a positive way by offering rewards, or in a negative way with catering staff who do not comply with requirements. Both methods can be effective and may be used by supervisors to achieve their goals. One of the most effective ways for a supervisor to motivate staff is to build a team and offer incentives for good performance.

However, staff may become indifferent to repeated schemes such as 'employee of the month'. A good

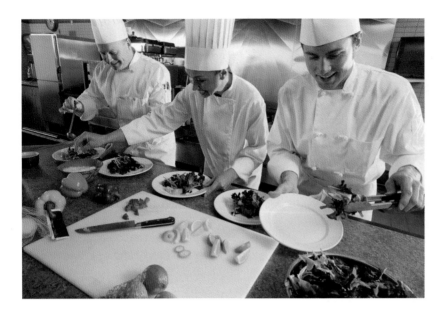

supervisor will attempt to introduce novelty and fun into the reward system.

The supervisory function and tasks

Certain leadership qualities are needed to enable the supervisor to carry out his or her role effectively. These qualities include the ability to:

- Communicate
- Initiate
- Make decisions
- Coordinate
- Mediate
- Motivate
- Inspire
- Organise.

Those under supervision should expect their supervisor to show:

- Consideration
- Understanding
- Loyalty
- Respect
- Cooperation
- Consistency.

The good supervisor is able to obtain the best from those for whom he or she has responsibility and can also completely satisfy the management of the establishment that a good job is being done.

The job of the supervisor is essentially to be an overseer. In the catering industry the name given to the

supervisor may vary: sous-chef, chef de partie, kitchen supervisor or section chef. In hospital catering the name would be sous-chef, chef de partie or kitchen supervisor. The kitchen supervisor will be responsible to the catering manager, while in hotels and restaurants a chef de partie will be responsible to the head chef. The exact details of the job will vary according to the different areas of the industry and the size of the various units, but generally the supervisory role involves three functions: technical, administrative and social.

Technical function

Culinary skills and the ability to use kitchen equipment are essential for the kitchen supervisor. Most kitchen supervisors will have worked their way up through the section or sections before reaching supervisory responsibility. The supervisor needs to be able 'to do' as well as know 'what to do' and 'how to do it'. It is also necessary to be able to do it well and to be able to impart some of these skills to others.

Administrative function

The supervisor or chef de partie will, in many kitchens, be involved with the menu planning, sometimes with complete responsibility for the whole menu but more usually for part of the menu, as happens with the larder chef and pastry chef. This includes ordering foodstuffs (which is an important aspect of the supervisor's job in a catering establishment) and, of course, accounting for and recording materials used. The administrative function includes the allocation of duties and, in all instances, basic work-study

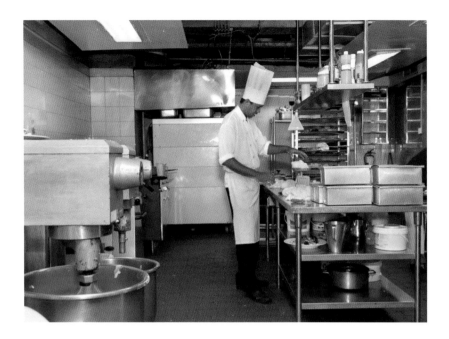

knowledge is needed to enable the supervisor to operate effectively. The supervisor's job may also include writing reports, particularly in situations where it is necessary to make comparisons and when new developments are being tried.

Social function

The role of the supervisor is perhaps most clearly seen in staff relationships because the supervisor has to motivate the staff under his or her responsibility. 'To motivate' could be described as the initiation of movement and action and having got the staff moving, the supervisor needs to exert control. Then, in order to achieve the required result, the staff need to be organised. Thus, the supervisor has a threefold function regarding the handling of staff; namely to organise, to motivate and to control. This is the essence of staff supervision.

Qualities in a good supervisor List the qualities you admire most in a good supervisor.

Elements of supervision

The accepted areas of supervision include: forecasting and planning, organising, commanding, coordinating and controlling. Each of these will be considered within the sphere of catering.

Forecasting

Before making plans it is necessary to look ahead, to foresee possible and probable outcomes and to allow for them. For example, if the chef de partie knows that the following day is her/his assistant's day off, she/he looks ahead and plans accordingly. When the catering supervisor in the hospital knows that there is a flu epidemic and two cooks are feeling below par, he/she plans for their possible absence. If there is a spell of fine, hot weather and the cook in charge of the larder foresees a continued demand for cold foods or when an end to the hot spell is anticipated, then the plans are modified.

For the supervisor, forecasting is the good use of judgement acquired from previous knowledge and experience. For example, because many people are on holiday in August fewer meals will be needed in the office restaurant: no students are in residence at the college hostel, but a conference is being held and 60 meals are required. A motor show, bank holidays, the effects of a rail strike or a wet day, as well as less predictable situations, such as the number of customers anticipated on the opening day of a new restaurant, all need to be anticipated and planned for.

Planning

From the forecasting comes the planning: how many meals to prepare; how much to have in stock (should the forecast not have been completely accurate); how many staff will be needed; which staff and when. Are the staff capable of what is required of them? If not, the supervisor needs to plan some training. This, of course, is particularly important if new equipment is installed. Imagine an expensive item, such as a new type of oven, ruined on the day it is installed because the staff have not been instructed in its proper use; or, more likely, equipment lying idle because the supervisor may not like it, may consider it is sited wrongly, does not train staff to use it, or for some similar reason.

As can be seen from these examples, it is necessary for forecasting to precede planning and from planning we now move to organising.

Organising

In the catering industry organisational skills are applied to food, to equipment and to staff. Organising in this context consists of ensuring that what is wanted is where it is wanted, when it is wanted, in the right amount and at the right time.

Such organisation involves the supervisor in the production of duty rotas, maybe training programmes and also cleaning schedules. Consider the supervisor's part in organising an outdoor function where a wedding reception is to be held in a church hall: a total of 250 guests require a hot meal to be served at 2 p.m. and in the evening a dance will be held for the guests, during which a buffet will be provided at 9 p.m. The supervisor would need to organise staff to be available when required, to have their own meals and maybe to see that they have got their transport home.

Calor gas stoves may be needed and the supervisor would have to arrange for these to be serviced and for the equipment used to be cleaned after the function. The food would need to be ordered so that it arrived in time to be prepared. If decorated hams were to be used on the buffet then they would need to be ordered in time so that they could be prepared, cooked and decorated over the required period of time. If the staff have never carved hams before, instruction would need to be given; this entails organising training.

Needless to say, the correct quantities of food, equipment and cleaning materials would also have to be at the right place when wanted and if all the details of the situation were not organised properly, problems could occur.

Commanding

The supervisor has to give instructions to staff on how, what, when and where; this means that orders have to be given and a certain degree of order and discipline maintained. The successful supervisor is able to do this effectively having made certain decisions and, usually, having established the basic priorities. Explanations of why a food is prepared in a certain manner,

why this amount of time is needed to dress up food, say for a buffet, why this decision is taken and not that decision, and how these explanations and orders are given, determine the effectiveness of the supervisor.

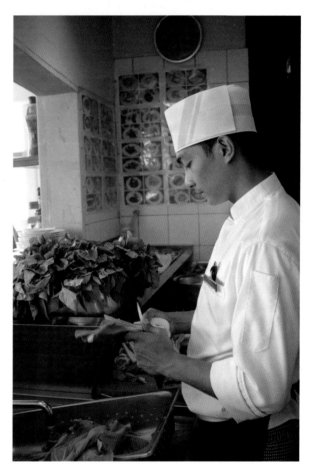

Coordinating

Coordinating is a skill required to get staff to cooperate and work together. To achieve this, the supervisor has to be interested in the staff, to deal with their queries, to listen to their problems and to be helpful. Particular attention should be paid to new staff, easing them into the work situation so that they quickly become part of the team or partie. The other area of coordination for which the supervisor has particular responsibility is in maintaining good relations with other departments.

However, the important persons to consider will always be the customers such as, for example, the patients or school children who will receive the service. Good service is dependent on cooperation between waiters and cooks, nurses and catering staff, stores staff, caretakers, teachers, suppliers and so on. The supervisor has a crucial role to play here.

Controlling

This includes controlling people and products, preventing pilfering as well as improving performance, checking that staff arrive on time, do not leave before time and do not misuse time in between. Controlling also involves checking that the product, in this case the food, is of the right standard, that is, of the correct quantity and quality; checking to prevent waste, and also to ensure that staff operate the portion control system correctly.

This aspect of the supervisor's function involves inspecting and requires tact; controlling may include inspecting the waste bin to observe the amount of waste, checking the disappearance of a quantity of food, supervising the cooking of the meat so that shrinkage is minimised and reprimanding an unpunctual member of the team.

The standards of any catering establishment are dependent on the supervisor doing his or her job efficiently and standards are set and maintained by effective control, which is the function of the supervisor.

Delegating

It is recognised that delegation is the root of successful supervision; in other words, by giving a certain amount of responsibility to others, the supervisor can be more effective.

The supervisor needs to be able to judge the person capable of responsibility before any delegation can take place. But then, having recognised the abilities of an employee, the supervisor who wants to develop the potential of those under his or her control must allow the person entrusted with the job to get on with it.

Delegating duties List the duties a sous chef or kitchen supervisor could or should delegate to a chef de partie.

Motivating

Since not everyone is capable of, or wants, responsibility, the supervisor still needs to motivate those who are less ambitious. Most people are prepared to work in order to improve their standard of living but there is also another very important motivating factor: most people wish to get satisfaction from the work they do. The supervisor must be aware of why people work and how different people achieve job satisfaction and then be able to act upon this knowledge. A supervisor should have received training that enables them to attempt to understand what motivates people, as there are a number of theories that she or he can use to stimulate ideas.

Motivation Think about yourself and what motivates you at work.

Symptoms of poor motivation

There are many symptoms of poor motivation; in general terms they reveal themselves as lack of interest in getting the job done correctly and within the required time. Although they may be indicators of poor motivation, the lack of efficiency and effectiveness could also be a result of the staff overworking, personal problems, poor work design, repetitive work, lack of discipline, interpersonal conflict, lack of training or failure of the organisation to value its staff. An employee may be highly motivated but may find the work physically impossible.

Money as a motivating factor How much does money feature in your motivation?

Employee welfare

People always work best in good working conditions and these include freedom from fear: fear of becoming unemployed, fear of failure at work, fear of discrimination. Job security and incentives such as opportunities for promotion, bonuses, profit sharing and time for further study encourage a good attitude to work. But as well as these tangible factors, people need to feel wanted and that what they do is important. The supervisor is in an excellent position to ensure that this happens. Personal worries affect individuals' performance and can have a very strong influence on how well or how badly they work. The physical environment will naturally cause problems if, for example, the atmosphere is humid, the working situation ill lit, too hot or too noisy, and there is constant rush and tear and frequent major problems to be overcome. In these circumstances, staff are more liable to be quick-tempered, angry and aggressive and the supervisor needs to consider how these factors might be dealt with.

Understanding

The supervisor needs to try to understand both men and women (and to deal with both sexes fairly), anticipate problems and build up a team spirit so as to overcome the problems. This entails always being fair when dealing with staff and giving them encouragement. It also means that work needs to be allocated according to each individual's ability; everyone should be kept fully occupied and the working environment must be conducive to producing their best work.

Communication

Finally, and most important of all, the supervisor must be able to communicate effectively. To convey orders, instructions, information and manual skills requires the supervisor to possess the right attitude to those with whom he or she needs to communicate. The ability to convey orders in a manner that is acceptable to the one receiving them is dependent not only on the words but on the emphasis given to the words, the tone of voice, the time selected to give them and on who is present when they are given. This is a skill that supervisors need to develop. Instructions and orders can be given with authority without being authoritative.

Thus the supervisor needs technical knowledge and the ability to direct staff and to carry responsibility so as to achieve the specified targets and standards required by the organisation; this he or she is able to do by organising, coordinating, controlling and planning but, most of all, through effective communication.

Supervisory skills

Supervisors need a wide range of technical, people and conceptual skills in order to carry out their work.

Technical skills

These are the skills chefs, restaurant managers and the like need in order to do the job. The supervisor must be skilled in the area they are supervising because they will be required in most cases to train other staff under them. Supervisors who do not have the required skills will find it hard to gain credibility with the staff.

People skills

Supervisors are team leaders; therefore they must be sensitive to the needs of others. They must be able to communicate effectively and be able to build a team to achieve the agreed goals: listening, questioning, communicating clearly, handling conflicts, and providing support and praise when praise is due.

Conceptual skills

A supervisor must be able to think things through, especially when planning or analysing why things are not going as expected. A supervisor must be able to solve problems and make decisions. For supervisors, conceptual skills are necessary for reasonably short-term

planning. Head chefs and hospitality managers require conceptual skills for long-term strategic planning.

Henry Mintzberg (*The Nature of Managerial Work*, Harper & Row, 1973) suggested that the supervisor has three broad roles:

1. Interpersonal: people skills
2. Informational: people and technical skills
3. Decision making: conceptual skills.

Supervisors and ethical issues

A supervisor must be consistent when handling staff, avoiding favouritism and perceived inequity. Such inequity can arise from the amount of training or performance counselling given, from the promotion of certain employees and from the way in which shifts are allocated. Supervisors should engage in conversation with all staff, not just a selected few, and should not single out some staff for special attention.

Ethical treatment of staff is fair treatment of staff. A good supervisor will gain respect if they are ethical.

Treating staff fairly As a supervisor, how would you treat staff fairly?

Confidentiality is an important issue for the supervisor. Employees or customers may wish to take the supervisor into their confidence and the supervisor must not betray this.

In business management, micromanagement is a management style where a manager closely observes or controls the work of his/her employees, generally used as a pejorative term. In contrast to giving general instructions on smaller tasks while supervising larger concerns, the micromanager monitors and assesses every step.

Micromanagement may arise from internal sources, such as concern for details, increased performance pressure, or insecurity. It can also be seen as a tactic used by managers to eliminate unwanted employees, either by creating standards they cannot meet, leading to termination of employment, or by creating a stressful workplace and thus causing the employee to leave.

Regardless of the motivation, the effect may be to demotivate employees, create resentment and damage trust.

Micromanagement can also be distinguished from management by worker-to-boss ratio. At any time when there is one worker being given orders by one boss, both people are rendered useless. When a boss can do a worker's job with more efficiency than giving the orders to do the same job, this is micromanagement.

Micromanagement is a counterproductive approach to dealing with the workforce and can be costly in many areas of the business.

A supervisor must be able to identify what staff are required and where they are required in order to cope with the level of business. At the same time labour costs must be kept to a minimum. The supervisor must therefore ensure adequate staffing at the lowest possible cost.

Micromanaging a kitchen Give a practical example of a head chef micromanaging a kitchen.

An important aspect is to be able to carefully analyse projected business in order to adopt the best staffing mix.

Job design and the allocation of duties also have to be considered; where jobs are simple and require little training, employment of casual labour can be justified. For more skilled staff, full-time employment has to be considered, with investment in staff development and training.

Often the supervisor has to write job descriptions. These documents are used for a number of purposes, which include:

- Deciding on the knowledge, experience and skills required to carry out the duties specified
- Allowing new staff to understand the requirements of their jobs
- Allowing new staff to develop accurate expectation of the jobs, identifying training needs
- Assisting in the development of recruitment strategies.

Leadership styles

Leadership style is the way in which the functions of leadership are carried out, the way in which the supervisor typically behaves towards members of the team.

There are many dimensions to leadership and many possible ways of describing leadership style.

Leadership

1. Explain what kind of leadership style you would adopt as a supervisory manager.
2. Name three leaders whom you are aware of – managers, executives, politicians, and so on – and why you consider them to be good leaders.

Supervisory styles

A supervisory style may be described as:

- **Dictatorial** A supervisor who is dictatorial is autocratic and often oppressive and overbearing.
- **Bureaucratic** A bureaucratic supervisor is one who follows official procedure and is very often office-bound. He/she sticks to the rules and operates within a hierarchical system.
- **Benevolent** A benevolent supervisor is kind, passionate, human, kind-hearted, good, unselfish, charitable.
- **Charismatic** A supervisor who is charismatic has a special charm that inspires loyalty and enthusiasm from the team.
- **Consultative** The consultative supervisor discusses issues with the team through team meetings.
- **Participative** A participative supervisor gets involved with the team, taking part in activities and issues and making an active contribution to the success or failure of the team.
- **Unitary** The unitary supervisor unites the team, bringing them together as a whole unit.
- **Delegative** The delegative supervisor entrusts others in the team to make decisions, assigning responsibility or authority to others.
- **Autocratic** This is where the supervisor holds on to power and all the interactions within the team move towards the supervisor. The supervisor makes all the decisions and has all the authority.
- **Democratic** The team has a say in decision making. The supervisor shares the decision making with the team. The supervisor is very much part of the team.

Laissez-faire

A genuine laissez-faire style is where the supervisor observes that members of the group are working well on their own. The supervisor passes power to the team members, allows them freedom of action, does not interfere but is available for help if needed. The word genuine is used because this is contrary to the type of supervisor who does not care, keeps away from trouble and does not want to get involved.

Reflect on your own practice Reflect on your leadership style. Consider what training you think you need to improve your ability to supervise and lead a team.

Continuous training

Supervisors and chefs should encourage continuous training to improve knowledge and skills and change attitudes. This can lead to many benefits for both the organisation and the individual.

Training and personnel development can help to:

- Increase confidence, motivation and commitment of staff
- Provide recognition, enhanced responsibility and the possibility of further career development
- Give a feeling of personal satisfaction and achievement and broaden wider opportunities
- Help to improve the availability and quality of staff.

Training is therefore a key element of improved organisational performance.

Training improves knowledge, skill, confidence and competence.

Main styles of training

The main styles of training are output training, task training, performance training and strategic training. Examples of each style are given in Table 1.8.

Training should be viewed as an investment in people. Training requires the cooperation of the managers and supervisors with a genuine commitment from all levels in the organisation.

There are different methods of training; as well as the formal methods such as attendance on training courses and working for qualifications there are the informal methods. People learn by doing and learn from close observation of 'role models' and from being in challenging situations which require initiative and positive leadership. A great deal can be learnt by shadowing a supervisor or work colleague. Having a good mentor also helps personal development. A good supervisor is also able to mentor and coach members of the team to achieve their goals and objectives.

Establishing and developing positive working relationships

In hospitality the supervisor is an important person who is responsible for developing good teamwork and acting as a catalyst in maintaining good relationships within the team.

As individuals working within an organisation we can achieve very little but working within a group we are able to achieve a great deal more. Teamwork is essential when working in a commercial kitchen. Good, effective teamwork is an important feature of human behaviour and organisational performance. Those managing the kitchen must develop effective groups in order to achieve the high standard of work that is required to satisfy both the organisation's and the consumer's needs.

Each member of a group must regard themselves as being part of that group. They must interact with one another and perceive themselves as part of the group. Each must share the purpose of the group; this will help build trust and support and will, in turn, result in an effective performance. Cooperation is therefore important in order for the work to be carried out.

People in groups will influence one another – within the group there may be a leader and/or hierarchical system. The pressures within the group may have a major influence on the behaviour of individual members and their performance. The style of leadership within the group has an influence on the behaviour of members within the group.

Table 1.8 Training styles

Style of training	Example
Output training	Investing in a new employee or new machine will endeavour to generate output as quickly as possible.
Task training	Involves selected individuals being sent on short training or college-based courses, i.e. hygiene courses, health and safety courses, financial training.
Performance training	Implemented when the organisation has grown substantially and becomes well established. Training is viewed positively, with a person responsible for overseeing training. Plans and budgets are now some of the tools used to manage the training process.
Strategic training	Implemented when the organisation recognises and practises training as an integral part of the management of people and the culture of the organisation.

Groups help to shape the work pattern of organisations as well as group members' behaviour and attitudes to their jobs.

> **Qualities in a good team** Write down what you admire in a good team.

The importance of teamwork

Two types of team can be identified within an organisation:

1. The 'formal' team is the department or section created within a reorganised structure to pursue specified goals
2. The 'informal' team is created to deal with a particular situation; members within this team have fewer fixed organisational relationships; these teams are disbanded once they have performed their function.

Both formal and informal teams have to be developed and led. Thought has to be given to relationships and the tasks and duties the team has to carry out.

Selecting and shaping teams to work within the kitchen is very important. This is the job of the head chef. It requires management skills. Matching each individual's talent to the task or job is an important consideration. A good, well-developed team will be able to do the following:

- Create useful ideas
- Analyse problems effectively
- Get things done
- Communicate with each other
- Respond to good leadership
- Evaluate logically
- Perform skilled operations with technical precision and ability
- Understand and manage the control system.

Maintaining the health of the team and developing it further demands constant attention. The individual members of a group will never become a team unless effort is made to ensure that the differing personalities are able to relate to one another, communicate with each other and value the contribution each employee or team member makes.

The chef, as a team leader, has a strong influence on his/her team or brigade. The chef in this position is expected to set examples that have to be followed. She/he has to work with the brigade, often under pressure, and sometimes dealing with conflict, personality clashes, change and stress. The chef has to adopt a range of strategies and styles of working in order to build loyalty, drive, innovation, commitment and trust in team members.

The team needs to identify its strengths and weaknesses, and develop ways to help those team members affected to overcome any weaknesses they may have.

> **Effective teams** List three teams you consider to be effective.

Successful team management

Changing situations, variable resources and constant compromise are the realities of working in busy commercial kitchens. Systems and methods of managing teams and solving daily problems provide the chef with a framework in which to operate. The team has to produce meals with the people and resources at its disposal. The chef in charge of a brigade has to know how to handle the staff and make the best use of their abilities. This is one of the most difficult aspects of the chef's job, as people's behaviour is affected by many factors, including their:

- Individual characteristics
- Cultural attributes
- Social skills.

All these have an important bearing on the complex web of relationships within the team. The team members must be supportive of each other. Effective relationships are developed by understanding and listening to individuals. It is important that team members respect and listen to each other, cooperate and value confidentiality. The chef must be able to give honest feedback to the team.

The chef must lead rather than drive, and encourage the team to practise reasonable and supportive behaviour so that any problems are dealt with in an objective way and the team's personal skills are harnessed to achieve their full potential. Every team has to deal with:

- Egos and the weaknesses and/or strengths of its individual members
- Self-appointed experts within the group
- Constantly changing relationships/circumstances.

The chef is able to manage the team successfully only by pulling back from the task in hand, however appealing he or she may find it. The chef must examine the processes that create efficient teamwork, finding out what it is that makes the team as a whole greater than the sum of its parts. To assist in this process, the chef must:

- Have a consistent approach to solving problems
- Take into account people's characters as well as their technical skills
- Encourage supportive behaviour in the team
- Create an open, healthy climate
- Make time for the team to appraise its progress.

Good team management Name three team managers you consider to be good managers. These may be managers in sport, kitchens, or restaurants. Why are they good managers? What can we learn from these managers?

Motivating a team

A chef must motivate his/her team by striving to make their work interesting, challenging and demanding. People must know what is expected of them and what the standards are.

Rewards are linked to effort and results. Any such factors must also work towards fulfilling the:

- Needs of the organisation, and
- Expectations of team members.

Improved performance should be recognised by consideration of pay and performance.

The chef in charge should attempt to intercede on behalf of his/her staff; this in turn will help to increase staff members' motivation and their commitment to the team. For the chef to manage his/her staff effectively, it is important to get to know them well, understand their needs and aspirations and attempt to help them achieve their personal aims.

If a chef is able to manage the team by coordinating its members' aims with the corporate objectives – by reconciling their personal aspirations with the organisation's need to operate profitably – she/he will manage a successful team and in addition will enhance his/her reputation.

Communication

Because communication pervades nearly everything we do, even small improvements in the effectiveness of our communicating are likely to have disproportionately large benefits. In the kitchen, most jobs have some communication component. Successful communication is vital when building working relationships. Training and developing the team is about

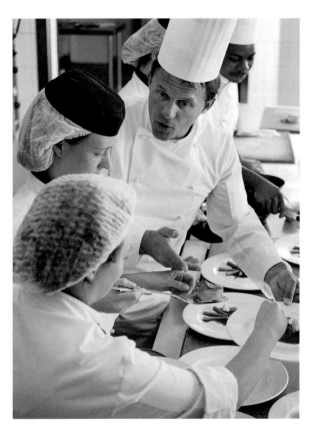

communicating. In work, the quality of our personal relationships depends on the quality of the communication system.

Breakdowns in communication can be identified by looking at the 'intent' and the 'effect' as two separate entities. It is when the intent is not translated into the effect that communication can break down. Such breakdowns affect staff and team relationships and individuals' attitudes towards and views of each other. Good relationships depend on good communication, and awareness of the potential gap between intent and effect can help clarify and prevent any misunderstanding within the group.

By bridging the gap between the intent and the effect you can begin to change the culture of the working environment: the processes become self-reinforcing in a positive direction; the staff begin to respect each other in a positive framework; they listen more carefully to each other, with positive expectations, hearing the constructive intent and responding to it.

As a chef/manager, the art is in achieving results through the team, communication being the key to the exercise. A great deal of the chef's time will be taken up with communicating in one way or another.

Communication, therefore, plays a major part in the chef/manager's role. Communication at work needs to be orientated towards action – getting something done.

Reflect on your communication skills How well do you communicate? Do you need to improve your communication skills? If so, how?

Diversity in the hospitality industry

The hospitality industry is becoming more diverse and, for this reason, the team must celebrate and welcome diversity and embrace equal opportunities.

Diversity in the kitchen can contribute positively to the development of the team, bringing to it a range of skills and ideas from different cultures. The free movement of labour within the European Union has meant that large numbers of people from different cultures now work together in the hospitality industry.

Diversity recognises that people are different. It includes not only cultural and ethnic differences but differences in gender, age, disability and sexual orientation, background, personality and work style.

Developing effective working relationships recognises values and celebrates these differences. Working relationships should be able to harness such differences to improve creativity and innovation and be based on the belief that groups of people who bring different perspectives will find better solutions to problems than groups of people who are the same.

Diversity List the advantages and benefits gained from a diverse workforce.

Minimising conflict in relationships

A conflict with the manager or with colleagues can easily get entangled with issues about work and status, both of which can make it difficult to approach the problem in a rational and professional way. One of the skills of the chef/manager is the need to identify conflict so that plans can be put in place to minimise it. The following are just some of the points that should be borne in mind:

- Conflict arises where there are already strained relationships and personality clashes between members of the team
- Conflict often occurs in a professional kitchen when the brigade is understaffed and under pressure, especially over a long period. Pressure can also come from, say, restaurant reviews and guides, when a chef is seeking a Michelin star or other special accolade
- Conflicts damage working relationships and upset the team and this will eventually show up in the finished product.

The chef and manager must also be aware of any insidious conflict that may be going on around them in less obvious places. Covert conflicts are those that take place in secret; they can be very harmful. Although this type of conflict is often difficult to detect, it will undermine the team's performance. Many conflicts start with misunderstandings or a small upset that grows and develops out of all proportion.

It is important to reflect on and analyse the nature of the conflict and individual attitudes to it. Conflicts can be very damaging and upsetting but there can also be some positive outcomes. A conflict can be a learning curve that a chef has to enter into; it has to be handled properly and focused on in order to achieve the desired outcome.

Prioritising the customer

Developing relationships within the team means that every member understands the goals and objectives of the team. One of the main goals is to satisfy the customer's demands and expectations. Good communication within the organisation assists in the development of customer care. The kitchen must communicate effectively with the restaurant staff so that they, in turn, can communicate with the customer. Any customer complaints must be handled positively: treat customers who complain well, show them empathy. Use customer feedback – good or bad – positively. This may further develop the team and help solve any problems within the team.

Good customer service List the most important factors you consider to be high priority in providing a good customer service programme.

In this chapter you have learned how to:

1. Apply and monitor good health and safety practices
2. Apply and monitor good health and safety training
3. Apply staff supervisory skills within a small team.

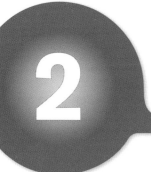

Supervising food safety

This chapter covers Unit 302: Supervising Food Safety in Catering, and Level 3 awards in food safety. In this section you will learn about:

1. The importance of food safety management procedures
2. The responsibilities of employers and employees in respect of food safety legislation and procedures for compliance
3. How the legislation is enforced.

 ## Food safety management procedures and legislation

Food safety legislation

Food safety means putting in place all of the measures needed to make sure that food and drinks are suitable, safe and wholesome through all of the processes; this ranges from selecting suppliers and delivery of food right through to serving the food to the customer.

It has never been more important than now for a chef or kitchen supervisor to have a sound understanding of the principles of food safety. It is also essential to have the knowledge to apply these principles effectively and to train and supervise others working in food areas to adopt the same high standards, so that the chef or supervisor will be **leading by example**.

In any food business, food safety procedures must be planned, organised and monitored. It involves protecting food from the time it is delivered through its storage, preparation cooking and serving to avoid the risk of causing illness or harm to the consumer. It is also essential for the business to comply with legal obligations, to avoid possible legal action or receiving notices served by local authority enforcement officers. Food safety management systems must be in place, with relevant documents forming part of this system. These must be available for inspection and could be used as part of a 'due diligence' defence.

Food safety legislation covers a wide range of topics including:

- Controlling and reducing outbreaks of food poisoning
- Registration of premises and vehicles
- Content and labelling of food
- Prevention of manufacture and sale of injurious food
- Food imports
- Prevention of food contamination and equipment contamination
- Training of food handlers
- Provision of clean water, sanitary facilities, washing facilities.

New food hygiene legislation affecting all food businesses came into force in the UK in January 2006. This new legislation originated in the European parliament; it replaced the existing 1990 Act and related regulations introduced after 1990, though most of the requirements of these earlier acts and regulations remain the same.

The most important and relevant regulations for food businesses are:

- The Food Hygiene (England) Regulations 2006;
  The Food Hygiene (Wales) Regulations 2006;
  The Food Hygiene (Scotland) Regulations 2006;
  The Food Hygiene (Northern Ireland) Regulations 2006

Regulation (EC) No 852/2004 on hygiene of foodstuffs. This gives details of the general hygiene requirements for all UK food businesses and all member countries of the EU.

The main difference introduced by the laws in 2006 was to provide a framework for EU legislation to be enforced in England (with similar requirements for Wales, Scotland and Northern Ireland) and the requirement to have an approved **food safety management procedure** in place with up-to-date permanent records available, including staff training records. All records must be reviewed and monitored regularly, especially if there is a change in procedures.

> *i* You will also find useful information about food hygiene legislation on the Food Standards Agency website – www.food.gov.uk
> Specific guidance topics include:
>
> - Food hygiene, a guide for business
> - Food Law, inspections and your business
> - Food hygiene legislation.

Before the introduction of the new legislation it had long been considered good practice for a food business to have a food safety management system in place. Now it is a **legal requirement** to have a system based on the seven principles of Hazard Analysis Critical Control Point (HACCP). (For more information about HACCP see page 64.) Such a system will:

- Identify, assess and monitor the critical control points in the kitchen procedures
- Ensure that corrective actions are put in place
- Ensure the systems are frequently verified, with accurate documentation available for inspection and ongoing review processes.

To simplify this process, especially for smaller businesses, the Food Standards Agency introduced a system called **Safer Food Better Business**, a straightforward food safety system involving a minimal amount of paperwork and no complicated jargon (see page 67).

See also the presentation 'Safer Food Better Business', provided on Dynamic Learning.

All food businesses must now have suitable and up-to-date food safety management based on HACCP and those responsible for food businesses must ensure that:

- Where a full HACCP system is established at least one person who has been trained in the principles of HACCP is involved in setting up the system
- The premises (and food vehicles) are registered with the local authority
- They can supply records of staff training commensurate with the different job roles
- Policies are in place for planning and monitoring staff training
- Appropriate levels of supervision are in place
- They provide adequate hygiene and welfare facilities for staff
- There is an adequate supply of materials and equipment for staff, including PPE (personal protective equipment)
- There is sufficient ventilation, potable water supplies and adequate drainage
- There are separate washing/cleaning facilities for premises, equipment and food as well as hand-washing facilities
- There are records of suppliers used
- There are systems for accident and incident reporting.

Employees also have food safety responsibilities. They must:

- Not do anything or work in such a way that would endanger or contaminate the food they work with
- Cooperate with their employers and the measures they have put in place to keep food safe
- Take part in planned training and instruction
- Maintain high standards of personal hygiene
- Report illnesses to supervisors or managers before starting work (see page 41)
- Report any breakages, shortages or defects that could affect food safety.

For a business to comply with the 2006 Act, food safety management system records are mandatory and will always include:

- Essential food business records confirming that reputable suppliers are used, supplier records, equipment and premises maintenance records, temperature controls, staff sickness records, cleaning schedules, pest audits
- Written documentation of recruitment, supervision, ongoing training, working practices and reporting procedures.

The main reason for adopting high standards of food safety is to prevent food poisoning. (In 2000 the Food Standards Agency committed to reducing the incidence of food poisoning across the UK.)

However, a food business can gain many more benefits by keeping food safety standards high. These include being compliant with food safety law, reducing food wastage and building a good reputation.

Good food safety standards Compile a list of all the advantages you can think of for a business to have good food safety standards. Also compile a list of disadvantages to a business not having good standards of food safety. You can check your lists with the suggestions in Appendix 1 provided on Dynamic Learning.

Unfortunately, food poisoning and food-borne illness cases in the UK remain unacceptably high. While food poisoning and food-borne illness caused by some specific pathogens have been reduced over the past few years, others have increased. It is also important to remember that only a very small proportion of food poisoning cases are ever reported and recorded so no one really knows the full extent of the problem.

See the chart of food poisoning outbreaks in Appendix 2.

Food safety legislation under the 2006 Act and previous 1990 (1995) Acts is enforced by local authorities through inspection by environmental health officers (EHOs) (environmental health practitioners (EHPs)) who are empowered to serve enforcement notices through criminal and civil courts. (The enforcement notices include the Hygiene Improvement Notice, Hygiene Prohibition Order and Hygiene Prohibition Notice.) Other legislation will be in place relating to working practices, procedures and training and may well involve bodies such as Trading Standards and the Health and Safety Executive.

Enforcement officers

Enforcement officers – EHOs (EHPs) – may visit food premises as a matter of routine, as a follow-up when problems have been identified or after a complaint. The frequency of visits depends on the type of business and food being handled, possible hazards within the business, the risk rating, any previous problems or convictions. Generally, businesses posing a higher risk will be visited more frequently than those considered low risk.

EHOs (EHPs) can enter a food business at any reasonable time without previous notice or appointment, usually, but not always, when the business is open. The main purpose of these inspections is to identify any possible risks from the food business and to assess the effectiveness of the business's hazard controls and also to identify any non-compliance of regulations so this can be monitored and corrected.

The role and powers of enforcement officers

In carrying out their role EHOs (EHPs):

- Offer professional food safety advice to food businesses on routine visits, information leaflets, and so on
- Advise on new food safety legislation
- Investigate complaints about the business
- Ensure food offered for sale is safe and fit for consumption
- Monitor food operations within a business and identify possible sources of contamination
- Ensure food safety law compliance
- Observe the effectiveness of the food safety management system
- Deal with food poisoning outbreaks
- Advise on and deliver food safety training
- Deal with non-compliance by formal action/ serving notices.

When dealing with non-compliance by formal action/ serving notices the EHOs (EHPs) have:

- Power to close premises
- Power to seize/remove food
- Power to instigate prosecution
- Power to seize records.

Issue of notices and orders for non-compliance

A Hygiene Improvement Notice

A Hygiene Improvement Notice will be served if the EHO (EHP) believes that a food business does not comply with regulations. The notice is served in writing and states the name and address of the business, what is wrong, why it is wrong, what needs to be done to put it right and the time in which this must be completed (usually not less than 14 days). This does not apply to cleaning. It is an offence if the work is not carried out in the specified time.

A Hygiene Emergency Prohibition Notice

A Hygiene Emergency Prohibition Notice is served if the EHO (EHP) believes that there is an imminent risk to health from the business. Risks would include serious issues such as sewage contamination, lack of water supply and rodent infestation. Serving this notice would mean immediate closure of the business for three days, during which time the EHO (EHP) must apply to magistrates for a Hygiene Emergency Prohibition Order to keep the premises closed. Notices/orders must be displayed in a visible place on the premises. The owner of the business must apply for a certificate of satisfaction before they can re-open.

A Hygiene Emergency Prohibition Order prohibits a person, that is, the owner/manager, from working in a food business.

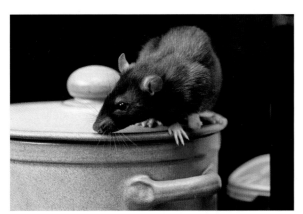

A rat infestation is an example of a hygiene emergency

Fines and penalties for non-compliance

Magistrates courts can impose fines of up to £5,000, a six-month prison sentence or both.

For serious offences, for example knowingly selling food dangerous to health, magistrates could impose fines of up to £20,000. In a Crown Court unlimited fines can be imposed and/or two years' imprisonment.

For more information on food safety legislation see Appendix 3.

Food safety legislation Complete the worksheet on food safety legislation, provided on Dynamic Learning.

Industry guide (to good hygiene practice)

The industry guide to good hygiene practice gives advice (in plain, easy-to-understand English) to food businesses on how to comply with food safety law.

Most industries have similar guides and whilst the guides have no legal force, food authorities must give them due consideration when they enforce the regulations.

It is the intention that industry guides will help business owners and managers to understand and use the information to meet legal obligations and to ensure food safety. Printed industry guides are available from HMSO Publications Offices or can be downloaded from www.archive.food.gov.uk.

Food Standards Agency

The Food Standards Agency was established in 2000 with a role 'to protect public health from risks which may arise in connection with the consumption of food and otherwise to protect the interest of customers in relation to food'. The agency is committed to put customers first, be open and accessible and be an independent voice on food-related matters. It provides information to public and government agencies on food safety and nutritional matters from 'farm to fork' and also protects consumers through enforcement and monitoring. The Food Standards Agency is responsible for:

- Research
- Food safety, contaminants, nutrition, additives and labelling
- Animal feeds
- The performance of local authority enforcements
- Meat and butchery hygiene.

A wide variety of information can be found on the Food Standards Agency website www.food.gov.uk. This includes:

- Various food safety topics
- Nutritional information
- Product and ingredient information (including food additives)
- Information on food and products causing concern and those that have been withdrawn from sale
- Academic papers and reports linked to food safety topics
- Relevant news and current information about food.

The Food Standards Agency also has a question answering service and provides free leaflets, DVDs and posters for food businesses as well as Safer Food Better Business packs on request.

2.2   Temperature control and avoiding food contamination

In this section you will learn about:

1. The importance of and methods for temperature control
2. Procedures to control contamination and cross-contamination
3. The importance of high standards of personal hygiene
4. Procedures for cleaning, disinfection and waste disposal
5. The importance of and methods for pest control
6. Outline requirements relating to design of food premises and equipment

Importance of temperature control

Effective use of temperatures (high or low) is one of the most useful means available to a food business to make food safe to eat and ensure that it remains safe. High temperatures can be effective in killing pathogens and bringing them to a safe level. Low temperatures are effective in preventing (or slowing) multiplication of harmful bacteria in food. Both are of great importance in reducing the likelihood of a food poisoning outbreak.

Legislation requires food businesses and food handlers to keep food safe and have sufficient temperature control equipment available for the levels of work being completed. Correct temperature control will also reduce wastage and retain the quality of food for longer. Recording temperatures will form part of a food safety management system and could be part of a due diligence defence.

Temperature control and equipment

It is important that food is kept out of the 'danger zone temperatures' (5–63°C) as much as possible (see page 51). When cooking and cooling foods, they must be taken through these danger zone temperatures quickly. Failure to do this can allow multiplication of dangerous bacteria and possibly the formation of spores.

Heat food quickly

Cook in smaller quantities, where appropriate, to allow for faster heating to safe temperatures.

Ensure that heat sources are adequate for the task and quantity. Make sure that heating and cool-ing equipment is in good repair and regularly serv-iced. Make use of thermostats to assist in achieving required food temperatures. Use sanitised and cali-brated temperature probes.

Cool food quickly

Cool food to refrigerator temperatures within 90 minutes (protect it from contamination).

Use blast chillers where appropriate. Break amounts down into smaller, thinner portions to allow quicker cooling. Use ice trays, ice packs, and so on. There is a wide variety of temperature control equipment available to a food business. This is listed in Table 2.1.

Table 2.1 Temperature control equipment available to a food business

Hot	Cold
Stoves, combi ovens, etc., bain marie, waterbaths, steamers, hot cabinets, thermal lamps, temperature probes, microwave equipment, thermal food flasks, heated trolleys, heat retaining pellets/mats, etc.	Refrigerators, freezers, blast chillers, chilled display equipment, trolleys and vehicles, thawing cabinets, computerised cold storage systems

Contamination of food

Contamination of food is a major hazard in any food-related operation. A contaminant is anything that is present in food that should not be there. Food con-taminants can range from inconvenient or slightly unpleasant, through to dangerous and even fatal. In any food business it is essential to protect food from contamination and remove or destroy contaminants already present (such as, for example, possible pathogens in raw poultry).

Contaminants could be:

- **Micro-organisms** such as pathogens, moulds, viruses
- **Physical** objects such as paperclips, fingernails, insects, packaging materials
- **Chemical** such as cleaning materials, disinfectants
- **Allergenic** such as nuts, wheat, dairy products.

Cross-contamination

Cross-contamination occurs when pathogenic bacteria (or other contaminants) are transferred from one place to another. This is often from contaminated food (usually raw food), equipment, areas or food handlers to ready-to-eat food. It is the cause of significant amounts of food poisoning and care must be taken to avoid it. Cross-contamination could be caused by:

- Foods touching, for example raw and cooked meat
- Raw meat or poultry dripping onto high-risk foods
- Soil from dirty vegetables coming into contact with high-risk foods
- Dirty cloths, dirty staff uniforms or dirty equipment
- Equipment used for raw then cooked food, for example chopping boards or knives
- Hands, touching raw then cooked food; not washing hands between tasks
- Pests spreading bacteria from their own bodies around the kitchen
- Different people touching hand contact surfaces, for example fridge or cupboard doors.

i Terms associated with cross-contamination

Source This is where bacteria comes from; for example raw meat and poultry, pests, dirty vegetables and unwashed hands.

Vehicle This is something that carries bacteria from the source to another place (often onto high-risk food). Vehicles could include dirty equipment, hands, cloths, pests.

Route This is the path the bacteria take from the source to another area, often onto high-risk foods where they can multiply to dangerous levels.

Cross-contamination Complete the cross-contamination worksheet provided on Dynamic Learning.

Ways of controlling cross-contamination

Separate working areas and storage areas for raw and high-risk foods are recommended. If this is not possible, keep them well away from each other and make sure that working areas are thoroughly cleaned and disinfected between tasks.

Cool food quickly to 8°C within 90 minutes and protect from contamination whilst cooling.

Vegetables should be washed before preparation and peeling and again afterwards. Leafy vegetables may need to be washed in several changes of cold water to remove all of the soil clinging to them.

Good personal hygiene practices by staff, especially frequent, effective hand-washing, are very important in controlling cross-contamination and will avoid the significant amounts of contamination caused by faecal–oral routes. (This is when pathogens normally found in faeces are transferred to ready-to-eat foods, resulting in cross-contamination and illness.) An obvious way that this could happen is when food handlers visit the toilet, do not wash their hands and then handle food.

Carefully control chemicals in food areas through COSSH (Control of Substances Hazardous to Health) control and staff training in correct use of cleaning chemicals

The use of swabbing procedures to monitor microbial presence is considered to be good practice.

Ensure that large and small equipment and utensils are kept in good repair and well maintained. Provide proper storage for equipment and utensils to protect them from contamination.

Areas and equipment should be smooth, impervious and easy to clean.

Check that there are good hand-washing facilities and that supplies are regularly checked (see page 42).

Put clear, strict policies in place for visitors to the kitchen such as, for example, restricted access, issue of white coats and hats, and so on.

Ensure that pest-control policies are in place, with regular audits and reports.

Control of waste (inside and outside) is important; waste can be a significant cause of cross-contamination. Use strong waste bins with lids. Kitchen waste bins should have a foot-operated lid and be lined with a suitable bag.

Much of the above can be achieved by setting high standards, effective supervision and planned staff training.

Colour-coded equipment

Colour-coded chopping boards are a good way to keep different types of food separate. Worktops and chopping boards will come into contact with the food being prepared, so need special attention when cleaning and disinfecting. Make sure that chopping boards are in good condition: cracks and splits trap bacteria and this could be transferred to food. As well as colour-coded chopping boards some kitchens provide colour-coded knives, cloths, cleaning equipment, storage trays, bowls and even staff uniforms to help prevent cross-contamination.

Personal hygiene

All humans can be a source of food poisoning bacteria and everyone working with food must be aware of the importance of personal hygiene in line with the tasks they complete. It is up to the supervisor to make staff aware of this and to lead by example.

Staphylococcus aureus may be present in the nose, mouth, throat, on skin and hair and could easily be transferred onto food where it could then multiply and cause illness. It is very important that hair, nose, ears, mouth and so on are not touched whilst preparing food. Cuts, burns and boils are also likely to be a source of bacteria so must be covered.

Anyone suffering from, or who is a carrier of, any disease that could be transmitted through food must not handle food. This would include: diarrhoea and/or vomiting or any food poisoning symptom, infected cuts, burns or spots, bad cold or flu symptoms.

Food handlers with any such illness, infection or wound must report this to their supervisor before starting work. They should also report any illness that had occurred on a recent holiday and illness of other members of their family.

All supervisors must be aware that food handlers can be **carriers** of dangerous pathogens that could get into the food they prepare. All known carriers must not handle food.

Convalescent carriers are recovering from an illness but still carry the bacteria and can pass it on to the food they handle.

Healthy carriers show no signs of illness but can still contaminate the food as above. These people can remain carriers for long periods or all of their lives.

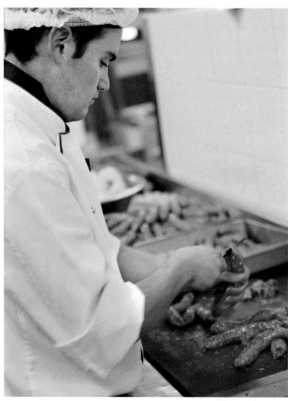

Food handling demands high standards of hygiene

Before starting a job involving food handling supervisors and head chefs must make all staff aware that they must practise high standards of personal hygiene; they must always arrive at work clean (daily bath or shower) and with clean hair.

They must also:

- Wear approved, clean kitchen clothing used only in the kitchen. This must completely cover any personal clothing
- Cover or contain hair in a suitable hat or net
- Keep nails short and clean; no nail varnish or false nails
- Remove jewellery and watches before handling food (a plain wedding band is permissible but could still trap bacteria)
- Avoid wearing cosmetics and perfumes

- Never smoke in food areas (ash, smoke and bacteria from touching the mouth area could get into food)
- Never eat food, sweets or chew gum when working with food. These may also transfer bacteria to food
- Always cover cuts, burns or grazes with a waterproof dressing, then wash hands thoroughly
- Report any illness to the supervisor as soon as possible.

Staff will also need to be instructed on the importance of frequent hand washing and how to do this properly. They need to know that contamination of food, equipment and surfaces from hands can happen very easily and care must be taken with hand washing to avoid this.

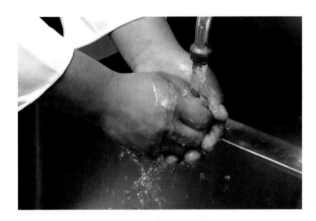

i Hand-washing procedure

1. Use a basin provided just for hand washing.
2. Wet hands under warm running water.
3. Apply liquid soap.
4. Rub hands together between fingers and thumbs.
5. Remember fingertips, nails and wrists.
6. Rinse off under the running water.
7. Dry hands on a paper towel and use the paper towel to turn off the tap.

Staff involved in food handling must know that thorough hand washing should take place:
- When they enter the kitchen, before starting work and handling any food
- After a break (using the toilet, in contact with faeces)

- Between different tasks but especially between handling raw and cooked food
- After touching hair, nose, mouth or using a tissue for a sneeze or cough
- After application or change of a dressing on a cut or burn
- After cleaning preparation areas, equipment or contaminated surfaces
- After handling kitchen waste, external food packaging, money or flowers.

Protective clothing

Protective clothing should be worn only in the relevant food areas. Clothing needs to be suitable for the work to be carried out, completely cover the wearers' own clothing, comfortable and washable at high temperatures. Jackets and coats should have press stud closures rather than buttons; any pockets should be on the inside. Hats or head covering should completely cover hair.

Protective clothing could actually be a cause of food contamination. If it becomes badly stained or dirty it must be changed for clean clothing. Staff must be provided with suitable areas or lockers to change and store their clothing and belongings.

Induction training Suggest the food safety topics that should be included in an *induction handbook* for new kitchen assistants who will have some food-handling duties.

Cleaning and disinfection

Clean food areas play an essential part in the production of safe food. Clean premises, work areas and equipment are essential to:
- Control the organisms that cause food poisoning
- Reduce the possibility of physical and chemical contamination
- Make accidents less likely, for example slips on a greasy floor
- Create a positive image for customers, visitors and employees
- Comply with the law
- Avoid attracting pests to the kitchen
- Create a pleasant and hygienic working environment.

Effective cleaning uses one or more of the following:
- **Physical energy:** human effort of the cleaner carrying out the task

- **Chemicals:** detergents
- **Mechanical methods**: machines
- **Turbulence**: movement of liquids
- **Thermal energy**: hot water and steam
- **CIP** (clean in place), for example for very large equipment.

When done properly cleaning is effective in removing dirt, grease, debris and food particles. Areas will look better, be tidier and it will be possible for work to be carried out more efficiently. However, cleaning alone is not effective in the removal of micro-organisms; for this **disinfection is required**. Disinfection is often carried out after the cleaning process but sometimes the two are done together, for instance when using a sanitiser. It is unlikely that disinfection will kill all micro-organisms but it will bring them to a safe level.

Disinfection may be completed with:

- Chemicals: use only those recommended for kitchen use
- Hot water: for example 82°C + for 30 seconds as occurs in a dishwasher
- Steam: use of steam disinfection is good for equipment and surfaces that are difficult to dismantle or reach, for example CIP.

All food contact surfaces, equipment and hand contact items (for example fridge handles) should be cleaned and disinfected regularly according to your cleaning schedule. Other areas and items may need thorough cleaning but not disinfection, for example floors and walls. It is important to clean and disinfect the cleaning materials after use.

Cleaning Complete the cleaning schedule worksheet provided on Dynamic Learning.

There is a wide range of cleaning products designed to complete different tasks.

Use of chemicals in cleaning

Chemicals used in cleaning and disinfection include:

- **Detergent:** this is designed to remove grease and dirt and hold them in suspension in water. It may be in the form of liquid, powder, gel or foam and usually needs to be added to water to use. Detergent will not kill pathogens (but the hot water it is mixed with may help to do this); however, it will clean and degrease so disinfectant can work properly. Detergents work best in hot water

- **Disinfectant:** this is intended to destroy bacteria when used properly. Disinfectants must be left on a cleaned grease-free surface for the required amount of time to be effective and usually work best in cool water (see below)
- **Sanitiser:** this cleans and disinfects and usually comes in spray form. Sanitiser is very useful for work surfaces and equipment especially between tasks
- **Steriliser:** this can be chemicals (or the action of extreme heat) and will kill all living micro-organisms.

For more information about disinfectants, refer to Appendix 4.

Terms associated with cleaning

Bactericide
A substance that destroys bacteria.

Biodegradable
A substance capable of being decomposed by bacteria and other living organisms.

Contact time
The time a chemical needs to be left on a surface to ensure it is effective; for example the time a disinfectant requires to achieve disinfection.

Detergent (surfactant)
A chemical used to remove dirt, grease and food particles. This does not kill bacteria.

Disinfectant
A chemical used to reduce micro-organisms to a safe level, for example bleach (also hot water 82°C + for 30 seconds) or steam.

Sanitiser
A detergent and disinfectant combined (but never mix it yourself).

Steriliser
A chemical used to destroy all micro-organisms, spores and toxins.

Sterilising
The process of destroying all micro-organisms, toxins and spores.

Dangers from chemicals

The supervisor must ensure that staff are aware of the possible dangers and hazards from cleaning chemicals. Recognised COSHH training for staff will increase awareness of the risks of the possible dangers from the chemicals they use as part of their job role. Staff must be made aware through ongoing training and supervision of the correct use of chemicals, use of PPE and of proper chemical storage procedures. Chemicals must be kept well away from food-preparation areas in separate and lockable storage; the chemicals must be kept in their original containers. Disposal of chemicals must be carried out in the correct manner according to company policy, health and safety regulations and advised COSHH procedures.

Clean as you go

As a food supervisor, it is important to train all staff in the importance of *clean as you go* and not allow waste to accumulate in the area where food preparation and cooking are being carried out. Staff need to understand that it is very difficult to keep untidy areas clean and hygienic and it is more likely that cross-contamination will occur in untidy areas.

To ensure that cleaning is effective staff must be properly trained, with emphasis given to use of the cleaning schedule, correct methods and use of chemicals and PPE.

As part of a food safety management system, cleaning of areas and equipment needs to be planned and recorded on a cleaning schedule. The cleaning schedule needs to include the following information:

- What is to be cleaned
- Who should do it (name if possible)
- How it is to be done and how long it should take
- When, time of day
- Materials to be used including chemicals, dilution, cleaning equipment, protective clothing to be worn
- Safety precautions necessary
- Signatures of cleaner and supervisor checking the work, also date and time.

Cleaning schedule A blank cleaning schedule is provided on Dynamic Learning. Fill in the schedule for a cold counter, salad bar or other area in your workplace.

Disposal of kitchen waste

Kitchen waste should be placed in suitable waste bins with lids (preferably with foot-operated lid). Bins should be made of a strong material, be easy to clean, pest proof and lined with a suitable bin liner. They should be emptied regularly to avoid waste build-up, as this could cause problems with multiplication of bacteria and attract pests. An over-full heavy bin is also much more difficult to handle than a regularly emptied bin. Waste should never be left in kitchen bins overnight (this needs to be part of *closing checks*).

Outside waste bins also need to be strong, pest proof and impervious with a closely fitting lid. Bins should stand on hard surfaces that can be easily hosed down and kept clean. Planned regular emptying of the bins and cleaning of the area should be recorded in the cleaning schedule/management system.

Dishwashing

The most efficient and hygienic method of cleaning dishes and crockery is the use of a dishwasher, as this will clean and disinfect items that will then air dry, so removing the need for cloths. The dishwasher can also be used to clean/disinfect small equipment such as bowls and chopping boards. The stages in machine dishwashing are: remove waste food, pre-rinse or spray, then load onto the appropriate racks. The wash cycle will run at 50–60°C using a detergent and the rinse cycle at 82–88°C. This very high rinse temperature will disinfect items and allow them to air dry so no drying cloths will be needed.

Dishwashing by hand

If items need to be washed by hand the recommended way to do this is:

- Scrape, rinse or spray off residue food
- Wash items in a sink of hot water; the temperature should be 50–60°C, which means rubber gloves should be worn. Use a dishwashing brush rather than a cloth. (The brush will help to loosen food particles and is not such a good breeding ground for bacteria)
- Rinse in very hot water; if rinsing is possible at 82°C for 30 seconds, it would disinfect the dishes
- Allow to air dry; do not use tea towels.

Before dishwashers were so widely used a double sink system of dishwashing was often used. Dishes were washed by hand in one sink using hot water and detergent, then loaded onto racks and plunged into a second sink of very hot rinse water (up to 80°C). The water in this sink was often heated by heating elements or pipes under the sink. Although this system can still be seen in some establishments it has fallen from favour because it is labour intensive, creates condensation problems and causes health and safety concerns (open sinks of very hot water).

Cleaning kitchen surfaces

Because kitchen surfaces are likely to come into direct contact with food it is essential that they undergo planned and recorded cleaning and disinfection. Details of two methods for cleaning kitchen surfaces are given in Table 2.2.

Avoiding hazards

Cleaning is essential to prevent hazards but if not managed properly can become a hazard in itself. Do not store cleaning chemicals in food preparation and cooking areas and take care with their use (*chemical contamination*). Make sure that items such as cloths and paper towel, fibres from mops do not get into open food (*physical contamination*). *Bacterial contamination* could occur by using the same cleaning cloths and equipment in raw food areas and then in high-risk food areas, or by not cleaning/disinfecting cleaning equipment properly.

Pests

When there are reports of food premises being forcibly closed down, an infestation of pests is often part of the reason. As pests can be a serious source of contamination and disease, they must be eliminated from food premises for food safety reasons and to comply with the law. Pests can carry food poisoning bacteria into food premises from their fur or feathers, feet or paws, saliva, urine and droppings. Other problems caused by pests include: damage to food stock and packaging, damage to buildings, equipment and wiring, blockages in equipment and piping.

Pests can be attracted to food premises because there is food, warmth, shelter, water and possible nesting materials; all reasonable measures must be put in place to keep them out. Staff must be made aware of possible signs that pests may be present and that any sightings must be reported to the supervisor or manager immediately.

Common pests that may cause problems in food areas are: rats, mice, cockroaches, wasps, flies, ants (pharaoh ants), birds and domestic pets.

Pest management needs to be planned as part of the food safety management system. You should allow a recognised pest control company to make regular visits to your premises because they will offer advice as well as deal with problems arising. Companies conducting a regular audit will provide a pest audit report, which should be kept and could be used as part of due diligence.

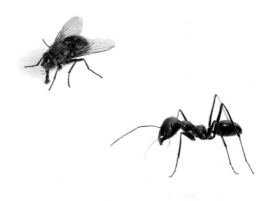

Possible diseases from pests

Pests in and around kitchens and food can result in contamination and disease. See Table 2.3.

Remember that pest infestations are the main reason for premises being closed and a common reason for prosecution. Contamination of food by pests is also a common reason for prosecution.

Table 2.2 Methods for cleaning kitchen surfaces

One of the following two methods is recommended for cleaning a kitchen surface:	
6 stage	4 stage
• Remove debris and loose particles • Main clean to remove soiling grease • Rinse using clean hot water and cloth to remove detergent • Apply disinfectant; leave for contact time recommended on container • Rinse off the disinfectant if recommended • Allow to air dry or use kitchen paper to dry	• Remove debris and loose particles • Main clean, use hot water and sanitiser • Rinse using clean hot water and cloth if recommended on instructions • Allow to air dry or use kitchen paper to dry

Table 2.3 Contamination and disease caused by rodents, birds and insects

Rodents and birds may cause contamination with:	Insects may cause contamination with:
Salmonella / Typhoid *Clostridium perfringens* *E. coli 0157* *Leptospirosis (Weil's)* *Cholera* *Trichinosis / parasites* *Campylobacter* *Listeria*	*Salmonella* *Clostridium perfringens* *E. coli 0157* *Dysentery*

The law requires there to be pest control in premises:

Regulation (EC) 852/2004 stipulates that:

'Effective pest control procedures must be implemented.'

'Food must be protected from contamination.'

Details of signs to look for as evidence of pests in your premises and advice about how to keep them out are given in Table 2.4.

Table 2.4 Signs of pest presence and how to keep them out

Pest	Signs that they are present	Ways to keep them out
Rats, mice	Sightings of rodent, droppings, unpleasant smell, fur, gnawed wires, etc. Greasy marks on lower walls, damaged food stock and packaging, paw prints and tail marks.	Wherever possible, block entry, e.g. no holes around pipe work, avoid gaps and cavities where rodents could get in. Sealed drain covers, wire guards on top of pipes and soil stacks, metal kick plates on doors. Make sure any damage to building, fixtures and fittings is repaired quickly. Check deliveries and packaging for pests. Cut back outside vegetation. Baits and traps, inside and outside.
Flies, wasps,	Sighting of flies and wasps, hearing them, dead insects (maggots).	Window / door screening / netting. Electronic fly killer.
Cockroaches	Sighting, dead or alive, also nymphs, eggs, lavae, pupae, egg cases. Live cockroaches often seen at night. Unpleasant smell.	No holes around pipes, windows, etc. Sealed containers, no open food left out. Regular checks of ducting pipe lagging, etc.
Ants	Sightings and present in food and food stores. The tiny, pale-coloured pharaoh ants are difficult to spot but can still be the source of a variety of pathogens.	No build-up of waste in kitchen. Outside waste not kept too close to kitchen. Dry goods in sealed containers. No open food left in kitchen or store rooms.
Weevils	Sightings of weevils in stored products, e.g. flour and cornflour. Very difficult to see – tiny black insects moving in flour, etc.	Effective stock control.
Birds	Sighting, droppings, in/outside storage areas and around refuse.	Block entry to building, use of screens, netting, etc. Make sure outside refuse bins have close fitting lids.
Domestic pets	These must be kept out of food areas as they carry pathogens on fur, whiskers, saliva, urine, etc.	Keep them out
Professional and organised pest management control, surveys and reports in place allow for organised management of pests		

Pest control measures can also introduce food safety hazards. Bodies of dead insects or even rodents may remain in the kitchen (physical and bacterial contamination). Pesticides, insecticides and baits could cause chemical contamination if not managed properly. Pest control problems are best managed by professionals.

Role of the supervisor in pest management

The role of a supervisor in pest management is mainly about good practice, good housekeeping and working with pest control contractors. These include:

- Reporting any damage to buildings and fittings and organising prompt repair
- Keeping entrances to the building clean and clear with undergrowth well cut back
- Keeping food areas clean (especially under and behind equipment and in corners) and not leaving out any traces of food or liquids overnight (part of the closing checks)
- Making sure refuse areas are regularly checked and cleaned and that refuse containers have tight-fitting lids and are emptied regularly
- Effective stock control and regular cleaning of storage areas. Keeping dry stores in sealed containers and off the floor. Checking deliveries for any possible signs of pests.

Pest control Draw a sketch of a kitchen or restaurant that you are familiar with; include all doors and windows in the sketch. Mark up any possible ways that pests could get in (name the type of pests). Suggest the measures available to prevent pests getting in through the areas you have marked.

Premises

Food premises must be planned to allow good food safety to take place. Suitable buildings with well-planned fittings, layout and equipment enable supervisors of food premises to plan for good food safety standards.

Certain basics need to be available if a building is to be used for food production such as, for example:

- There must be electricity supplies and preferably gas supplies
- Potable (clean and drinkable) water and efficient effluent drainage
- Suitable road access for deliveries and refuse collection

- Surrounding areas and buildings should not be sources of contamination by pests, chemicals, smoke, odours or dust.

Layout

When planning food premises a linear workflow should be in place, as shown in the example below.

Example of a linear workflow

Delivery → storage → preparation → cooking → hot holding → serving.

This means there will be no cross-over of activities that could result in cross-contamination. There must be adequate storage areas; the availability of sufficient refrigerated storage is especially important.

Appropriate staff hand washing and drying facilities suitable for work being carried out must be provided.

Clean and dirty (raw and cooked) processes should be well segregated. Cleaning and disinfection should be planned, with separate storage for cleaning materials and chemicals.

All areas should allow for efficient cleaning, disinfection and pest control.

Personal hygiene facilities must be provided for staff as well as changing facilities and storage for personal clothing and belongings.

Lighting and ventilation

Lighting (natural and artificial) must be sufficient for tasks being completed, to allow for safe working and so that cleaning can be carried out efficiently.

Good ventilation is essential in food premises to prevent excessive heat, condensation, circulation of air-borne contaminants, grease vapours and odours. If ventilation is poor, working conditions may be unpleasant and the likelihood of contamination greater. Ventilation systems should flow from clean areas to dirty areas.

Drainage

Drainage must be adequate for the work being completed without causing flooding. If channels, grease traps and gullies are used they should allow for frequent and easy cleaning. The direction of drainage must be from clean to dirty.

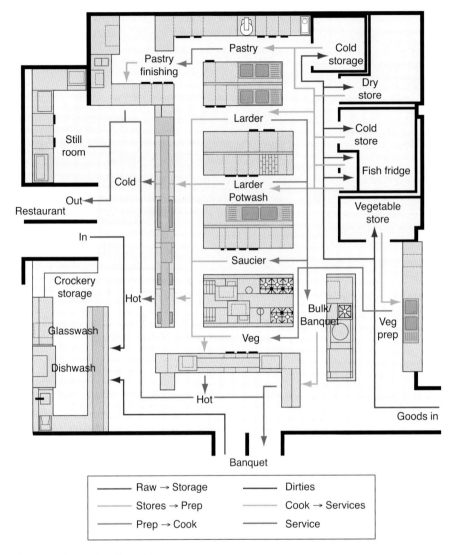

Example of a kitchen floor plan

Floors

These need to be durable and in good condition; they must be impervious, non slip, and easy to clean. Where necessary the floor must allow for efficient drainage into gullies. Suitable materials are: non-slip quarry tiles, epoxy resins, industrial vinyl sheeting, and granolithic flooring. Where the materials allow, edges between floor and walls should be coved to prevent debris collecting in corners.

Walls

Walls need to be impervious, smooth, easy to clean, non toxic and preferably light in colour. Suitable wall coverings are: plastic cladding, stainless steel sheeting, ceramic tiles, epoxy resin or rubberised painted plaster or brickwork. Walls should be coved where they join the floor. Lagging and ducting around pipes should be sealed and gaps sealed where pipes enter the building to eliminate pests.

Ceilings

Design often includes suspended ceilings so pipe work and wiring can be concealed. However, care must be taken to prevent pests from getting into these areas. Ceiling finishes must resist build-up of condensation which could encourage mould; they should be of a non-flaking material and be washable. Non-porous ceiling panels and tiles are frequently used and may incorporate lighting; non-flaking paints are also useful. Once again, edges should be coved where possible.

Windows and doors

Windows and doors make it possible for pests to enter the building so should be fitted with suitable screening, strip-curtains, metal kick plates, and so on. Doors and windows should also fit well into their frames, again to stop pests gaining access. Door handles and windows handles need to be included in the cleaning schedule as they are hand-contact surfaces and could be a cause of cross-contamination.

Fittings and surfaces

Surfaces and equipment in food areas should be smooth, impervious, corrosion-resistant, non-toxic and easily allow effective cleaning and disinfection to take place. All should be of suitable quality for the work to be done, kept in good repair and be regularly maintained. Surfaces and equipment are likely to come into direct contact with food, so planned cleaning and disinfection recorded in the cleaning schedule is essential. Sinks for washing food must have hot and cold *potable* water.

Kitchen flooring As a supervisor of a large kitchen you are concerned about the poor state of the very old kitchen flooring and wish to make a case to management for a new kitchen floor.

What are the points you would raise about the importance of good flooring? What problems could occur if the floor is not replaced?

2.3 Food safety hazards and controlling food safety

In this section you will learn about:

1. The importance to food safety of microbial, chemical, physical and allergenic hazards

2. Methods and procedures for controlling food safety to include critical control points, critical limits and corrective actions

3. The requirements for monitoring and recording food safety procedures

4. Methods for and the importance of evaluating food safety controls and procedures.

Food safety hazards

In any food business there are going to be food safety hazards, which could be any of the following:

- **Microbial hazards (micro-organisms)** such as pathogens causing food poisoning or food-borne illness; also spores and toxins (see below), moulds, viruses, parasites, etc. These could be the cause of food poisoning or food-borne illness.

- **Physical hazards**: objects such as machine parts, paperclips, fingernails, insects, packaging materials, coins, buttons and blue plasters getting into food. These could cause a wide range of reactions including distaste, choking, nausea, broken teeth and cuts to the mouth.

- **Chemical hazards** from various chemicals such as kitchen cleaning materials, disinfectants, insecticides, rodenticides, degreasers, agricultural chemicals and beer line cleaners. These could cause a range of problems including skin or eye irritation, breathing problems, burning and vomiting.

- **Allergenic hazards** may come from nuts, wheat products, dairy products, shellfish, mushrooms and soft fruits. Reactions may be serious such as, for example, anaphylactic shock, breathing difficulties, rashes, irritation and swelling.

All of these food safety hazards are cause for concern and care must be taken not to allow contamination of food from them. When implementing the food safety management system all types of hazard needs to be considered and controls put in place to make them safe.

All of the above hazards are of concern in a food business but probably of the greatest concern is food poisoning from **microbial sources**.

Food poisoning

This is an acute intestinal illness that is the result of eating foods contaminated with pathogenic bacteria and/or their toxins. Food poisoning may also be caused by eating poisonous fish or plants, chemicals or metals. Symptoms of food poisoning are often similar and may include: diarrhoea, vomiting, nausea, fever, headache, dehydration and abdominal pain.

Food-borne illness

This is an illness caused by pathogenic bacteria and/or their toxins and also viruses, but in this case pathogens do not need to multiply in the food; they just need to get into the intestine where they start to multiply. Only tiny amounts are needed and may be transmitted person to person, in water or airborne as well as through food. Symptoms of food-borne illness are wide and varied and include: severe abdominal pain, diarrhoea, vomiting, headaches, blurred vision, flu symptoms, septicaemia and miscarriage.

At-risk groups

Food poisoning and food-borne illness can be unpleasant for anyone, but for some the illnesses can be very serious or even fatal.

These high-risk groups include:
- Babies and the very young
- Elderly people
- Pregnant women
- Those with an impaired immune system
- Those who are already unwell.

Pathogenic bacteria

The most common cause of food poisoning and food-borne illness is bacteria, though not all bacteria are harmful. Some are essential to maintain good health, for example in the digestive system; some are used in the manufacture of medicines and others in food production, for example in making cheese and yoghurt.

The bacteria that can be harmful and cause food poisoning are referred to as pathogenic bacteria. These are dangerous once they get into food because they are not visible to the human eye and the appearance, smell and taste of the food may remain unchanged.

It is not possible to completely eliminate pathogenic bacteria from food premises as they are to be found widely in the environment, including in raw foods, dirty vegetables, animal pests and humans to name just a few. They can very easily be transferred onto hands, surfaces, cooked foods, equipment and cloths; this is called *cross-contamination*. Bacteria may be carried from one place to another in the kitchen, for example on hands or equipment; these are referred to as *vehicles* of contamination.

Multiplication of bacteria

Once bacteria (pathogens) are present in food, given the right conditions (see below) they are able to multiply by dividing into two. This is called *binary fission*.

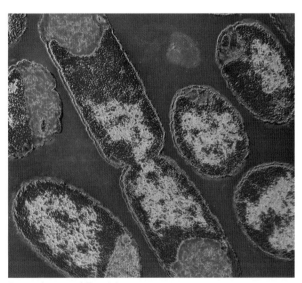

Binary fission of E. coli bacteria

The conditions needed for bacteria to multiply in this way are:
- **Time**: given the conditions they need, bacteria can divide by binary fission every 10–20 minutes.
- **Warmth**: the optimum temperature for bacteria to multiply is 37°C (body temperature). This is when binary fission occurs most quickly; but some form of bacterial multiplication can occur between the temperatures of 5°–63°C, the temperature range called the **Danger Zone**.
  - Different bacteria prefer slightly different temperature ranges for growth (multiplication); for example, *Clostridium perfringens* grow best at 45°C while *Listeria monocytogenes* grow most

efficiently at 30°C but can still multiply at fridge temperatures. In a fridge running below 5°C, bacteria would multiply very slowly or not at all and there would be no multiplication at freezer temperatures, though these temperatures would not actually kill bacteria.

- **Food (nutrients)**: a wide selection of foods, especially protein-rich foods such as meat, fish, and dairy foods, supports the growth of bacteria. Foods with high concentrations of sugar, salt or acids such as vinegar do not support bacterial growth. This is why sugar, salt and vinegar are often used to preserve foods.

- **Moisture**: bacteria need water to support their life cycle and processes. The amount of water in food is referred to as aw (water activity). Other than dried foods most food contains some moisture and a wide variety of foods contains enough water to support bacterial multiplication.

- **Oxygen requirement**: some bacteria need oxygen in order to multiply; this group of bacteria is referred to as *aerobes*. Some can multiply only where there is no oxygen and these are called *anaerobes*. Others can multiply with or without oxygen and are called *facultative anaerobes*.

- **pH**: this is a measure of how acid or alkaline a food or liquid may be. The scale runs from 1–14. Acid foods are below 7 on the scale; 7 is neutral; above 7 and up to 14 is alkaline. Bacteria multiply best around a neutral ph and most bacteria cannot multiply at a pH below 4, so foods such as citrus fruits would not support bacterial multiplication.

The phases bacteria go through in their multiplication are shown in the bacterial growth curve chart.

Bacterial growth curve

Lag phase: when bacteria first enter suitable conditions for growth no immediate growth takes place; the bacteria are getting used to their surroundings.

Log phase: in the presence of ideal conditions bacteria will multiply rapidly.

Stationary phase: bacteria are multiplying but some are also dying off. There may also be competition between different bacteria for survival so numbers stay the same.

Decline phase: bacteria start to die off and numbers decrease.

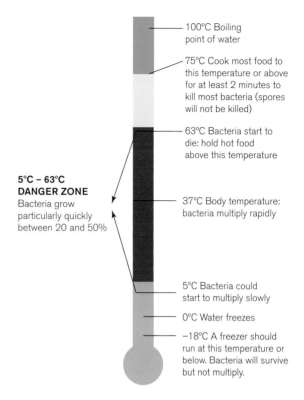

5°C – 63°C DANGER ZONE Bacteria grow particularly quickly between 20 and 50%

100°C Boiling point of water

75°C Cook most food to this temperature or above for at least 2 minutes to kill most bacteria (spores will not be killed)

63°C Bacteria start to die: hold hot food above this temperature

37°C Body temperature: bacteria multiply rapidly

5°C Bacteria could start to multiply slowly

0°C Water freezes

−18°C A freezer should run at this temperature or below. Bacteria will survive but not multiply.

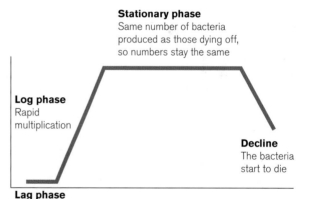

Stationary phase Same number of bacteria produced as those dying off, so numbers stay the same

Log phase Rapid multiplication

Decline The bacteria start to die

Lag phase No multiplication

Bacterial growth curve chart

Some common food poisoning bacteria

Salmonella

Salmonella used to be the most common cause of food poisoning in the UK but since measures were put in place to reduce salmonella in chickens and in eggs, food poisoning from this source has reduced. The sources of salmonella are the human and animal gut and excreta; but salmonella is also found in pests such as rodents, insects, terrapins and birds as well as domestic pets and has been associated with sewage and untreated water supplies. Food sources of salmonella could be: raw meat and poultry, raw eggs, untreated milk and shellfish. Salmonella poisoning can also be passed on through human carriers (someone carrying salmonella but not showing any signs of illness). There are different types of salmonella that can cause illness. For more information about salmonella, refer to Appendix 5, provided on Dynamic Learning.

Staphylococcus aureus

The main source of this organism is the human body. It may be present on skin, hair and scalp, nose and throat. Cuts, spots, burns and boils will also be a source of this organism. When *Staphylococcus* multiplies in food, a toxin (poison) is produced which is very difficult to kill, even with boiling temperatures. To avoid food poisoning from this organism, food handlers need to maintain very high standards of personal hygiene and always report any illness they have (or have had) to their supervisor before handling food.

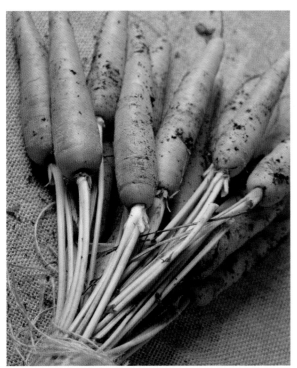
Clostridium perfringens may be present on dirty vegetables

Clostridium perfringens

Clostridium perfringens can be present in human and animal faeces and raw meat, poultry and dirty vegetables (also insects, soil, dust and sewage). A number of food poisoning incidents from this organism have occurred when large amounts of meat have been brought up to cooking temperatures slowly, then allowed to cool slowly for later use by reheating. *Clostridium perfringens* can produce spores during this heating and cooling. Spores are very resistant to any further cooking and facilitate the survival of bacteria in conditions that would usually kill them.

Bacillus cereus

This is another organism that can produce spores and it can also produce two different types of toxins, making it a dangerous pathogen. It is often associated with cooking rice in large quantities, cooling it too slowly and then reheating. The reheating temperatures would not be enough to destroy spores and toxins. It has also been linked with other cereal crops, spices, soil and vegetables.

Clostridium botulinum

This is a spore-forming organism that fortunately is rare in the UK. Symptoms can be very serious, even fatal. Sources tend to be intestines of fish, soil and vegetables.

Organisms causing food-borne illness

Some different organisms from the above are said to cause *food-borne illness*. These do not multiply in food but use food to get into the human gut, where they then multiply and cause a range of illnesses, some of them serious. They include:

- *Campylobacter*: it is found in raw poultry and meat, sewage, animals, insects and birds. (This now causes more food-related illness than any other organism.)
- *E. coli*: present in the intestines (and excreta of animals and humans), raw meat and can be present on raw vegetables.
- *Listeria*: this organism is of concern because it can multiply (slowly) at fridge temperatures, that is, below 5°C. It has been linked with chilled products such as unpasteurised cheeses, pate and prepared salads, as well as cook/chill meals.

Table 2.5 Food poisoning and food-borne disease: pathogenic bacteria

Major food poisoning pathogens	Sources of bacteria	Preferred temp. for growth	Illness onset time	Symptoms	Can it form spores?
Salmonella	Raw meat/poultry, raw egg, intestines of humans and animals, sewage/water, carriers, pets and pests	7–45°C	12–36 hours	Stomach pain, diarrhoea, vomiting, fever (1–7 days)	No
Clostridium perfringens	Animal and human intestines and excreta. Soil and dust, insects and raw meat	15–50°C	12–18 hours	Stomach pain and diarrhoea; vomiting is rare (12–48 hours)	Yes
Staphylococcus aureus toxin in food is heat resistant	Humans – mouth, nose, hair, skin, boils, cuts, burns, etc.	7–45°C	1–7 hours	Stomach pain and vomiting, flu-like symptoms, maybe some diarrhoea, lowered body temperatures (6–24 hours)	No
Clostridium botulinum	Soil, intestines of fish and animals	7–48°C	2 hours–8 days (usually 12–36 hours)	Difficulty with speech, breathing and swallowing. Double vision, nerve paralysis. Death	Yes
Bacillus cereus i) toxin in food is heat resistant	Cereals, especially rice, dust and soil	3–40°C	1–5 hours	Vomiting, abdominal pain, maybe some diarrhoea (12–24 hours)	Yes
ii) toxin in intestine	Cereals, especially rice, dust and soil		8–16 hours	Stomach pain, diarrhoea, some vomiting (1–2 days)	

Destroying pathogens

The majority of pathogenic bacteria will be destroyed by temperatures of 70°C + (but spores and toxins will not be destroyed by these temperatures). To destroy pathogens in food effectively this temperature must reach the centre of the food and must be held for long enough (usually 2 minutes is recommended), before the temperature drops. Processes such as disinfection and sterilisation will also kill bacteria.

Controlling pathogens

It is a food handler's responsibility to keep food areas clean and hygienic at all times. Food handlers should work in a clean and tidy manner – *clean as you go* – and not allow waste to build up. Spills must be cleaned up straight away. All kitchen staff need to be aware of protecting food from bacteria and preventing bacterial growth by keeping food clean, cool and covered. The

supervisor needs to check and regularly monitor that good practices are in place and always lead by example.

Care must be taken with kitchen cloths: they provide an ideal growing area for bacteria. If dish cloths are used, different cloths for different areas will help to reduce cross-contamination and it is certainly necessary to use different cloths in raw food and cooked food areas. Use of disposable cloths or paper kitchen towel is the most hygienic way to clean food areas.

If tea towels are used treat them with great care: remember that they can easily spread bacteria so don't allow them to be used as an 'all purpose cloth', and don't allow any members of staff to place cloths on their shoulder (this may transfer bacteria from the neck or hair to equipment and food).

Toxins

Toxins (poisons) can be produced by some bacteria as they multiply in food: these are called *exotoxins*. They

Table 2.6 Food-borne illnesses and viruses

Bacteria or virus	Sources	Preferred temp. for growth	Illness onset time	Symptoms	Can it form spores?
Campylobacter Jujuni	Raw poultry/meat, untreated milk or water, pets and pests. Birds	28–46°C	2–5 days	Headache, fever, bloody diarrhoea, abdominal pain (mimics appendicitis)	No
E. coli 0157	Intestines of cattle and humans. Water, raw milk, raw meat, undercooked mince. Salad items. Sewage	4–45°C	1–8 days (usually 3–4 days)	Stomach pain, fever, bloody diarrhoea, nausea. Has caused kidney failure and **death**	No
Listeria monocytogenes	Pate, soft cheeses made from unpasturised milk; raw vegetables and salads. Cook-chill meals	0–45°C	1 day–3 months	Meningitis, septicaemia, flu-like symptoms, still births	No
Norovirus	Air borne, environment, person to person. Does not grow in food – viruses grow only in living cells	N/A	24–48 hours	Severe vomiting and diarrhoea	No
Typhoid / paratyphoid	Long-term carriers (food handlers need 6 negative faecal samples before returning to work). Sewage, untreated water. Also dirty fruit/ vegetables	N/A	8–14 days	Fever, nausea, enlarged spleen, red spots on abdomen. Severe diarrhoea. Some fatality	No
Shigella sonni Shigella flexneri (dysentery)	Infected carriers, sewage, water supplies, contaminated food, shellfish (faecal–oral routes)	N/A	12 hours–7 days but usually 1–3 days	Bloody diarrhoea with mucus. Fever, abdominal pain, nausea, vomiting	No
Hepatitis A	Carriers, blood, urine, faeces, sewage, untreated water, shellfish, salads, dirty vegetables	N/A	15–50 days	Nausea, vomiting, abdominal pain, jaundice	No

are very heat resistant and would not be killed by the normal cooking processes that kill bacteria (it would need prolonged cooking at boiling temperatures or above), so once formed, toxins often remain in the food and can cause illness. Some bacteria produce toxins as they die, usually in the intestines of the person eating the food. These are called *endotoxins*. Toxins are further identified as *neurotoxins*, that is they affect the nervous systems, and *enterotoxins* affecting the intestines.

Spores

Some bacteria are able to form spores when the conditions surrounding them become hostile, for example as temperatures rise, or in the presence of chemicals such as disinfectant. A spore forms a protective 'shell' inside the bacteria, protecting the essential parts from the high temperatures of normal cooking, disinfection, dehydration, and so on. Once spores are formed the outer cell disintegrates and the organism cannot divide and multiply as before but simply survives until conditions improve, for example high temperatures drop to a level where cells can reform and multiplication can start again. Prolonged cooking times and/or very high temperatures are needed to kill spores. Food canning processes use *Botulinum Cook* – 121°C for 3 minutes or a tested alternative time/temperature combination to kill any spores that may be present.

Time is very important in preventing the formation of spores. When you bring large amounts of food, such as meat for stewing, slowly to a cooking temperature it allows time for spores to form; these are then very difficult to kill. An effective control is to bring food up to cooking temperature quickly, possibly by cooking in smaller quantities, and always cool food quickly.

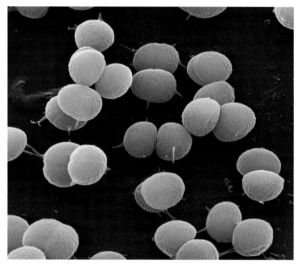

Bacterial spores forming

Pathogens Complete the worksheet about pathogens, provided on Dynamic Learning.

Requirements for multiplication of different pathogens

The temperature requirements for the multiplication of the following pathogens are:

- **Psychrophiles** prefer temperatures below 20°C for multiplication (for example, *Listeria* and *Bacillus cereus*)
- **Mesophiles** prefer temperatures of 20–50°C for multiplication – optimum 37°C (for example, *salmonella* and *Staphylococcus aureus*)
- **Thermophiles** multiply most rapidly above 45°C (for example, *Clostridium perfringens*).

The oxygen requirements for the multiplication of the following pathogens are:

- **Obligate aerobe** multiplies only where there is oxygen present (for example, *Bacillus cereus*)
- **Faculative anaerobe** can multiply with or without oxygen (for example, *salmonella* and *Staphylococcus aureus*).
- **Obligate anaerobe** can multiply only in the absence of oxygen.

Toxins (poisons) are produced by some bacteria and can be very resistant to heat/cooking:

- **Exotoxins** are produced when bacteria are multiplying (for example in *Staphylococcus aureus* and *Bacillus cereus*)
- **Endotoxins** are produced when the bacteria die; this is often in the intestine of the consumer (for example, *Bacillus cereus* and *Clostridium perfringens*).

Competition The rate at which bacteria multiply and survive may be partly dependent on other bacteria that are present, as they will compete for the same conditions and nutrients.

Viruses are even smaller than bacteria and can be seen only with a powerful microscope. They multiply only on living cells, not on food, though they may be transferred into the body on food or drinks and may live for a short time on hard surfaces such as kitchen equipment. Viruses can easily be passed from person to person and are sometimes associated with shellfish that come from contaminated water.

Moulds are usually associated with food spoilage (see page 57) rather than food poisoning, but it is now known that some moulds can produce toxins called *mycotoxins* (see page 56). Unlike bacteria, moulds will grow on acid, alkaline, sugary and salty foods. They grow best between 20–30°C, but will also grow at fridge temperatures.

Poisoning from metals

Occasionally metal elements may accidentally get into food. This may be from old water pipes, food placed in unsuitable metal containers, or crops sprayed with the wrong concentrations of chemicals containing metals.

Lead: this may be present in old piping or old toys (now unusual), paint, batteries and pottery glazes. If it gets into the food or water supply it could cause lead poisoning, presenting as fatigue, headaches and appetite loss as lead accumulates in the brain and blood.

Tin: contamination used to occur when acidic foods were stored over a long period in tin cans. Modern canning processes avoid this but always transfer food from open cans into another container to save in the fridge.

Copper poisoning: this has been recorded when copper has come into contact with milk and milk products; copper can also react with fats and oils. Make sure copper pans and food containers are lined with a material that is safe for food use.

Zinc: this is used to galvanise metals; do not use galvanised metal containers for any sort of food storage as it can react with the food and cause illness.

Cadmium: this is used to plate fittings in cookers and fridges. Modern units do not use it where it can come into direct contact with food, but in older units make sure that food (particularly acidic food) does not directly touch the fittings.

Antimony: this is used on equipment and utensils with enamel coatings. To avoid a reaction from this do not use enamelled items that are chipped or cracked.

Poisoning from fish and vegetable items

Scombrotoxic fish poisoning (SFP): this is associated with the consumption of contaminated **fish** of the Scombroid family (including tuna, mackerel, herring, marlin and sardines). The poison builds in the fish especially in storage above 4°C. It is a chemical intoxication and symptoms occur within 10 minutes to 3 hours after eating the affected fish. Symptoms include rash on the face/neck/chest, flushing, sweating, nausea, vomiting, diarrhoea, abdominal cramps, headache, dizziness, palpitations and a sensation of burning in the mouth. Symptoms are usually gone within 12 hours. Although most cases are not serious enough for hospital attention, in some cases they are severe and urgent medical attention is necessary, when antihistamine drugs may be used.

These toxins are very heat resistant and are not affected by normal cooking. Scombrotoxins are thought to be responsible for up to 70 per cent of food poisoning from fish in the UK.

Paralytic fish poisoning: this is a very dangerous form of fish poisoning. It occurs when some

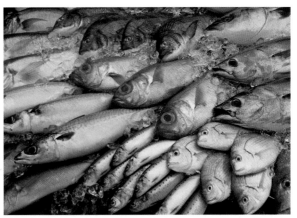

Toxins can build up in fish such as tuna or herring if they are not stored correctly

Bivalve shellfish such as, for example, mussels feed on poisonous plankton. The poison can survive normal cooking temperatures. Symptoms after eating affected shellfish may be nausea, vomiting, lowered temperature, diarrhoea and also a numbness of the mouth, neck and arms which can lead to paralysis and death within 2–12 hours.

Red kidney beans (black kidney beans): every year there are a number of reported cases of mild poisoning from the toxin in red kidney beans (haemagglutin). Poisoning occurs when the beans are not boiled rapidly at temperatures to kill the toxin, that is, rapid boiling for 10 minutes or more. After this initial rapid cooking at high temperatures the heat can then be reduced to finish the cooking process. The symptoms of this poisoning include nausea, vomiting, pain and diarrhoea. The symptoms usually disappear within a few hours. You may experience problems in failing to get kidney beans hot enough if cooking in very large quantities or if using a 'slow cooker'.

Poisoning from mycotoxins

Some moulds can produce toxins as they grow; these are called mycotoxins. They can cause serious illness and have been linked with cancers. Mycotoxins are invisibly present in mouldy food over a much wider area than the visible mould. Mycotoxin-producing moulds can tolerate a wide range of acid/alkaline conditions, low water activity and temperature ranges from −6 to 35°C. Mycotoxins are heat resistant and can withstand very high temperatures.

A wide range of foods may be affected by mycotoxin-producing moulds, but the foods most frequently affected are: cereal crops and products, nuts and fruit products such as juices, dried fruit and jams.

Food parasites

A variety of parasites can live on plants or animals from where they get their food. They present in different forms, for example worms, eggs, lice or grubs. They can usually be destroyed by thorough cooking or very high temperature food preservation methods. In most cases they will also be killed by freezing.

High-risk foods

Some foods support the rapid growth of bacteria more than others when given the required conditions; these are referred to as high-risk foods. They are usually foods that are ready to eat, have a high protein and moisture content and will not go through a cooking process that kills bacteria. They include:

- Cooked meat, poultry and products made from these

    (Protect from contamination, and store at 1–4°C)
- Eggs and egg-based products, especially where raw egg is used, for example fresh mayonnaise

    (Eggs may contain pathogens, cook thoroughly and wash hands well after handling. Use pasteurised egg in items such as mayonnaise and mousses)
- Milk, cream and custards

    (Keep custards hot – above 63°C – or cool quickly and refrigerate. Keep milk and cream under refrigeration as much as possible)
- Stock, sauces, gravy and soup

    (Keep these hot – above 63°C – or cool quickly and refrigerate)
- Shellfish and seafood products

    (Use a reputable supplier, cook or reheat thoroughly to kill bacteria. Throw away shellfish with broken shells, and mussels or clams that don't open when cooked)
- Cooked rice

    (Rice can contain the spores of *Bacillus cereus* which would not be killed by normal cooking temperatures. If rice is cooled slowly in a warm kitchen these spores germinate and multiply enough to cause food poisoning. Keep cooked rice above 63°C for service or cool quickly. Avoid cooking rice in very large quantities.)

Clean-sanitise-disinfect

Cleaning and disinfection play an essential role in the control of pathogens.

Clean and sanitise worktops and chopping boards before working on them and do this again after use, especially when they have been used for raw foods. (See page 41.) A good way to clean and disinfect chopping boards after use is by putting them through a dishwasher with a high rinse temperature (usually 82°C+). For effective cleaning of surfaces see page 42 in Section 2 of this chapter.

Small equipment, such as knives, bowls, spoons and tongs, could also be the cause of cross-contamination; it is important to wash them thoroughly (once again a dishwasher does this well). This is especially important when they are used for a variety of food and for raw foods.

Food spoilage and food preservation

Most foods, once harvested, slaughtered, fished or manufactured, have a limited life and will eventually deteriorate. The deterioration may be caused by moulds, yeasts, enzymes or bacteria. Spoilage of food could also be due to exposure to oxygen, moisture or chemicals, damage by pests or by poor handling and bad storage.

Unlike bacterial contamination that is impossible to detect in a normal kitchen situation, food spoilage can usually be detected by organaleptic observation, that is, the spoilage can be observed by sight, smell, taste, touch, and so on.

Food spoilage includes mouldy, slimy, dried up, over-wet fresh foods, blown cans and vac packs and food with freezer burn.

Food spoilage and food preservation Complete the worksheets on food spoilage and food preservation, provided on Dynamic Learning.

Over many years different methods have been developed to prolong the natural life of various foods and keep them fresh. These include:

- Use of heat: cooking, canning, sterilisation, UHT, pasteurisation
- Use of heat and sealing: canning, bottling, cooking then vacuum packaging
- Use of low temperatures: chilling, freezing
- Exclusion of air: vaccum packaging
- Changing gases surrounding food: modified atmosphere packaging (MAP)

- Removal of moisture: dehydrated foods
- Use of acids, sugar or salt concentrations (see above)
- Smoking: used on meat and fish (but this will offer only limited preservation)
- Preservatives: for example nitrates and nitrites.

Food preservation will often combine methods to ensure effective preservation. For example, smoked fish may be vacuum packed and will also be refrigerated; milk is pasteurised but also stored under refrigeration.

Careful use and control of temperature is essential in producing safe, high-quality food for customers.

High temperatures

Normal cooking temperatures of 75°C + will kill most pathogens (but not toxins and spores). Use of heat to make foods safe and to preserve them is one of the most useful procedures available in food production and manufacture. Table 2.7 shows some temperatures commonly used to make food safe.

Table 2.7 Temperatures used to make food safe and for food preservation

Cooking **75°C for 2 minutes**	This is the most common of 'heat treatments' for food. Cooked food does generally keep for longer than raw equivalents. However, treat cooked items with care as once foods have been cooked they may then be in the 'high risk' category. Normal cooking, i.e. to 75°C for 2 minutes at the core of the food, will kill most pathogens but not spores and toxins.
Pasteurisation **72°C for 15 seconds**	This involves heating food to a temperature similar to cooking temperatures but for a very short time, i.e. milk is heated to 72°C for 15 seconds then rapid cooling takes place. These temperatures will kill most pathogens, bringing them to a 'safe level'. Toxins and spores will not be killed. Because relatively low temperatures are used, milk that has been pasteurised will spoil more quickly than milk preserved by some of the methods described below and must be kept at refrigerator temperatures. Pasteurisation is also used for liquid egg, cream, ice cream, some fruit juices and wine. Because of the relatively low temperatures used the taste of the product remains mostly unchanged, though vitamin content is reduced by about 25 per cent. Unpasteurised milk products can legally be sold in the UK, as long as they are clearly labelled as such.
Sterilisation **100°C for 15–30 minutes**	The sterilisation of milk and other food items destroys all micro-organisms. Sterilisation involves heating to 100°C for 15–30 minutes by applying steam and pressure. Because very high temperatures are used over a relatively long time some caramelisation occurs; taste is altered and vitamin content is significantly reduced. Unopened sterilised milk lasts much longer than pasteurised milk. Liquid or semi-liquid food such as soup, stock and sauces sold in pouches also go through a sterilisation process. These foods have a long shelf life and do not need refrigerated storage.
UHT **135°C for 1 second**	UHT or Ultra Heat Treatment gives milk a long shelf life without the need for refrigeration (until the package is opened). The milk is heated under pressure to very high temperatures, i.e. 135°C, for just 1 second, then cooled rapidly and sealed in sterile containers. UHT is also used for cream.
Canning **121°C for 3 minutes**	Canning is an efficient method of food preservation using very high temperatures, along with sealing the food in a can (pouch or bottle). A concern with canning is the survival of anaerobic bacteria, especially *Clostridium botulinum* which is particularly dangerous, as food poisoning from this organism can be debilitating and even fatal. This is because any surviving anaerobic bacteria could thrive inside a can where there is no oxygen; also sources of *Clostridium botulinum* include some fish and vegetables, foods that are frequently canned. To overcome this, canned food is subjected to 'botulinum cook'; this is a time/temperature combination, e.g. 121°C for 3 minutes or a time/temperature combination calculated to be as effective as this dependent upon the acidity and texture of the food.

Table 2.8 Important temperatures when dealing with food

For most fridges a running temperature of 1–4°C is recommended			
Food stored in a freezer	**−18 to −23°C**	Ambient food storage, e.g. cans, dry foods grains, general grocery items	**Cool and well ventilated**
Raw meat/poultry Raw fish and shellfish	**1 to 4°C**		
Cooked meats/meat products Cooked fish/fish products Dairy products/fats Eggs Salad items, herbs, leafy vegetables Cooked foods/high-risk items	**(Storage of large amounts of meat e.g. in butchers' fridges a temperature of −1 to +1°C is recommended)**	Unless told otherwise, probe cooked hot food to a core temperature of:	**75°C +**
		Most cooked fish (EHO may advise higher temperature than this)	**63°C**
		Reheating food Reheating food (Scotland – legal requirement)	**75°C +** **82°C +**
		Food held for service	**63°C +**

* Although the law states 'foods which support growth of pathogens or formation of toxins must not be stored above 8°C' it is recognised best practice to store below 5°C

Methods and procedures for controlling food safety

Food delivered to food businesses will be taken through a number of stages before it reaches the customer. Careful control at each stage (*Critical Control Points*) is essential to keep food safe and wholesome.

Food deliveries and storage

For food to remain in best condition and be safe to eat it is essential that correct storage is in place and procedures are fully understood by kitchen staff. Full documentation systems needs to be completed for all kitchen deliveries in line with the food safety management system. This will ensure food is stored correctly and will be available for inspections by EHO and if necessary as part of due diligence. Only approved suppliers should be used who can assure that food is delivered in the best condition, in suitable packaging, properly date coded and at the correct temperature. Ensure that you carry out the following:

- Check all deliveries, then move to the appropriate storage area as soon as possible and chilled/ frozen food within 15 minutes of delivery
- Use a food probe to check the temperature of food deliveries; chilled food should be below 5°C, (reject it if above 8°C); frozen foods should be at or below 18°C (reject if above 15°C)
- Many suppliers will now supply a printout of temperatures at which food was delivered (save these printouts in kitchen records; they could be an important part of due diligence)

- Dry goods should be in undamaged packaging, well within best before dates, be completely dry and in perfect condition on delivery
- Remove food items from outer boxes before placing the products in the fridge, freezer or dry store. Remove outer packaging carefully, remaining fully aware of any possible pests that may have found their way into packaging
- Segregate any unfit food from other food until it is thrown away or collected by the supplier. This is to avoid any possible contamination to other foods.

Raw meat and poultry: wherever possible, store in fridges just for meat and poultry storage running at temperatures between 1°C and 4°C (butchers' fridges −1°C to +1°C). If not already packaged, place on trays, cover well with cling film and label. If it is necessary to store meat or poultry in a multi-use fridge make sure it is covered, labelled and placed at the bottom of the fridge running below 5°C and is well away from other items.

Fish: a specific fish fridge is preferable (running at 1–4°C). Remove fresh fish from ice containers and place on trays, cover well with cling film and label. If it is necessary to store fish in a multi-use fridge make sure it is well covered, labelled and placed at the bottom of the fridge well away from other items. Remember that odours from fish can permeate other items such as milk or eggs.

Dairy products/eggs: pasteurised milk and cream, eggs and cheese should be stored in their original containers in fridges running at 1–4°C. Sterilised or UHT milk can be kept in the dry store following the storage instructions on the label. After delivery eggs should be stored at a constant temperature and a fridge is the best place to store them. Prevent eggs from touching other items in the fridge.

Frozen foods: store in a freezer running at −18°C or below. Make sure that food is wrapped or packaged. Separate raw foods from ready-to-eat foods in the freezer and never allow food to be re-frozen once it has thawed. In a specific ice cream freezer ice cream can be kept at −12°C or below for up to one week before use.

Cooked foods: these include a wide range of foods such as, for example, pies, pate, cream cakes, desserts and savoury flans. They will usually be 'high-risk foods' so correct storage is essential. For specific storage instructions see the labelling on the individual items, but generally, keep items below 8°C and preferably below 5°C. Store carefully, wrapped and labelled, where possible in a fridge used only for high-risk items. If a multi-use fridge needs to be used, store well away from and above raw foods to avoid any cross-contamination.

Fruit, vegetables and salad items: storage conditions will vary according to type; for example sacks of potatoes, root vegetables and some fruit can be stored in a cool, well-ventilated store room, but salad items, green vegetables, soft fruit and tropical fruit would be better in refrigerated storage. If possible a specific fridge running at 8–10°C would be ideal to avoid any chill damage.

Multi-use fridges

If food cannot be stored in separate specific fridges and needs to be stored in multi-use fridges it is absolutely essential that all staff know the correct procedures to store the food and this should become part of ongoing staff training. Posters, pictures and charts near the fridge may help with this. Keep the fridge running at 1–4°C. Ensure that you:

- Store raw foods such as meat, poultry and fish at the bottom of the fridge in suitable deep containers to catch any spillage. Cover with cling film and label with the commodity name and the date. Do not allow any other foods to touch these raw foods
- Store other items above raw foods, again they should be covered and labelled. Keep high-risk foods well away from raw foods

- Never overload the fridge: to operate properly cold air must be allowed to circulate between items
- Wrap strong-smelling foods very well, as the smell (and taste) can transfer to other foods, for example milk
- As with other foods, check date labels and use strict stock rotation procedures.

Make sure that fridges are cleaned regularly; this needs to be part of the cleaning schedule. The procedure should be:

- Remove food to another fridge
- Clean according to cleaning schedule using a recommended sanitiser (a solution of bicarbonate of soda and water is also good for cleaning fridges)
- Remember to empty and clean any drip trays, and clean door seals thoroughly
- Rinse, then dry with kitchen paper
- Make sure the fridge front and handle are cleaned and disinfected to avoid cross-contamination
- Make sure the fridge is down to a temperature of 1–4°C, before replacing the food in the proper positions (see above). Check dates and condition of all food before replacing.

Defrosting

If you need to defrost frozen food, place it in a deep tray, cover with film and label with what the item is, and the date when defrosting was started. Place at the bottom of the fridge where thawing liquid can't drip onto anything else. Defrost food completely (no ice crystals on any part), then cook thoroughly within 12 hours. Make sure that you allow enough time for the defrosting process. It may take longer than you think! (A 2 kg chicken will take about 24 hours to defrost at 3°C.)

Dry (ambient) food stores

A dry or ambient food store is an area to store foods that generally have a longer shelf life than those needing refrigerated or frozen storage (though the dry stores area may also have areas for refrigerated and freezer storage).

Items usually kept in the dry stores would include:

- Rice, dried pasta, cereal products, spices and dried herbs, sugar, flour and grains. (Retain packaging information as this may include essential allergy and storage advice)

- Packaged goods such as biscuits, canned goods, bottled items, chocolate/cocoa, tea and coffee
- Fruit and vegetables not requiring refrigeration (for example sacks of potatoes and onions).

Refrigerated storage may also be available for items needing temperature-controlled storage. The room should be large enough to allow for correct storage of stock. It needs to be cool (10–15°C would be ideal), well ventilated, a light colour, well lit, protected to prevent entry of pests and easy to clean/disinfect efficiently.

When fitting out the room, surfaces for walls, ceilings and floors need to be smooth, impervious and easy to clean. Edges where walls join the floor or ceiling should be coved if possible to prevent build-up of debris in corners. Remember that:

- Doors should be protected by metal kick plates and a plastic or chain curtain to prevent pests from gaining entry (but also check packaging of deliveries for possible pests)
- Windows should be well protected with wire gauze or netting and food items should not be stored in direct sunlight from windows (greenhouse effect – see page 62)
- Shelves/racking must be made of a non-corrosive, easy-to-clean material, for example

tubular stainless steel. Shelving must be deep enough to store the items required and the bottom shelf should be well raised from the floor to allow for ease of cleaning underneath. Never store items directly on the floor as this would prevent effective cleaning from taking place.

Where possible, store dry goods in covered containers on wheels, or in smaller sealed containers on shelves, or in bins to stop pests getting into them, but make sure the stock is rotated effectively, that is, first in – first out; this will ensure that existing stock is always used first. When new packages of dry stock are delivered do not empty them into the container on top of what is already being stored. These should be kept in clean, covered containers.

To avoid any possible cross-contamination, store high-risk (ready-to-eat) foods well away from any raw foods such as dirty vegetables and make sure all items remain covered.

Canned products: cans are usually stored in the dry store area and once again rotation of stock is essential. Canned food will carry best before dates and it is not advisable to use after this date. 'Blown' cans must never be used and do not use badly dented or rusty cans. Once opened transfer any unused canned food to a clean bowl, cover and label it and store in the fridge for up to 2 days.

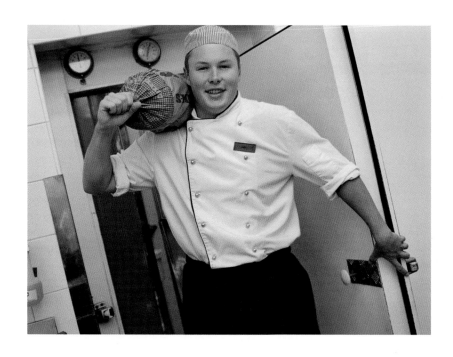

Using cling film

Cling film is a very useful product for storing food hygienically, protecting from cross-contamination and preventing food from drying out. However, because cling film seals in moisture it can encourage growth of moulds on food. Do not leave cling film-wrapped or covered foods in direct light, as it can increase temperature of the food inside. This is referred to as 'the greenhouse effect' and also applies to glass or Perspex display cabinets.

Because of concerns about migration of chemicals into food it is recommended that foods are never cooked or reheated when wrapped in cling film unless a film specifically recommended for this is used.

First in – first out

This term is used to describe stock rotation and is applied to all categories of food. It simply means that foods already in storage are used before new deliveries (providing stock is still within recommended dates and in sound condition). Food deliveries should be labelled with delivery date and preferably the date by which they should be used. Use this information along with food labelling codes (see below). Written stock records should form a part of a food safety management system.

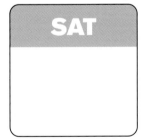 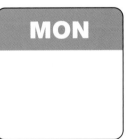

Example of a date labelling system

Food labelling codes

USE BY dates appear on perishable foods with a short life. Legally, the food must be used by this date and not stored or used after it.

BEST BEFORE dates apply to foods that are expected to have a longer life, for example dry prod-ucts or canned food. A best before date advises that food is at its best before this date and to use it after the date is still legal but not advised. These foods are usually stored at ambient temperature.

Storing food correctly The following foods have just been delivered. Write instructions for a new member of staff about the correct way to store these items.

Frozen chicken breasts (need defrosting for tomorrow), sirloin steaks, lamb's liver, bacon. Fresh whole sole, smoked haddock and live crabs. Butter, eggs, cream, strawberries, bread rolls, onions, salad leaves, potatoes, rice, canned tomatoes, flour, ice cream.

Food preparation

Food should not be prepared too far in advance of cooking. If food is prepared a significant time before it is to be cooked control measures must be in place to ensure that this is safe. Preparation areas for raw and cooked food should be well separated, as should dirty and clean processes. Food being prepared should be out of temperature control (for example refrigeration or cooking processes) for only the shortest time possible. Avoid handling food unnecessarily; use disposable gloves, tongs, slices and spoons, where possible. High standards of personal hygiene are essential for those handling food; approved kitchen clothing must be worn and changed if it becomes dirty or badly stained, as this could contaminate food and equipment. It is essential to develop and monitor 'clean as you go' methods of work to help avoid microbial and physical contamination of food. Also take care when preparing food not to allow any chemical contamination from sanitiser sprays, disinfectants and other kitchen chemicals, and be aware of allergenic contamination. Do some foods that pose an allergenic risk need to be prepared in a separate area or eliminated altogether?

Use of colour-coded equipment is very useful in food preparation areas to avoid cross-contamination. Items in frequent use include colour-coded chopping boards, knife handles, bowls, aprons, cloths and trays.

Use of temperature

Cooking is one of the best measures available to destroy and control bacteria in food. The usual recommendation is to cook to a core temperature of 75°C for at least 2 minutes but slightly lower temperatures for a longer time can be as effective. Also dish specifications or personal preference may require lower temperatures than this such as, for example, rare beef and some fish dishes. However, avoid undercooked dishes when dealing with the groups of people who are vulnerable to the effects of food poisoning. The most usual way to check if required core temperatures (the temperature in the centre of the food) have been achieved is with a calibrated and disinfected temperature probe, but you may also make visual checks; for example look at the amounts of steam and in a cooked chicken check that no part is pink and that juices running off it are clear.

Staff should be aware of the danger zone temperatures and the need to heat food through these temperatures quickly to avoid formation of spores. It is also good practice to use lids on cooking pans to prevent heat escaping and to stir food frequently to keep temperatures even.

Low temperatures

As bacteria can only multiply very slowly at low temperatures (see danger zone diagram), it is good practice to keep fridges running between 1–4°C. The legal requirement is at or below 8°C.

Fridge and freezer temperatures should be checked and recorded at least once daily; keep the recorded temperatures as part of food safety management records. Cold food can be kept out of temperature control for up to 4 hours on any single occasion, for example a buffet. This time includes preparation time and food must be disposed of at the end of the 4 hours.

Temperature probes

Electronic temperature probes are extremely useful in food production to measure the temperature in the centre of both hot and cold food. They are also very useful for recording the temperature of deliveries and checking uniformity of food temperatures in fridges. Make sure the probe is clean and disinfected before use (disposable disinfectant wipes are useful for this). Place the probe into the centre of the food, making sure it is not touching bone or the cooking container. Allow the temperature to 'settle' before reading. Check regularly that probes are working correctly (calibration). This can be done electronically but a simple and low-cost check is to place the probe in icy water; the reading should be within the range −1°C to +1°C. To check accuracy at high levels place the probe in boiling water and the temperature reading should be in the range of 99°C to 101°C.

If probes read outside of these temperatures they need to be repaired or replaced.

Record when temperature probes have been checked for accuracy and store this with food safety records.

Infra red thermometers

These are also very useful in kitchen areas and give instant readings as they work by measuring radiant energy. They are very hygienic to use as they do not actually touch the food so there is no chance of cross-contamination or damaging the food. For safety reasons, keep the infra red away from your eyes.

Data loggers

These will record information about the temperatures of refrigeration over a set period. They record highs and lows of temperature in individual or different fridges/freezers and can provide a graph of trends. Systems are available that record all refrigerator, chill unit and freezer temperatures in a business and send the information to a central computer.

Holding temperatures

Hot, cooked food being held for service must not fall below 63°C. Make sure that there is adequate equipment to keep food above this temperature, check the temperature frequently and record it. Hot food kept out of this temperature for more than 2 hours must be thrown away (this includes the time in the kitchen). Make sure that equipment for keeping food hot, for example bains marie or hot cabinets, is pre-heated and clean/disinfected; do not over fill food containers and allow all of the food to be used from them before topping up. Use lids on open containers to keep the heat in.

For cold food being held for service or displayed there are similar rules.

The food being held for service should not be above 5°C (legal requirement 8°C). Make sure that there is adequate refrigeration with display cabinets at the correct temperature, check the temperature and keep a record. Cold food kept above 8°C for 4 hours on one occasion must be thrown away (this includes the preparation time).

Cooling cooked food

When food is cooled either to be served cold or to be reheated it must be done carefully and quickly, to avoid the formation/germination of spores and to reduce the risk of cross-contamination as food is cooling.

It is recommended that food is cooled to 8°C within 90 minutes; this is best done in a blast chiller. If this is not available, food in containers can be plunged into ice water baths or placed on trays and surrounded with ice or ice packs may be used. Place cooling food in the coolest place available; fans can also be useful to speed up cooling time.

To allow food to cool more quickly it is recommended that:

- Items such as soups, stews and sauces are placed in small containers; also use shallow containers; increased surface area allows the food to cool more quickly
- Smaller joints of meat are cooked because these will cool more quickly. A maximum weight of 2.5 kg is recommended.

Reheating

Reheating should be done thoroughly and quickly to a core temperature of at least 75°C (Scottish law requires a temperature of 82°C). Reheated food should also be served quickly and never reheated more than once.

Serving food

Food must also be protected when it is being served. Do not keep food unprotected and out of temperature control in service areas longer than necessary. Make sure that all service equipment and surfaces are suitable for food service and are clean. Staff training in food safety is essential for food service staff as well as for those preparing the food.

HACCP and food safety management systems

For some time it has been considered good practice for all food businesses to have a food safety management system in place. From January 2006 this became law.

Article 5 of the Food Hygiene (England) Regulations 2005 gave effect to the EU Regulations and states that:

> *Food Business operators shall put into place, implement and maintain a permanent procedure based on the principles of hazard analysis critical control point (HACCP). Food handlers must receive adequate instruction and/or training in food hygiene to enable them to handle food safety. Those responsible for HACCP based procedures in the business must have enough relevant knowledge and understanding to ensure the procedures are operated effectively.*

This gave strength to the Food Standards Agency's commitment to significantly reduce food poisoning cases by 2020.

The advantages of implementing HACCP are:

- It is needed to comply with EU legislation
- Risks are reduced, so less risk of civil action
- System is internationally recognised
- Demonstrates due diligence
- A proactive system where action can be taken before problems occur
- Generates a food safety culture, all staff are involved in procedures
- Less food will be wasted
- Assists with local authority (enforcement officer) inspections
- Ensures correct records are kept and documentation is in place.

As stated all systems must be based on HACCP, Hazard Analysis Critical Control Point. This is an internationally recognised food safety management system that looks at identifying the critical points or stages in any process and identifying hazards that could occur, that is what could go wrong, when, where, how.

Controls are then put in place to deal with the risks – *making possible risks safe*.

Controls are carried out. If something goes wrong, do staff know what to do about it? What checks are in place and what should be done to put things right?

Procedures are kept up to date – confirm that they are still working.

Documents and records are kept that show the system is working and is regularly reviewed. A wide range of documents is used as part of the HACCP system.

Pre-requisites

Before setting up a new HACCP system certain pre-requisites need to be considered, that is, what needs to be in place:

- **Suppliers** should be approved suppliers and wherever possible they should provide written specifications

- **Traceability,** systems in place along with suppliers to trace the source of all foods
- **Premises, structure and equipment,** records that premises are properly maintained. A flow diagram needs to be produced showing the process from delivery to service avoiding any cross-over of procedures that could result in cross-contamination
- **Storage and stock control,** raw ingredients to finished product. Effective stock control, stock rotation and temperature-controlled storage must be in place
- **Staff hygiene,** protective clothing, hand-washing facilities, toilets and changing facilities need to be provided. A policy for personal hygiene needs to be established, with appropriate training on the standards to be achieved
- **Pest control,** a written pest control policy ideally as part of a pest management system and involving a recognised contractor
- **Cleaning/disinfection/waste,** a documented system in place that includes cleaning schedules and how waste removal will be managed
- **Staff training,** records of all staff training with dates completed.

Setting up HACCP

A team of people suitably trained in HACCP procedures will be established to set up the system. If the business is small just one person may be responsible. There are also a number of specialist HACCP consultancy companies which can complete and monitor the procedure.

The hazards identified and the controls put in place will be essential to food safety and safe production methods such as, for example, core cooking temperatures, possible multiplication and survival of bacteria, time food spends in danger zone and cooling food.

Food handlers must receive food safety training and effective supervision commensurate with the tasks being completed. Staff training records must be kept.

There must be awareness that physical and chemical hazards could occur at any stage in the process, and controls must include these hazards.

The HACCP system involves seven stages

The system needs to provide a documented record of the stages all food will go through right up to the time it is eaten and may include: purchase and delivery, receipt of food, storage, preparation, cooking, cooling,

Conduct a hazard analysis
Decide which operations, processes, products and hazards to include. Prepare a flow diagram, identify the hazards and specify the control measures.

Determine the critical control points (CCPs)
Control measures must be used to prevent, eliminate or reduce a hazard to an acceptable level.

Establish critical limits
Must be measurable, e.g. temperature, time, pH, weight and size of food. Set a target limit and a critical limit; the difference between the two is called the tolerance.

Establish a system to monitor control of each CCP
What are the critical limits? How, where and when will the monitoring be undertaken? Who is responsible for monitoring?

Establish corrective actions when monitoring indicates that a particular CCP is not under control
Deal with any affected product and bring the CCP and the process back under control.

Establish procedures for verification to confirm that the HACCP system is working effectively
Validation: obtain evidence that the CCPs and critical limits are effective. Verification: ensure that the flow diagram remains valid, hazards are controlled, monitoring is satisfactory, and corrective action has been, or will be, taken.

Establish documentation and records of all procedures relevant to the HACCP principles and their application
This will be proportionate to the size and type of business. Documentation is necessary to show that food safety is being managed. Managers need records when auditing; enforcement officers and external auditors will also need to see them.

The seven principles of HACCP

hot holding, reheating, chilled storage and serving. Once the hazards have been identified, corrective measures are put in place to control the hazards and keep the food safe.

The system must be updated regularly, especially when new items are introduced to the menu or systems change (for example a new piece of cooking equipment). Specific, new controls must be put in place to include them.

A flow diagram will need to be produced for each dish or procedure, showing each of the stages (critical control points) that need to be considered for possible hazards.

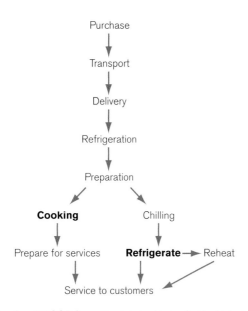

Example of an HACCP flow diagram: cooking a fresh chicken

When dealing with fresh chicken it is necessary to recognise the possible hazards at all of the identified stages.

Cooking a fresh chicken

Hazard: pathogenic bacteria are likely to be present in raw chicken.

Control: the chicken needs to be cooked thoroughly to 75°C + to ensure pathogens are killed.

Monitor: check the temperature where the thigh joins the body with a calibrated temperature probe (75°C +), make sure no parts of the flesh are pink and juices are running clear – neither red nor pink.

Hot holding: before service the chicken must be kept above 63°C; this can be checked with a temperature probe.

Or chill and refrigerate: chill to below 10°C within 90 minutes. Cover, label and refrigerate below 5°C.

Documentation: temperatures measured and recorded. Hot holding equipment checked and temperature recorded. Record any corrective measures necessary.

For the cold storage of the chicken after cooking/chilling

Hazard: cross-contamination, multiplication of micro-organisms in cooked chicken.

Control: protect from cross-contamination, store below 5°C.

Monitor: check temperature of the chicken is below 5°C.

Corrective action: if the chicken has been above 8°C for 4 hours or more it should be thrown away. Investigate why the temperature control has not worked so it can be put right if there is a fault.

Documentation: Record temperatures at least once a day and record any corrective action.

HACCP worksheet Complete the HACCP worksheet provided on Dynamic Learning.

Due diligence

'Due diligence' is the main defence available under food safety legislation. It means that a business took all reasonable care and precaution and did everything reasonably practicable to prevent the offence or food poisoning outbreak, that it exercised all due diligence. To prove due diligence, accurate written documents are essential and could include:

- Staff training records, with topics covered, and dates
- Temperature records (delivery, cooking and cold storage)
- Details of suppliers and contractors
- Pest control policy and audits
- Cleaning schedules and deep clean reports
- Maintenance schedules
- Records of equipment faults, breakdown and repairs
- CCP monitoring activities (only CCPs to avoid excessive paperwork)
- Deviations, corrective actions and recalls
- Modifications to the HACCP system
- Customer complaints/investigation results
- Calibration of instruments
- Pre-requisite programme records.

Table 2.9 Example HACCP control chart

Process steps	Hazards	Controls	Critical limit	Monitoring	Corrective action
Purchase	Contamination, pathogens, mould or foreign bodies present	Approved supplier			Change supplier
Transport and delivery	Multiplication of harmful bacteria	Refrigerated vehicles		Check delivery vehicles, date marks, temperatures	Reject if > 8°C or out of date
Refrigerate	Bacterial growth Further contamination – bacteria, chemicals, etc.	Store below 5°C Separate raw and cooked foods Stock rotation	Food below 5°C	Check and record temperature twice a day Check date marks	Discard if signs of spoilage or past date mark
Prepare	Bacterial growth Further contamination	No more than 30 minutes in 'danger zone' Good personal hygiene Clean equipment, hygienic premises		Supervisor to audit at regular intervals Visual checks Cleaning schedules	Discard if > 8°C for 6 hours
Cook	Survival of harmful bacteria	Thorough cooking	75°C	Check and record temperature/ time	Continue cooking to 75°C
Prepare for service	Multiplication of bacteria Contamination	No more than 20 minutes in 'danger zone'	2 hours	Supervisor to audit at regular intervals	Discard if > 8°C for 2 hours
Chill	Multiplication of bacteria Contamination	Blast chiller	90 minutes to below 10°C	Supervisor to audit at regular intervals	Discard if > 20°C for 2 hours
Refrigerate	Multiplication of bacteria Contamination	Store below 5°C Separate raw and ready-to-eat foods	8°C for 4 hours	Check and record temperature twice a day	Discard if > 8°C for 4 hours
Reheat	Survival of bacteria	Reheat to 75°C in centre	75°C (82°C in Scotland)	Check and record temperature of each batch	Continue reheating to 75°C

Safer Food Better Business

The HACCP system described above may seem complicated and difficult to set up for a small or fairly limited business. With this in mind the Food Standards Agency launched its **Safer Food Better Business** system for England and Wales. This is based on the principles of HACCP but in an easy-to-understand format with pre-printed pages and charts to enter the relevant information such as temperatures of individual dishes. It is divided into two parts. The first part is about safe methods, for example avoiding cross-contamination, personal hygiene, cleaning, chilling and cooking. The second part covers opening and closing checks, proving methods are safe, recording safe methods, training records, supervision, stock control and the selection of suppliers and contractors.

Once the basic information has been recorded, for example suppliers and staff training, the actual diary pages are very easy to complete and just need confirmation that opening and closing checks have been completed and have been dated and signed. The only other entries in the diary are the recording of problems, any occurring and what will be done about them. If no problems occur that day nothing needs to be entered. This is called 'management by exception' or 'exception reporting'.

A copy of Safer Food Better Business is available free from www.food.gov.uk.

A similar system called **CookSafe** has been developed by the Food Standards Agency (Scotland) and **Safe Catering** in Northern Ireland.

Scores on Doors

This is another strategy that has been piloted by the Food Standards Agency to raise food safety standards and help reduce the incidence of food poisoning. The piloted areas tested various schemes where a star rating of food safety was awarded based on the following three criteria taken from the Food Standards Agency's statutory risk-rating system:

- Level of compliance of food hygiene practices and procedures
- Level of compliance relating to structure and cleanliness of premises
- Confidence in management of the business and food safety controls.

The intention is to place the given star rating in a prominent position on the door or window of premises, but it is not mandatory to do so.

After the successful pilot scheme the Food Standards Agency decided on a standard system for England and Wales based on 0 to 5 stars. For more information about Scores on Doors, refer to Appendix 6.

It is expected that the **Scores on Doors** scheme will have a lasting positive impact on food safety standards. No matter how good the food in a particular establishment, few people will want to eat there if the food safety score is low!

2.4 Food safety training and communicating food safety procedures

In this section you will learn about:

1. The requirements for induction and ongoing training of staff
2. The importance of effective communication on food safety procedures.

Effective planning of food safety is essential to ensure that high standards are maintained, there is compliance with the 2006 Food Safety laws and the proceeding legislation and to avoid the possibility of food safety related problems. The supervisor (head chef) plays a key role in implementing and managing food safety procedures and is an important link between management and the actual food operation. Although supervisors may not be the policy makers it is likely that they will be involved in devising, setting and managing the day-to-day food safety procedures. This will involve implementing the food safety management system (HACCP or similar) including:

- Overseeing formal and informal staff training
- Managing the various temperature controls and recording

- Putting measures in place to avoid contamination of food and cross-contamination
- Setting required standards for personal hygiene and requirements for protective clothing
- Monitoring standards for premises and equipment and safe disposal of waste
- Monitoring and managing the correct storage of food and rotation of stock
- Managing cleaning and disinfection of premises and equipment and the proactive control of pests.

Communication

Effective communication of food safety matters to staff is of great importance and can be achieved through induction procedures, ongoing staff training, supervision, mentoring, information posters, leaflets, films, information/training from EHO (EHP), and by making food safety issues part of staff meetings, briefings and handovers. Effective communication to staff of food safety standards and requirements must be ongoing and consistent.

Because the supervisor is part of the day-to-day food operation, he or she is the obvious person to communicate food safety matters to business owners, managers, other departments, suppliers, contractors and enforcement officers. Keeping of up-to-date and accurate records will help towards effective communication.

Food safety training

As well as being a legal requirement, food safety training for staff 'commensurate' to their job roles is essential in any food business. The person responsible for food safety management of a business must also be responsible for staff training. The supervisor will frequently monitor and manage the training for staff and make sure that training records are accurate and up to date and kept for possible inspection. Specific training sessions, both formal and informal, may be delivered by the supervisor to meet the need of the actual business and specific staff as well as satisfying legal requirements. Planned retraining and refresher sessions are also essential at all levels.

Training methods

Appropriate training can take place in house or with a training provider. The training methods chosen will depend on the type of business, the activities carried out and the previous training in which staff have taken part. Training could take place in the following ways:

- Food safety management companies which undertake part or all of the food safety requirements for a business including training at different levels
- Working towards gaining accredited food safety qualifications
- Online or computer package training, often with end tests and certification
- Food safety training packs that could include books, workbooks, DVDs and activities
- Use of a variety of materials now widely available, for example posters, leaflets, films, interactive games and puzzles
- Training delivered by the EHO (EHP).

Just one or a selection of these methods could be used. Some training materials are now available in a number of different languages with visual explana-

tions. There are also training materials in the Safer Food Better Business packs.

Food safety qualifications

Awarding bodies that give accreditation to food safety qualifications include: CIEH, RSPH, City & Guilds, EDI and Highfield. Courses are available at colleges and universities, through independent training providers, local authorities and adult education centres. Training and testing for these can also take place in the workplace. The different levels for these qualifications are most usually:

- Level 1: often completed in the workplace for those new to food handling tasks or those employed on non complex or limited tasks
- Level 2: this is the most popular food safety qualification and is designed for those handling a wide variety of foods including 'open' and high-risk foods
- Level 3: a qualification for supervisors of food premises (food operations) and for those completing more complex tasks and requiring a greater depth of knowledge
- Level 4: a management-level qualification that may also be completed by more senior supervisors and anyone requiring a high-level food safety qualification.

Induction

Induction of new staff plays a very important role in ensuring that food safety standards are fully met and that new employees completely understand the requirements of their job role. Supervisors must ensure that induction of all new staff is planned, well organised, and recorded. Induction procedures need to be linked with planned supervision, mentoring and ongoing staff training. Induction is a good time to establish the high standards required in the job role.

Monitoring, control and auditing

Because food safety must be organised and planned it is necessary to complete monitoring, control and auditing procedures.

Control

This involves making sure that the agreed and recorded food safety policies are taking place in the day-to-day operations of the kitchen. This could be implemented by training, staff meetings, spot checks, posters and information sheets, training-update sheets and short information films.

Monitoring

This involves the supervisor and others checking (and recording where appropriate) that controls are being adhered to and are working properly. Many monitoring procedures will be part of the food safety management system (such as monitoring fridge temperatures or the cleaning schedule). Other methods of monitoring may include visual inspections, *organoleptic* checks of food stocks, checklists, walk-through checking procedures, checking that required tasks are completed, for example temperature recording. In some establishments bacterial monitoring is completed by swabbing surfaces, equipment or processes to establish specific pathogens that may be present, that is, total viable counts (TVCs).

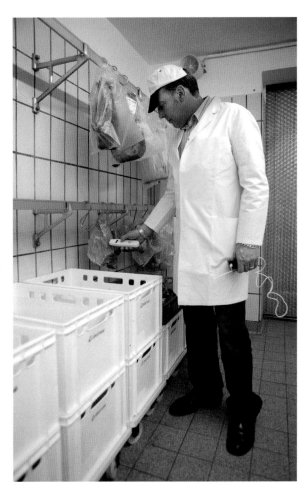

(Swabbing kits are available from food safety management/equipment companies for checking and recording the levels of bacteria on a surface or piece of equipment. This may be done at regular intervals and the findings used to improve cleaning and disinfection of areas. The findings always provide a good tool for staff trainings and meetings).

Auditing

This is often a more formal procedure taking the form of an inspection. This could be done by an internal auditor (that is, part of the organisation) or an external auditor or consultant may be used, but it should be someone who is not part of carrying out or monitoring the day-to-day systems. Auditing is often used to verify that the HACCP or similar system is working properly.

Working with the EHO (EHP)

Because supervisors are familiar with the operational procedures of the food operation they are in a very good position to liaise with the EHO (EHP) on specific and more general food safety matters (see page 37).

It is of absolute importance that the supervisor cooperates fully with the EHO (EHP) in the event of any problems occurring such as a suspected food poisoning outbreak linked with the business.

In such an event, follow the instructions from the EHO (EHP) specifically. The supervisor may be requested:

- Not to allow cleaning of the kitchen until after the EHO (EHP) inspection
- To provide a list of all kitchen staff and their duties (plus any illnesses they may have reported)
- To stop trading or remove food from sale and keep samples of any suspect food.

All food safety-related records will need to be made available.

An inspection visit As a supervisor of a large kitchen, list the documents and records you would have available for an EHO (EHP) inspection visit.

Why are these documents important?

How would these documents be essential as part of a 'due diligence' defence?

In this chapter you have learned about:

1. The importance of food safety management procedures

2. The responsibilities of employers and employees in respect of food safety legislation and procedures for compliance

3. How the legislation is enforced

4. The importance of and methods for temperature control

5. Procedures to control contamination and cross-contamination

6. The importance of high standards of personal hygiene

7. Procedures for cleaning, disinfection and waste disposal

8. The importance of and methods for pest control

9. Outline requirements relating to design of food premises and equipment

10. The importance to food safety of microbial, chemical, physical and allergenic hazards

11. Methods and procedures for controlling food safety

12. The requirements for monitoring and recording food safety procedures

13. Methods for and the importance of evaluating food safety controls and procedures

14. The requirements for induction and ongoing training of staff

15. The importance of effective communication on food safety procedures.

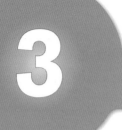

Practical gastronomy

This chapter covers Unit 303: Practical Gastronomy. In this chapter you will:

1. Explore the influences on eating and drinking cultures from the chef's perspective

2. Investigate the supply and use of commodities.

Influences on eating and drinking cultures

Gastronomy

Over the years there have been a number of definitions of gastronomy. In very simple terms it is the study of how food influences habits and the influence of history and location in society.

Choosing what to eat is a complex development process which we learn from childhood and the way we are socialised into food habits through family and relationships. This is how our taste for certain foods is developed.

Taste

Why do we eat what we eat, select one dish from the menu in preference to another, choose one particular kind of restaurant or use a takeaway? Why are these dishes on the menu in the first place? Is it because the chef likes them, the customer or consumer wants them, or is this the only food available? What dictates what we eat?

Hospitality reflects the eating habits, history, customs and taboos of society, but it also develops and creates them. You have only to compare the variety of eating facilities available on any major high street today with those of a short while ago.

Taste affects food choice and is based on biological, social and cultural perspectives. The perception of taste results from the stimulation of the taste cells that make up the taste buds. Taste is not specific to individual foods but to the balance between four main types of chemical compound.

Taste preferences Reflect on your own taste preferences and how they have been developed.

Factors affecting what we eat

There are many factors influencing our choice of what we eat. These include our individual preferences, our relationships and emotional needs. Other factors such as what is acceptable to us as food, images of food, as well as the needs and preferences of people we eat with also affect our choice.

The individual

Everyone has needs and wishes, which are met according to their own satisfaction.

Tastes and habits in eating are influenced by three main factors:

- Upbringing
- Peer-group behaviour
- Social background.

For example, children's tastes are developed at home according to the eating patterns of their family, as is their expectation of when to eat meals. Teenagers may frequent hamburger or other fast-food outlets and adults may eat out once a week at an ethnic or high-class restaurant, steakhouse or gastro pub.

How hungry an individual feels will affect their choice of what, when and how much to eat – although some people in the Western world overeat and food shortages cause under-nourishment in poorer countries.

Everyone ought to eat enough to enable body and mind to function efficiently; if you are hungry or thirsty it is difficult to work or study effectively.

Health considerations may influence an individual's choice of food, either because they need a special diet for medical reasons or (as the current emphasis on healthy eating shows) because of a belief that everyone needs a nutritionally balanced diet. Many people nowadays feel it is healthier to avoid eating meat or dairy products. Others are vegetarian or vegan for moral or religious reasons.

Relationships

Eating is a necessity, but it is also a means of developing social relationships. You should also consider the needs and preferences of the people you eat with. This applies in the family or at your place of study or work. The provision of suitable foods and dishes for pupils at school mealtimes in an appropriate environment can be a means of developing good eating habits and fostering social relationships. For people at work, it is in canteens, dining rooms and restaurants that relationships may develop.

Often the purpose of eating, either in the home or outside it, is to be sociable and to meet people, or to renew acquaintances, or provide the opportunity for people to meet each other. Frequently there is a reason for the occasion (such as birthday, anniversary, wedding or awards ceremony), requiring a special party or banquet menu, or it may just be for a few friends who choose to have a meal at a restaurant.

Business is often conducted over a meal, usually at lunchtime but also at breakfast and dinner. Eating and drinking help to make work more enjoyable and effective.

Using food to build relationships Consider how you use food and have learnt how to use food to build relationships.

Emotional needs

Sometimes we eat not because we need food but to meet an emotional requirement:

- For sadness or depression: in eating a meal we may comfort ourselves or give comfort to someone else; after a funeral, people eat together to comfort one another
- For a reward or treat, or to give encouragement to oneself or to someone else; an invitation to a meal is a good way of showing appreciation.

Ideas about food

People's ideas about food and meals and about what is and what is not acceptable vary according to:

- Where and how they were raised
- The area in which they live and its social customs.

Different societies and cultures have conflicting ideas about what constitutes good cooking, a good chef and about the sort of food a good chef should provide. The French tradition of producing fine food and their chefs being highly regarded continues to this day – whereas other countries traditionally may have less interest in the art of cooking, and less respect for chefs.

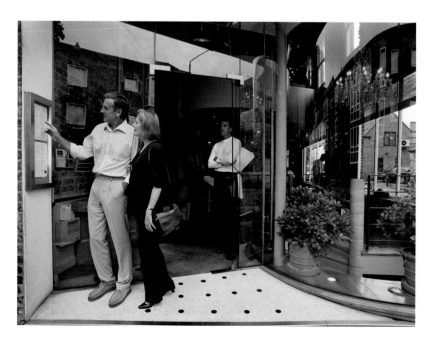

Individuals' ideas of what constitutes a snack, a proper meal or a celebration will depend on their backgrounds, as will their interpretation of terms such as lunch or dinner. One person's idea of a snack may be another person's idea of a main meal; a celebration for some will be a visit to a hamburger bar; for others, a meal at a fashionable restaurant.

The idea of what is 'the right thing to do' when eating varies with age, social class and religion. To certain people it is right to eat with the fingers, while others use only a fork. Some will have cheese before the sweet course; others will have cheese after it. It is accepted that children and, sometimes, elderly people need to have their food cut up into small pieces and that people of some religions do not eat certain foods. The ideas usually originate from practical and hygiene reasons, although sometimes the origin is obscure.

Images of food

Fashions, fads and fancies affect foods and it is not always clear if catering creates or copies these trends.

Nutritionists inform us about foods that are good and necessary in the diet, what the effect of particular foods will be on the figure and how much of each food we require. This helps to produce an 'image' of food. This image changes according to research, availability of food and what is considered to constitute healthy eating.

What people choose to eat says something about them as a person; it creates an image. We are what we eat, but why do we choose to eat what we do when there is choice? One person will perhaps avoid trying snails because of ignorance of how to eat them or because the idea is repulsive, while another will select them deliberately to show off to other diners. One person will select a dish because it is a new experience; another individual will choose it because they have previously enjoyed eating it. The quantity eaten may indicate a glutton or a gourmand; the quality selected, a gourmet.

Crop failure or distribution problems may make food scarce or not available at all. Foods in season are now supplemented by imported foods so that foods out of season at home are now available much of the time. This means that there is a wide choice of food for the caterer and the customer.

Effects of images on food choice Think about your images of food and how they affect your food choice.

Food is available through shops, supermarkets, cash and carry, wholesalers and direct suppliers. It is now possible for people at home and caterers to purchase, prepare, cook and present almost every food imaginable due to rapid air transport and food preservation. Food spoilage and wastage are minimised; variety and quality are maximised.

It is essential that food looks attractive, has a pleasing smell and tastes good, since individuals are less likely to eat food that does not meet these criteria, even if it is nutritious. Remember that people's views on what is attractive and appealing will vary according to their background and experience.

Money, time and facilities

Money, time and facilities affect what people eat – the economics of eating affects everyone.

How much money an individual has available or decides to spend on food is crucial to their choice of what to eat. Some people will not be able to afford to eat out; others will be able to eat out only occasionally, while for others, eating out will be a frequent event. The money that individuals allocate for food will determine whether they:

- Cook and eat at home
- Use a takeaway (for example, fish and chips, Chinese)
- Go to a pub, eat at a pizza restaurant or at an ethnic or other restaurant.

The amount of time people have to eat at work will affect whether they use any facilities provided, go out for a snack or meal during their lunch break, or take in their own food to the workplace.

The ease of obtaining food, the use of convenience and frozen food, and the facility for storing foods have led to the availability of a wide range of foods in both the home and catering establishments. It is possible to freeze foods that are in season and use them throughout the year, so eliminating spoilage in the event of a glut of items.

The media

The media influences what we eat: television, radio, newspapers, magazines and literature of all kinds have an effect on our eating habits.

Healthy eating, nutrition, hygiene and outbreaks of food poisoning are publicised; experts in all aspects of health, including those extolling exercise, diet and environmental health, state what should and should not be eaten.

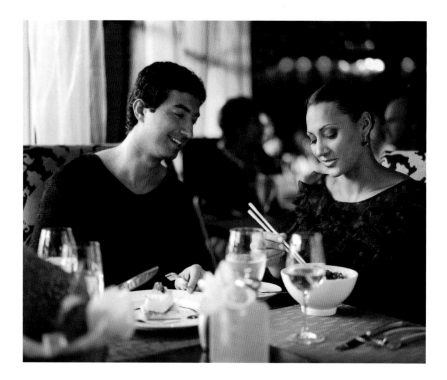

Information given about the content of food in packets and the advertising of food influences our choice. The media contributes to our knowledge about eating and foods alongside our learning on this topic from the family, teachers, at school meals, at college, and through the experience of eating abroad.

The influences on our choice of food that are listed in Table 3.1 are separated for convenience but in reality they overlap. Only when sufficient food is available for survival can people begin to derive pleasure from eating food.

Impact of media on food choice Explain how the media affects people's food choices.

Cultural influences on our choice of food

Cultural variety

The differing races and nations of the world represent a great variety of cultures, each with their own ways of cooking. Knowledge of this is essential for those working in the catering industry because:

- There has been a rapid spread of tourism, creating a demand for a broader culinary experience
- Many people from overseas have opened restaurants using their own foods and styles of cooking

- The development of air cargo means perishable foods from distant places are readily available
- The media, particularly television, has stimulated an interest in worldwide cooking.

Food and religion Explain how food is used in religion to symbolise events, meanings and its symbolic use in ceremonies.

Food and celebrations

Food is used every day to express a range of emotions: love, happiness, joy, satisfaction, and so on. Food is used in celebrations to convey these emotions in all parts of the world, regardless of culture or religion. Food can unite and strengthen community bonds and help to maintain a common identity amongst groups of people. Different countries use food in different ways to help celebrate special occasions such as Christmas, New Year, weddings and birthdays.

Christmas

In Britain it is traditional to serve roast turkey, Christmas pudding and mince pies as part of the festivities, but in other countries different foods are eaten. Some examples of different types of food eaten at Christmas include:

- France: black and white pudding, which is sausage containing blood

Table 3.1 Influences on choice of food

Media	Transport	Religion
TV Books Newspapers Journals	Transport of foods by sea, rail and air Transport of people	Taboos Festivals Pork, beef, shellfish, alcohol, halal, kosher
Geographical	**Historical**	**Economic**
Climate Indigenous fish, birds, animals, plant life Soil, lakes, rivers, seas, terrain	Explorations Invasions Establishment of trade routes	Money to purchase Goods to exchange
Sociological	**Political**	**Cultural**
Family School Workplace Leisure Fashion and trends	Tax on food Policies on 'food mountains' Export and import restrictions	Ethnic Tribal Celebrations
Psychological	**Physiological**	**Scientific**
Appearance of food Smell Taste Aesthetics Reaction to new foods	Nutritional Healthy eating Illness Additives	Preservation Technology Shorter ripening times Reduction in fat content in livestock Increased resistance to pests/disease Increased use of fertilisers Increased yields Increased shelf life GM foods Irradiated foods Intensive farming Ready meals – chilled, frozen, sous-vide

- French Canada: desserts include doughnuts and sugar pie
- Germany: gingerbread biscuits and liqueur chocolates
- Nicaragua: chicken with a stuffing made from a range of fruits and vegetables including tomato, onion and papaya
- Russia: a feast of 12 different dishes, representing Christ's disciples.

New Year

Traditional New Year foods around the world include:

- Greece: a special sweet pastry baked with a coin inside it
- Japan: up to 20 dishes are cooked and prepared one week before the start of the celebrations. Each food represents a New Year's wish; for example, seaweed asks for happiness in the year ahead
- Scotland: haggis (sheep's stomach stuffed with oatmeal and offal), gingerbread biscuits and scones
- Spain: 12 grapes, meant to be put into the mouth one at a time at each chime of the clock at midnight.

Lunar New Year

In many Asian countries, the New Year doesn't start on January 1, but with the first full moon in the first Chinese lunar month. Traditional New Year's food includes:

- China: fish, chestnuts and fried foods
- Korea: dumpling soup
- Vietnam: meat-filled rice cakes and shark fin soup.

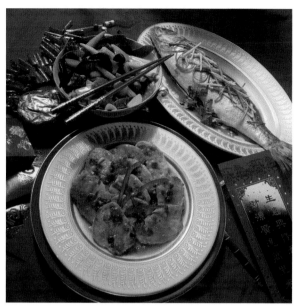

A celebration meal in China

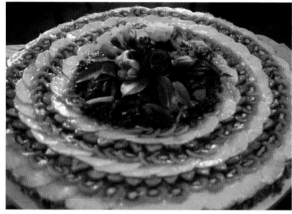

A fruit-topped wedding cake from Italy

Weddings

Around the world, weddings share common ground – no matter what the religion or culture, the typical wedding is a joint celebration for the families that involves a wedding cake and traditional foods. Foods that feature prominently in weddings include:

- China: roast suckling pig, fish, pigeon, chicken, lobster and a type of bun stuffed with lotus seeds are commonly served. It is especially important to offer both lobster and chicken: the lobster represents the dragon and the chicken the phoenix so including both on the menu is thought to harmonise the Yin and Yang of the newly joined families

- Indonesia: foods served depend on the region and religion but could include spicy rice dishes like nasi goreng, dim sum, sushi or even Western recipes like beef Wellington
- Italy: food is a very important part of an Italian wedding. Bowtie-shaped twists of fried dough, sprinkled with sugar, represent good luck. A roast suckling pig or roast lamb is often the main dish, accompanied by pastas and fruits. Traditional wedding cakes in different regions of Italy include one made from biscuits and another topped with fruit
- Korea: noodles are served, because they represent longevity
- Norway: the traditional wedding cake is made from bread topped with cream, cheese and syrup
- Britain: the honeymoon has been said to originate from a time when the father of the bride gave the groom a moon's (month's) worth of mead (alcoholic beverage made from honey) before the bride and groom left after the ceremony.

Birthdays

The custom of the birthday party originated in medieval Europe, when it was supposed that people were vulnerable to evil spirits on their birthdays. Friends, family members, festivities and presents were thought to ward off the spirits. Traditional birthday foods from around the world include:

- Australia: birthdays are often celebrated by sharing a decorated birthday cake with lit candles, which the person celebrating the birthday blows out while making a wish
- England: a cake may be baked containing symbolic objects which foretell the future. If your piece of cake has a coin, for example, you will one day be wealthy
- Ghana: the child's birthday breakfast is a fried patty made from mashed sweet potato and eggs. Traditional birthday party fare includes a dish made from fried plantain (a kind of banana)
- Korea: for their first birthday, the child is dressed and sat before a range of objects including fruit, rice, calligraphy brushes and money. Whichever item the child picks up predicts their future; for example, picking up the rice indicates material wealth. After this ceremony, the guests eat rice cakes
- Mexico: a papier-maché container in the shape of an animal (piñata) is filled with lollies and other treats. The child who is celebrating his or her

birthday is blindfolded and hits at the piñata until it breaks. The treats are shared among the guests

- Western Russia: the birthday boy or girl is given a fruit pie instead of a cake.

> **The effect of diversity on planning menus** Explain why a chef should understand the implications of different cultures when planning menus.

Consumer behaviour

Consumer behaviour examines the relationship between how individuals make decisions about how to spend their available resources on food, goods and services (their resources being their money, time and effort) and how producers such as the hospitality industry act to meet or create their needs and wants. For example:

- Who buys what
- When they buy
- Why they buy
- How they buy
- Where they buy
- How often they buy.

Consumer decision making

Here are some examples of the types of factors affecting the consumer purchasing process, that is, why consumers buy certain foods and services:

- **Cultural:** cultural trends and norms, customs, religion, myths, symbolism, local, regional, national preferences, habits
- **Economic:** income, prices, taxes
- **Marketing:** advertising and promotion, distribution, restaurant/hotel location, size, product, portfolio and layout
- **Physiological:** heredity, allergy, taste, food acceptability/intolerance
- **Political:** EU legislation, food policy, Common Agricultural Policy
- **Psychographic:** personality, self-concept, lifestyle, values, attitudes, beliefs, emotions, mood, preferences, significance of food
- **Social:** social class, reference groups, household size, family life cycle stage, demography, educational level
- **Technical:** food processing and preparation methods, cooking and storage options, packaging materials and type, nature of ingredients
- **Other:** seasonality, perishability, portability.

Source: Suzan Green, 'Consumer product management' in Proudlove, 2010, *The Science and Technology of Foods*, Forbes Publications

Depending on individual products, dishes, types of restaurants and the circumstances of the consumer, all of these factors will have some bearing on what is selected, the quality, when and how often.

An example of four basic stages in choosing food is shown in Table 3.2.

Table 3.2 Example of four basic stages in choice

1	Noticing	I'm hungry That looks tasty
2	Choosing	I feel like a snack I like that brand/flavour
3	Acting	I'll buy that to eat now Just a small portion will do
4	Assessing	I prefer the item I usually buy That was good value for money

Consumers may be conscious of all or none of these stages. Sometimes decision, purchases and consumption experiences are done on autopilot. Sometimes one stage may dominate – I'm hungry.

The consumer and society

Lifestyles are actual patterns of behaviour and are constructed by measuring consumers' activities, interests and opinions, which affect their food choice. See Table 3.3.

Table 3.3 Factors affecting lifestyles

Activities	Work, hobbies, social events, vacation, entertainment, club membership, community, shopping, sports
Interests	Family, home, job, community, recreation, fashion, good, media, achievements
Opinions	Themselves, social issues, politics, business, economics, education, products, future, culture
Demographics	Age, education, income, occupation, family size, dwelling, geography, stage of life cycle

Source: Reprinted with permission from *Journal of Marketing*, published by the American Marketing Association, Plummer, 38:1, 1974, 'The concepts and application of life style segmentation'

More people are consuming more varied food and drink products on more occasions than ever before. For an explanation of the relationship between cultural values and consumer food choice see Table 3.4.

Devise a weekly menu plan Using these cultural values and consumer food choice factors devise a week's menus for a sports team of your choice for breakfast, lunch and dinner.

Table 3.4 Cultural values and consumer food choice

Core cultural values	Food production
A more casual lifestyle with less formality	Destructuring of meal occasions and more individual autonomy over what is eaten, multiple product choices consumed at the same meal time by different people and less formal meals and meal times
Pleasure seeking and novelty – a desire for products and services which make life more fun	Constant innovation and product differentiation in all aspects – taste, texture, portion size, packaging, advertising, branding, product concepts, etc. Food as entertainment
Consumerism – increased concern over value for money with rising expectations about quality and performance	Rise in 'grocerant' products – restaurant-style food available to take home, for 'eating out, staying in'. Increase in functional foods, e.g. energy drinks, vitamin-enriched products
Instant gratification – living for today and intolerance of non-immediate availability	Rise in treats, indulgence and luxury items, super-premium lines. More convenient access and availability through wider distribution of food
Simplification – a removal of time and energy spent on 'unnecessary' things or tasks	More pre-prepared, pre-packaged, processed and added-value lines for consumption at once or after microwaving to cut down effort in product selection, preparation, cooking and clearing away
Time conservation – time has to be used effectively	Pre-/part-prepared complete or partially ready meals
Concern with appearance and health, youth, keeping fit and looking good	Expansion/creation of calorie-light product meals. Increase in low-fat, low-calorie, low-salt, high-fibre products and substitutes. More product innovation in the areas of functional foods and nutraceuticals. Meat reduction and meat substitutes (mycoprotein, soya, tofu). Eat yourself healthy campaign – 'five fruits and vegetables a day', Mediterranean 'superfoods' (e.g. garlic, olive oil, red wine, red peppers, sun-dried tomatoes, pasta, rice, fish and shellfish)

Source: Proudlove, 2010, *The Science and Technology of Foods* (Forbes)

3.2 The supply and use of commodities

Suppliers

Most companies find that 80 per cent by value of their purchases of goods and services come from 20 per cent of their suppliers.

Suppliers of food include:

- **Producers:** the producers of the food, for example the farmers, also sell their produce direct through farm shops or to supermarkets or large catering companies
- **Wholesalers:** wholesale suppliers buy from the producers, food manufacturers, and so on and sell to the caterer. Cash and carry wholesalers are an example of this type of operation
- **Retailers:** large retail supermarkets stock a wide range of ingredients. This type of buying may be suitable for a small restaurant operation.

Purchasing consortiums

Purchasing consortiums are organisations set up to negotiate prices for goods and commodities for hospitality companies to enable them to obtain the best possible price for the desired quality.

Centralised or decentralised purchasing

Whether you decide to centralise or decentralise the purchasing procedure will depend on the size of the business.

Well-managed centralised buying reduces costs by consolidating quantities to achieve lower prices from your suppliers and reducing overall stock levels through using central facilities.

Centralisation should avoid duplication of administrative effort at each site, thereby reducing errors and bringing further savings. Equally important is that centralisation will often allow a buyer to specialise. A purchasing consortium operates a similar principle as centralised buying.

Decentralised buying is about local control where:

- Sites/operations are some distance apart
- Purchasing is bound up with other functions, that is, part of a specialist unit requiring different types of ingredients
- Corporate culture stresses the need for people at the sharp end of the operation to have maximum control, where the chef responsible for the ordering reports directly to the client he or she is serving.

In a small company where there is a need to purchase only a limited number of commodities and ingredients, the purchase department may well be the chef or one person and an assistant. In a large organisation with several hundred employees, however, it would not be unusual to have ten or more people in the purchasing department.

The overall size of the firm, either in turnover or employment terms, can be a major factor as can the total value of the purchases. The main determinants tend to be the type of business, the complexity of the ingredients and the commodities.

Buying and negotiation

Buying and negotiation involves selecting suppliers and negotiating terms. It may include the selection of speciality ingredients and the buyer will need to understand the importance of quality as well as securing value for money. Other important aspects of buying and negotiating include research, and seeking out local, regional and national suppliers.

Follow-up and expediting

The chef or purchaser needs to develop a good working relationship with their suppliers. They must have close contact with quality management, sales planning and sales support staff and will be involved with delivery and quality targets, as well as detailed specifications (traceability).

Purchase research

Purchase research is undertaken by an individual or group that looks beyond the day-to-day requirements and considers alternative ingredients sources of supplier, long-term price trends or at improving supplier appraisal. Those involved in purchase research must have up-to-date knowledge of future marketing plans and menu design.

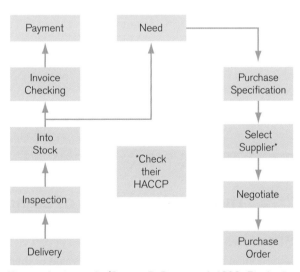

The purchasing cycle (Source: D. Drummond, 1998, *Purchasing and Costing in the Hospitality Industry*, Hodder Arnold, reproduced by permission of Hodder Education)

Knowing the market

Since markets vary considerably, in order to do a good job when purchasing commodities a buyer must know the characteristics of each market.

A market is a place in which ownership of a commodity changes from one person to another. This exchange of ownership could occur while using the telephone, on a street corner, in a retail or wholesale establishment, or at an auction.

It is important that a food and beverage purchaser has knowledge of the items to be purchased, such as:

- Where they are grown
- Seasons of production
- Approximate costs
- Conditions of supply and demand
- Laws and regulations governing the market and the products
- Marketing agents and their services
- Processing
- Storage requirements
- Commodity and product, class and grade.

The buyer

This is the key person who not only makes decisions regarding quality, amounts required, price and what will satisfy the customers but also makes a profit. The wisdom of the buyer's decisions will be reflected in the success or failure of the operation. The buyer must be knowledgeable about the products and must have the necessary skills to deal with sales people, suppliers and other market agents. The buyer must be prepared for hard and often aggressive negotiations.

The responsibility for buying varies from company to company according to its size and management policy. Buying may be the responsibility of the chef, manager, storekeeper, buyer or buying department.

A buyer must have knowledge of the company's internal organisation, especially the operational needs, and be able to obtain the products needed at a competitive price. Buyers must also acquaint themselves with the production procedures and how these items are going to be used in the production operations, in order that the right item is purchased. For example, the item required may not always have to be of prime quality, such as, for instance, tomatoes for use in soups and sauces.

A buyer must also be able to make good use of market conditions. For example, if there is a glut of fresh salmon at low cost, has the organisation the facility to make use of extra salmon purchases? Is there sufficient freezer space? Can the chef make use of salmon by creating a demand for the product on the menu?

Buying methods

Buying methods depend on the type of hospitality operation and the market they serve. Purchasing procedures are usually formal or informal. See Table 3.5.

Table 3.5 Informal and formal methods of buying

| Informal buying | This usually involves oral negotiations, talking directly to sales people, face to face or using the telephone. Informal methods vary according to market conditions. |
| Formal buying | Known as competitive buying, formal buying involves giving suppliers written specifications and quantity needs. Negotiations are normally written. |

Both methods of buying have advantages and disadvantages. Informal methods are suitable for casual buying, where the amount involved is not large, and speed and simplicity are desirable. Formal contracts are best for the purchase of commodities over a long period of time; prices do not vary much during a year once the basic price has been established. Prices and supply tend to fluctuate more with informal methods.

Selecting suppliers

The selection of suppliers is an important part of the purchasing process. First, consider how a supplier will be able to meet the needs of your operation. Consider:

- Price
- Delivery
- Quality/standards.

You may obtain information on suppliers from other purchasers. Buyers should be encouraged to visit suppliers' establishments. When interviewing prospective suppliers, you need to question how reliable a supplier will be under competition and how stable under varying market conditions.

Principles of purchasing

A menu dictates an operation's needs for commodities; basing potential purchasing decisions on the menu, the buyer searches for a market that can supply the company. After locating the right market, the buyer investigates the various products that are available and may meet the company's needs. The right product of the right quality must be obtained to meet those needs. Other factors that might affect food production include:

- Type and image of the establishment
- Style of operation and system of service
- Occasion for which the item is needed
- Amount of storage available (dry, refrigerated or frozen)
- Finance available and supply policies of the organisation
- Availability, seasonality, price trends and supply.

In making your choice as a buyer, you should also take into account the skill of the employees, catering assistants and chefs who work at the establishment. You should consider the condition of the product and the processing method for which it is to be used, the suitability of the product to produce the item or dish required, and the storage life of the product.

Buying tips

As a buyer you should:

- Make sure that you have an up-to-date and sound knowledge of all commodities, both fresh and convenience, to be purchased.
- Be aware of the availability of the different types and qualities of each commodity.
- When buying fresh commodities, be aware of part-prepared and ready-prepared items available on the market.
- Keep a sharp eye on price variations. Buy at the best price you can to ensure the required quality and also an economic yield. The cheapest item may prove to be the most expensive if waste is excessive. When possible, order by number and weight. For example, 20 kg plaice could be 80 × 250 g plaice, 40 × 500 g plaice, or 20 × 1 kg plaice. It could also be 20 kg total weight of various sizes and this makes efficient portion control difficult. Some suppliers (for example butchers, fishmongers) may offer a portion-control service by selling the required number of a given weight of certain cuts. For example, 100 × 150 g sirloin steaks, 25 kg prepared stewing beef, 200 × 100 g pieces of turbot fillet, 500 × 100 g plaice fillets.
- Organise an efficient system of ordering, ensuring that you keep copies of all orders for cross-checking, whether orders are given in writing, verbally or by telephone.

- Compare purchasing by retail, wholesale and contract procedures to ensure the best method is selected for your own particular organisation.
- Explore all possible suppliers: local or markets, town or country, small or large.
- Keep the number of suppliers to a minimum. At the same time have at least two suppliers for every group of commodities, when possible. The principle of having competition for the caterer's business is sound.
- Issue all orders to suppliers fairly, allowing sufficient time for the order to be implemented efficiently.
- Request price lists as frequently as possible and compare prices continually to make sure that you buy at a good market price.
- Buy perishable goods when they are in full season, as this gives the best value at the cheapest price. To help with purchasing the correct quantities, it is useful to compile a purchasing chart for 100 covers from which items can be divided or multiplied according to requirement. An indication of quality standards can also be incorporated in a chart of this kind.
- Deliveries must all be checked against the orders given for quantity, quality and price. If any goods delivered are below an acceptable standard they must be returned, either for replacement or credit.
- Containers can account for large sums of money. Ensure that all containers are correctly stored, returned to the suppliers where possible and the proper credit given.
- All invoices must be checked for quantities and prices.
- All statements must be checked against invoices and passed swiftly to the office so that payment may be made in time to ensure maximum discount on purchases.
- Foster good relations with trade representatives because you can gain much useful up-to-date information from them.
- Keep up-to-date trade catalogues, visit trade exhibitions, survey new equipment and continually review the space, services and systems in use in order to explore possible avenues of increased efficiency.

Quality assurance

Quality assurance of suppliers is anything you need to do to give you confidence that you will receive the goods you want, performing as specified at the time you want them. Carry out a supplier appraisal. Consider, for example:

- Are they financially stable?
- Do they have the ability to deliver?
- Do they understand what you want?
- Are they easy to deal with?

How good are your existing suppliers? Formal measurement is called 'vendor rating', which gives a good guide in helping to review the purchasing base.

Setting up a vendor rating system involves:

- Writing down the (preferably measurable) qualities you expect from a good supplier
- Recording performance
- Looking at results from time to time and
- Acting on them.

Good purchasing procedures Good purchasing is an important aspect of operation control. Explain good purchasing procedures and how these contribute to an overall operational control policy.

An example of a vendor rating system is shown in Table 3.6.

Table 3.6 An example of a vendor rating system

	Maximum	Achieved
Quality achievement	20	20
Price	20	5
Delivery on time	20	20
Packaging temperature	20	12
Efficient paperwork	10	8
Good communication	10	6
Total	100	71

Source: Defra, *Putting it into Practice*, 2008, reproduced under the terms of the click-use licence

Table 3.6 shows that the problems relate to the supplier's price, packaging, paperwork, and how the purchaser should measure these objectively.

Quality can be measured at goods inwards. Price may be measured from competitive tenders, delivery performance from orders and delivery notes, and so on.

These assessments should be done on a regular basis, at least every six months. Inform suppliers how they are being measured. If improvements are required from suppliers, set them a time limit in which to improve.

How many suppliers can you afford?

It takes time to research a supplier, to establish relationships and to set up the purchasing system in order to get the best out of your main suppliers; you will need to develop and educate suppliers about your needs, listen to any suggestions they have, track their performance and correct any problems.

One approach is to move towards single sourcing. This involves bringing together the requirements from all parts of the business in order to make larger, more regular orders from fewer suppliers. Where you purchase the same ingredients from two or more suppliers, consider choosing one main supplier. In other areas, where purchases are small in value, think about buying from a distributor who handles a range of goods. With fewer suppliers you can afford more time for each one. They will respond well to more personal contact and the possibility of larger orders. The danger of this approach is that if you have fewer suppliers you are more dependent on their performance. Some hospitality companies do not adopt this approach, as it is often considered to be too high a risk.

Free trade This means governments have to treat local and foreign producers in the same way, for example by not creating barriers to importing goods, services or people from other countries, or giving national businesses and farmers an advantage over foreign firms by offering them financial support. In practice, truly free trade has never existed and the reduction of trade barriers is always subject to intense political negotiation between countries of unequal power.

Ethical trade This involves companies finding ways to buy their products from suppliers who provide good working conditions and respect the environment and human rights.

Fair Trade This encourages small-scale producers to play a stronger role in managing their relationship with buyers, guaranteeing them a fair financial return for their work. Some corporate buyers help to set up schools and health centres on the farms in countries where the food is produced.

World Trade Organisation The WTO was created in 1944 to liberalise world trade through international agreements. Based in Geneva, the WTO has 140 member countries, some of which have much more power than others. Some poor countries cannot afford to keep any staff in Geneva.

Globalisation This is the rapid integration of trade and culture between the world's nations. With a more open market, goods and, by association, cash can now travel across the globe much more freely. This greater global trade has been able to happen for the following reasons:

- Governments have changed laws that, in the past, restricted economic trade
- New technologies have enabled faster communication
- Travel and transport costs have been reduced
- Western companies have looked abroad for investment.

Sustainable food

This is food which is purchased, consumed and prepared with as little impact on the environment as possible, for a fair price, and which makes a positive contribution to the local economy.

i Simple guidelines to follow when purchasing food

- Use local, seasonal and available ingredients as standard to minimise goods transport, storage and energy use.
- Specify produce from farming systems that minimise harm to the environment such as certified organic.
- Limit foods of animal origin such as meat, dairy products, eggs, as livestock farming is one of the most significant contributors to climate change. Promote meals rich in fruit, vegetables, pulses and nuts.
- Ensure that meat, dairy and egg products are produced to high environmental and animal welfare standards.
- Exclude fish species identified as most 'at risk' by the Marine Conservation Society and specify fish only from sustainable sources.

- Buy Fair Trade certified products and drinks imported from poorer countries to ensure a fair deal for disadvantaged producers.
- Avoid bottled water. Serve plain, filtered tap water. This will minimise transport and packaging waste.

Source: Defra, *Putting it into Practice*, 2008, reproduced under the terms of the click-use licence

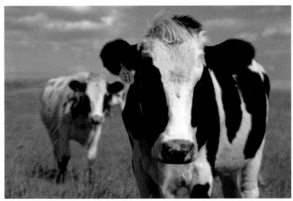

Are your meat and dairy products produced to high animal welfare standards?

A sustainable food policy Design a poster or leaflet to explain a sustainable food policy.

Building relationships with suppliers

Areas to investigate with a supplier are:

- Where do they source goods from at the moment, for example country of origin, farms, and so on?
- What do they buy in season? Most fruit and vegetable wholesalers will be able to show you their 'buying plan', which will show you where and when they buy in the UK and from abroad. When fresh produce is in season it is at its most abundant and therefore at its cheapest.
- What are the production strengths of your region? Some regions are better at growing things than others. For example, Sussex has a good reputation for its South Downs lamb, salad production and fresh sweetcorn, whereas Kent is known for apples, soft fruit and brassicas. As with seasonality, local abundance makes these items more affordable.
- Can they supply more fresh items? Using frozen goods increases the likelihood that the goods in question have travelled a considerable distance within the UK or have come from abroad. Blast freezing also uses a considerable amount of energy and storing frozen goods is less energy efficient than storing chilled fresh goods.

- What are the delivery arrangements? Can you, the purchaser, manage with less frequent deliveries?
- Are they willing to arrange producer visits and visit your team at work? Supplies are an important part of building the food culture in your organisation and seeing how food is produced first-hand is something that most teams find interesting and inspiring.

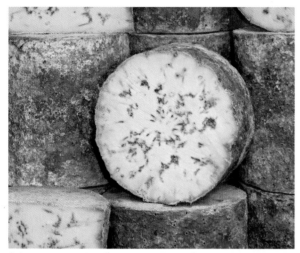
Stilton: an example of a regional British food product

Taking a team approach to sustainability

Ask all the team in the kitchen to review the menu to see what changes can be made to favour more seasonal produce.

Organise a visit to a farm and producer in your local area whose produce you use. This helps your team of chefs to understand the products better. Take photographs to promote the food within your organisation and local press.

Organise promotions that reflect seasonality or celebrate your success in obtaining local produce. Celebrate seasonal produce with special menu items, new recipes to celebrate a new ingredient or new source of supply.

Get the chefs to sit down together and eat seasonal food, to learn about food and ingredients. Invite the producer or farmer to explain how the food is produced.

Measuring success of sustainability

Key success indicators for sustainability are:
- Percentage of food sourced locally, nationally and abroad

- Decrease in food wastage
- Reduction in food miles
- Financial contribution to the local economy
- Increase in recycling
- Increase in food sales.

Technologies and 'food miles' bring with them implications for greenhouse gas emissions and their consequent effects on the climate.

Consider for example:
- **Meat:** According to figures from the United Nations, animal farming globally produces more greenhouse gas emissions than all of the cars, lorries and planes' carbon emissions in the world put together.
- **Dairy:** Research by the Danish Institute of Agricultural Research found that organic milk has more Omega 3, a higher content of some vitamins and more antioxidants.
- **Food miles:** This refers to the distance the food travels from producer to consumer. Eating according to the seasons has disappeared for most people in the developed world. You can buy asparagus and strawberries all year round thanks to refrigeration, heated greenhouses and, of course, global food transportation.

Speciality foods

Areas through the country and throughout the world are known for speciality foods, many of which are grown and produced locally and feature on menus in the area. Examples of these foods are Evesham asparagus, Kent strawberries, Somerset cider, local cheeses such as Dorset Blue and Stilton, Isle of Wight rhubarb, South Downs lamb and Cornish lobster.

Local speciality foods List the local speciality foods in your area.

Several of these foods go back centuries and are part of the area's local heritage. This heritage is the important part of tourism for the region. The experience of food and drink and taste is an important part of tourism. Many tourists will visit a local area to sample the food and drink and expect to see it on real menus. Local chefs are able to promote themselves through their creative menus which display local heritage and the speciality foods from the region.

Methods of sourcing ingredients

Visit local producers, farms, dairies, factories. Speak to other chefs in the area: visit other restaurants, taste their dishes and assess what they have to offer. Use the internet to research ingredients and suppliers.

You may also find information about ingredients and suppliers from:

- **Directories:** Trade organisations produce directories of suppliers.
- **Company representatives:** Invite company representatives to see you and ask them to bring samples of their produce.
- **Trade shows:** Attend local and national trade shows, where there are always suppliers present. Country and regional shows are also good venues to meet producers and growers.
- **Media:** Always read local newspapers. Listen to local radio and farming news. Refer to the trade press, where there is always information on new products. Often these products are tested and evaluated by specialist panels of consumers.

Assessing commodities and ingredients

When deciding to purchase a commodity or ingredient, it is important to assess whether it is suitable for your needs and whether it will satisfy the demands of your menu. Ensure that you check:

- **Quality and flavour:** Is the commodity or ingredient affordable? Is it cost-effective? Will it give the number of portions required? Will it give the yield required?
- **Terms of supply:** What are the terms of supply, for example delivery times, payment requirements, and so on?
- **Supply meets demand:** Is the supplier able to regularly supply to your requirements? Can they supply the quantity required on a regular basis?
- **Hygiene, hazard analysis critical control points:** Visit the supplier before committing to purchase. Inspect the supplier premises for hygiene. Do they have a HACCP policy? How effective is the policy? Do they have appropriate records?
- **Supplier's reputation:** What reputation does the supplier have? Who are they already supplying to? What do these restaurants, hotels, catering establishments think of the supplier and the produce? Are they reliable? What type of packaging do they use? How efficient are they?

Ethical considerations

What kind of production methods are used to produce the commodities, for example free range farming, factory farming. What state are the animals kept in? How well are the animals looked after? How energy efficient are the production methods? How green are the transport methods used? Are they environmentally friendly?

How are the supplier's employees treated? Do they have an equal opportunity policy, a health and safety policy, and a welfare policy for staff?

What are their employees' working conditions like? Do they receive a fair wage?

Monitor and control receipt of goods

Staff responsible for receiving goods should be trained to recognise the items being delivered and to know if the quality, quantity and specific sizes, and so on are those ordered. This skill is acquired by experience and by guidance from the departmental head, for example the head chef, who will use the items.

Purchasing specifications detailing the expected standards of the goods to be delivered assist in this matter. However, the chef, supervisor, storekeeper, food and beverage manager, or whoever is responsible for controlling receipt of goods, needs to check that the specification is adhered to. If the establishment does not have a system of purchasing specifications, a check must still be made when goods are delivered that the expected standards have been achieved. In the event of goods being unsatisfactory, they should not be accepted.

Receipt of goods

Receipt of deliveries must be monitored to ensure that goods delivered correspond with the delivery note and there are no discrepancies. It is essential that items are of the stipulated size or weight, since this could affect portion control and costing; for example, 100 g fillets of plaice will need to be that weight and melons to be used for four portions should be of the appropriate size.

It is necessary to ensure that effective control can be practised. This means that:

- Delivery access and adequate checking and storage space are available
- These areas are clean, tidy and free from obstruction
- Staff are available to receive goods.

It is important that the standard of cleanliness and temperature of the delivery vehicles are also satisfactory. If these are not up to the required standard, the supplier must be told at once.

Temperatures

Vehicles over 7.5 tonnes must have an internal temperature of 5°C or below when being used to deliver food outside their locality. For local deliveries of food the temperature of vehicles under 7.5 tonnes should be 8°C or under.

On receipt, goods should be transferred as soon as possible to the correct storage area. Frozen items should be stored at the optimum temperatures, as shown in Table 3.7.

Table 3.7 Optimum storage temperatures for frozen items

Commodity	Temperature (°C)
Meat	−20
Vegetables	−15
Ice cream	−18 to −20

Refrigerator temperatures should be 3–4°C and larders provided for cooling of food should have a temperature of no higher than 8°C.

It is essential that a system of reporting non-compliance with the procedures of the establishment is known. Every place of work will have a security procedure to ensure that goods are stored safely. It is important that staff are aware of the system and to whom they should report any deviation.

Control storage of goods

If control of stock is to be effective, there should be ample storage space with adequate shelving bins, and so on, to enable the correct storage of goods. The premises must be clear and easy to keep clean, well lit and well ventilated, dry, secure and safe. Space should be available for easy access to all items which should not be stored at too high a level. Heavy items should be stored at a low level.

Stock rotation is essential so as to reduce waste; the last items in are the last items to be issued. Any deterioration of stock should be identified, action taken and reported. In order to keep a check on stock, there is a need for a system of documentation which states:

- The amount in the stores
- The amounts issued, to whom and when
- The amounts below which stock should not fall.

Shelf life and justification on 'use by date' information should be complied with. As a guide to storage, consider the points given in Table 3.8.

Persons responsible for controlling the storage of stock, in addition to checking the personnel using the stores and those working as storekeepers, must also check the correct storage temperatures of storerooms, refrigerators, deep freezes, and so on. The policy of the establishment may be to keep records of temperature checks.

Details of recommended storage temperatures for a range of food items are given in Table 3.9.

Table 3.8 Guide to storage

Item	Storage conditions and time
Canned goods	Store up to 9 months. Discard damaged, rusted, blown tins
Bottles and jars	Store at room temperature. Store in refrigerator once opened
Dry foods	Dry room temperature. Humid atmosphere causes deterioration
Milk and cream	Refrigerate and use within 3 days
Butter	Up to 1 month refrigerated
Cheese	According to the manufacturer's instruction. Soft cheese should be used as soon as possible
Salads	Keep longer if refrigerated or in a dark, well-ventilated area
Meat and poultry	Up to 1 week in refrigerator
Meat products	For example, sausages and pies, refrigerated for up to 3 days
Fish	Use on day of purchase ideally or up to 12 hours if refrigerated
Ice cream	Deep freeze for a week
Frozen foods	Six months: meat −18°C; fruit and vegetables −12°C

Table 3.9 Storage temperatures

Temperature (°C)	Food item
8	Soft cheese, whole
5 or below	Cut cheese
5	Cooked foods Smoked and cured fish Smoked and cured meat Sandwiches and rolls containing meat, fish, eggs (or substitutes), soft cheeses or vegetables
8 below	Desserts containing milk or milk substitutes (with pH value of 4.5 or more) Vegetables and fruit salads Pies and pastries containing meat, fish or substitute, or vegetables into which nothing has been added after cooking Cooked sausage rolls Uncooked or partly cooked pastries and dough products containing meat or fish or substitutes Cream cakes

Checking stock

An essential aspect of the supervisory role is the full stock audit and spot-check of goods in the stores, to assess deterioration and losses from other causes. Spot-checks by their very nature are random; stock audits will occur at specified times during the year. Some establishments have a system of daily records of stock-in-hand.

Control the issue of stock and goods

To supervise the issuing of stock, a system of control is needed so that a record of each item – how much, to whom and when – is kept. This enables a check to be made so that only authorised persons can obtain goods, the amount of items issued can be controlled and it is known how much of each item is used over a period of time.

This should help to avoid over-ordering and thus having too much stock on the premises. It should also diminish the risk of pilfering.

Having documentation enables accurate records to be available so that action can be taken to control the issue of goods.

To be effective the requisition document should include the date, the amount of the item or items required, and the department, section or person to whom they are to be issued. Usually a signature of the superior, for example chef, chef de partie or supervisor, is required. It may be desirable to draw a line under the last listed item so that unauthorised items are not then added.

Implement the physical stock-take

The purpose of a physical stock-taking procedure is to check that the documentation of existing stock tallies with the actual stock held on the premises. The reason for this exercise is to prevent capital being tied up by having too much stock in hand. It also provides information regarding the accuracy of the system and thus indicates where modifications could be made.

At the same time as the physical stock-take, details of discrepancies may become apparent that would then be investigated. Items such as returned empties, damaged stock and credit claims will be reconciled so that an accurate record is made for use by appropriate staff. This may mean that both the storekeeper and the manager responsible will take action on the stock-take details. It is for this reason that records must be accurate, legible and carefully maintained in order to achieve the aim of the exercise.

To be effective, every item should be recorded, indicating the appropriate detail such as weight, size, and so on, and the number of items in stock.

Design a documentation system Explain why it is important to keep accurate documentation. Design a documentation system for a simple storekeeping process for a small organisation which does not have a sophisticated computer system.

In this chapter you have:

1. Explored the influences on eating and drinking cultures from the chef's perspective

2. Investigated the supply and use of commodities.

4 Vegetables and vegetarian dishes

This chapter covers Unit 304: Advanced Skills and Techniques in Producing Vegetable and Vegetarian Dishes.

In this chapter you will learn to produce starters, main courses, accompaniments and garnishes.

Vegetables

Vegetables, like fruits, are the edible products of certain plants. They share several characteristics: they are savoury rather than sweet; we add salt to them; and, in most countries, they are associated with poultry, meat or fish as part of a meal or as an ingredient. Some vegetables are botanically classed as fruits: tomatoes are berries, and avocados are drupes, but both are commonly used as vegetables because they are not sweet.

Composition

Flavour accounts for a very small percentage of a vegetable's composition. Most contain at least 80 per cent water, the remainder being carbohydrate, protein and fat. Squashes, in particular, contain a high percentage of water, while potatoes contain a great deal of starch, which is used by the vegetables as a reserve food supply. Invert sugars are also a food source, and sucrose is present in corn, carrots, parsnips, onions and so on.

When vegetables age, the woody lignin increases, water evaporates and sugars become concentrated – old raw carrots appear to be sweeter than young ones, for example. But sugars change as soon as the vegetable is separated from the plant. (A good example is corn, which is often rushed straight from the stalk to the pot in order to preserve its taste.)

Quality

When choosing vegetables you should obviously avoid those that are limp and wilting, discoloured or damaged by harvesting. Leaf vegetables need careful picking over to avoid serving garden pests on the plate. Vegetables should be prepared for the pot as simply as possible. Wash them just before cooking, don't soak them and, as they lose nutrients through peeling and cutting, they should be peeled only thinly (vitamins are usually found just under the skin).

Storage

Many root and non-root vegetables that grow underground can be stored over winter in a root cellar or other similarly cool, dark and dry place, to prevent the growth of mould, greening and sprouting. Care should be taken in understanding the properties and vulnerabilities of the particular roots to be stored. These vegetables can last through to early spring and be almost as nutritious as when fresh.

During storage, leafy vegetables lose moisture and vitamin C degrades rapidly. They should be stored for as short a time as possible in a cool place in a container, such as a plastic bag or a sealed plastic container.

Storage points:

- Store all vegetables in a cool, dry, well-ventilated room at an even temperature of 4 to 8°C, which will help to minimise spoilage. Check vegetables daily and discard any that are unsound.
- Remove root vegetables from their sacks and store in bins or racks.
- Store green vegetables on well-ventilated racks.
- Store salad vegetables in a cool place and leave in their containers.
- Store frozen vegetables at −18°C or below. Keep a check on use-by dates, damaged packages and any signs of freezer burn.
- The fresher the vegetables the better the flavour, so ideally they should not be stored at all. However, as in many cases storage is necessary, then it should be for the shortest time possible.
- Green vegetables lose vitamin C quickly if they are bruised, damaged, stored for too long or overcooked.
- If vegetables are stored at the incorrect temperature micro-organisms may develop.
- If vegetables are stored in damp conditions moulds may develop.
- To prevent bacteria from raw vegetables passing on to cooked vegetables, store them in separate areas.
- Thaw out frozen vegetables correctly when necessary and never refreeze them once they have thawed out.

Preservation

Vegetables may be preserved using various methods, including:

- Canning: certain vegetables are preserved in tins – artichokes, asparagus, carrots, celery, beans, peas, tomatoes, mushrooms, truffles.
- Drying: the seeds of legumes (peas and beans) have their moisture content reduced to 10 per cent.
- Freezing: many vegetables, such as peas, beans, sprouts, spinach and cauliflower, are deep frozen.

Cooking

On contact with air certain vegetables tend to discolour, regardless of whether they are cooked or raw. This is because certain enzymes cause oxidisation. This activity can be halted by the addition of an acid, which is why cooks plunge celeriac – and apples – into acidulated water (water with a little lemon juice added) after peeling them.

Blanching helps to preserve colour, especially in green vegetables, but some vegetables' dyes are lost in the cooking process. Purple broccoli contains both chlorophyll (green) and anthocyanin (purple), the latter being water soluble, so cooked broccoli always looks green. Red cabbage reacts like litmus paper – it turns blue in the presence of an alkali (the lime in tap water), so you need to add a dash of acid, such as vinegar, to preserve the colour.

Approximate times only are given in the recipes in this chapter for the cooking of vegetables, as quality, age, freshness and size all affect the length of cooking time required. Young, freshly picked vegetables will need to be cooked for a shorter time than vegetables that have been allowed to grow older and that may have been stored after picking.

As a general rule, all root vegetables (with the exception of new potatoes) are started off by cooking in cold salted water. Those vegetables that grow above the ground are started in boiling salted water; this is so that they may be cooked as quickly as possible for the minimum period of time so that maximum flavour, food value and colour are retained.

Methods of cookery

All vegetables cooked by boiling may also be cooked by steaming. The vegetables are prepared in exactly the same way as for boiling, placed into steamer trays, lightly seasoned with salt and steamed under pressure for the minimum period of time in order to conserve maximum food value and retain colour. High-speed steam cookers are ideal for this purpose and also because of the speed of cooking they offer; batch cooking (cooking in small quantities throughout the service) can be practised instead of cooking large quantities prior to service, refreshing and reheating.

Many vegetables are cooked from raw by the stir-fry method, a quick and nutritious method of cooking.

Plant structure and cooking vegetables

Plant texture is determined by both the cell wall structure and the inner water pressure, or turgor, of the tissue. The application of heat, whether by boiling, baking or stir-frying, tenderises the food by weakening the cell walls and extracting water. First, heat denatures the proteins that make up the cell membranes, which thereby lose the selective permeability that regulates the cells' water content. Water leaks from the cells, the tissue loses turgor, and the plant becomes wilted and flabby. Even boiled vegetables, surrounded by water as they are, lose water during cooking, as weighing before and after will demonstrate.

Then there are the changes in the cell walls. While cellulose is not affected by heat, the hemicelluloses and pectins are; some hemicelluloses dissolve. In addition, the distribution of the pectic substances is altered: the amount of soluble pectin increases at the expense of the insoluble protopectins, and the walls lose still more of their 'cement'. The result: substantially weakened cell walls and more tender tissue.

The problem in cooking vegetables, of course, is how to make the tissue tender without making it too soft. Usually we take the common-sense approach of sampling the food during cooking and stopping when it is tender but still firm. In some cases colour can be used to indicate that a vegetable is cooked. One possible generalisation is that leaf vegetables, with their relatively thin, exposed and delicate layer of tissue, need only a minute of two of heating, while stem and root vegetables may require many times that amount. Experience and personal taste remain the best guides.

Potatoes

Potatoes are one of the most interesting vegetables you will find and, at long last, those selling them are becoming aware that the variety matters.

The first thing you need to know about a potato is whether it is floury or waxy. This determines how you must cook it. It also helps if you have some idea of the dry matter content. High dry matter means a floury potato – good for mashing, good for frying – but if you're the sort of person who leaves potatoes boiling in the pan for 20 minutes before looking at them, you may be disappointed when you take off the lid and see that your supper has turned into potato soup.

Waxy potatoes are great for boiling – they don't fall apart if you boil for too long (within reason) and they are good cold. Examples are Pink Fir and immature Jersey Royal, and there are lots more.

Floury potatoes are the best for mashing, for baking and for eating cold – but you must cook them carefully because overcooking will cause them to disintegrate. If you steam them, the timing isn't quite so critical, but you must still not overcook them or the texture will be lost. The cut surface of a perfectly cooked floury potato will have a beautiful white floury finish if you've got it right.

Good-flavoured mid- and main-crop potatoes include Golden Wonder, Kerr's Pink, British Queen, King Edward, Red King Edward, Binji, Pink Fir and Edzell Blue. Charlotte is good when young but not so good later on. Yukon Gold is a fine-flavoured potato with yellow flesh. Desiree is another yellowish-fleshed potato – a good all-rounder but its flavour is not quite as good as that of the other varieties listed above.

Shetland Black is good if you can get it – bluish-coloured flesh and a sweet flavour.

Congo is quite like Salad Blue; it has blue flesh but tastes more buttery.

Best for chips are probably Golden Wonder and Maris Piper, with Desiree a close third.

Vegetarian and vegan catering

This information has been adapted from the technical brief on vegetarian and vegan catering prepared by HCIMA, now the Institute of Hospitality, in 1993.

Introduction

People choose to eat vegetarian or vegan food for a variety of reasons. This includes the following:

- Vegetarians have religious beliefs, ethical and ecological views against meat eating; this includes Jews and Muslims without access to kosher or halal meat and those who choose vegetarian foods for health reasons.
- Demi-vegetarians are people who choose to exclude red meat from their diet.
- Vegans will not eat any animal food or by-product because they consider it cruel to do so. Veganism is living entirely on the products of the plant kingdom.

Within the above groups, the foods that are avoided by each sector are as follows.

Lacto vegetarians

This group eats milk and cheese but not eggs, whey or *anything* that has been produced as a result of an animal being slaughtered, that is: meat, poultry, fish or any by-products such as fish oils, rennet, cochineal.

Ovo-lacto vegetarians

Ovo-lacto vegetarians include eggs otherwise as for lacto vegetarians.

Demi-vegetarians

This group usually chooses to exclude red meat, though they may eat it occasionally. White poultry and fish are generally acceptable.

Vegans

Vegans avoid *all* animal products and by-products including milk, cheese, yoghurt, eggs, fish, poultry, meat and honey. They eat only items or products from the plant kingdom.

These groups of people are generally more interested in a diet lower in fat and higher in fibre.

All vegan recipes in this chapter are marked with the ✿ icon.

Special points for consideration

Protein

In a meat eater's diet, meat, poultry and fish provide a considerable amount of the daily protein intake. Protein cannot be destroyed by cooking but, more importantly, it *cannot* be stored in the body. Any vegetarian or vegan meal must therefore contain an adequate source of protein to replace meat protein.

Amino acids

Protein is made up of amino acids. Human protein tissue and animal proteins contain all the 'essential' amino acids (the body can manufacture the non-essential amino acids). Vegetable proteins, however, contain fewer of the essential amino acids. The lack of some amino acids in one plant is compensated for by another.

Protein complementing

This means combining various plant proteins in one dish or meal to provide the equivalent amino acid profile of animal protein. Putting together 60 per cent beans (or other pulses) or nuts with 30 per cent grains or seeds and grains and 10 per cent green salad or vegetables, makes the ideal combination.

Best sources of vegetarian protein

The best sources of vegetarian protein are cheese, eggs, milk, textured vegetable protein (TVP) followed by tofu, soya beans, all other pulses and nuts. Seeds: sesame, sunflower and pumpkin. Cereals (preferably wholegrain): millet, wheat, barley and oats. Vegans exclude cheese, eggs and milk as a source of protein and substitute soya milk, soya cheese and soya yoghurt. All other items above are acceptable.

In protein equivalent terms (all cooked weights)

50 g meat = 75 g fish
= 50 g (hard) cheese
= 100 g soft or cottage cheese
= 2 eggs
= 100 g nuts
= 50 g peanut butter
= 150 g pulses (lentils, peas, beans)
= 75 g seeds

Pulses, nuts, seeds and to a lesser extent tubers and roots contain significant protein. Leaves, stems, buds and flowers are almost all water and have an insignificant protein content.

A dish such as ratatouille, made from 'water' vegetables, is suitable only as a side dish. 'Vegetable' curries, hotpots and similar dishes should all include a recognisable and good vegetable protein source.

A vegetarian menu: excluded items
Rennet- or pepsin-based cheeses
These should be excluded from a vegetarian menu (rennet is an enzyme from the stomach of a newly killed calf; pepsin is from pigs' stomachs).

Replace these items with approved 'vegetarian' cheeses or non-rennet cheeses such as cottage and cream cheese (not suitable for vegans, unless made with soya milk). Check to ensure ready-made vegetarian dishes include vegetarian cheese.

Battery farm eggs
Battery farm hens may have been fed fish meal; also strict vegetarians consider battery rearing of hens is cruel.

Replace these items with free-range eggs.

Strict vegetarians will eat only free-range eggs; this is impractical for most manufacturers and caterers, so clear labelling is important so as not to mislead.

Whey
Whey is a by-product of cheese making and therefore may contain rennet. Whey may be found in biscuits.

Crisps may contain whey as a processing aid; this need not be stated on the label. Some muesli may also contain whey.

Check all product labels of items bought in and used in the production of a vegetarian choice.

Cochineal
Cochineal, or E120, is made from the cochineal beetle.

This is often present in glacé cherries and mincemeat. Choose an alternative red colouring.

Alcohol
Some wines or beers may be 'fined' using isinglass (a fish product) or dried blood. Some ciders contain pork to enhance their flavour.

Check with the wholesaler or manufacturer, where possible, if in any doubt before use in cooking or serving to a vegetarian.

Meat or bone stock and animal-based flavourings
Meat or bone stock for soups or sauces; animal-based flavourings for savoury dishes.

Replace these items with stock made from vegetables or yeast extract (Tastex, Barmene, Marmite), or bought vegetable stock cubes/bouillon; soy sauce, miso, Holbrook's Worcester Sauce (which is anchovy free).

Animal fats
Animal fats (suet, lard or dripping), ordinary white cooking fats or margarine. (Some contain fish oil.) Bought-in pastry may contain lard or fish oil margarine.

Replace these items with Trex and Pura white vegetable fats, 100 per cent vegetable oil margarines, Suenut or Nutter (available from health food stores), White Flora.

Oils containing fish oil
Replace these items with 100 per cent vegetable oil (sunflower, corn, soya, groundnut, walnut, sesame, olive) or mixed vegetable oil.

Note: Fish oils may well be 'hidden' in margarine and products such as biscuits, cakes and bought-in pastry items. Check suitability before using.

Setting agents
Gelatine, aspic, block or jelly crystals (for glazing, moulding, in cheesecakes and desserts). Some yoghurts are set with gelatine as are some sweets, particularly nougat and mints.

Replace these items with agar-agar (a fine, white odourless powder), gelozone, apple pectin. Other gums are also used as substitutes, for example, alginates (produced from seaweed), other pectins, xanthan gum and the tree gums tragacanth and carob bean gum.

Animal-fat ice cream

Replace animal-fat ice cream with vegetable-fat ice cream.

Note that many additives contain meat products: look on the label for 'edible fats', 'emulsifiers', 'fatty acids' and the preservative E471. The safest course is to ask the manufacturer of any bought-in product you wish to use.

Claims about vegetarian dishes

Never claim that a food or dish is vegetarian if you have used a non-vegetarian ingredient.

If you knowingly mislead a customer into believing you have a suitable vegetarian choice on offer, you can be prosecuted under the Trade Descriptions Act 1968 and/or the Food Safety Act 1990.

Salads

Simple salads are made up of one main ingredient – for example, a tomato salad, in which the tomatoes are peeled, sliced, sprinkled with a little finely chopped onion or shallot and dressed with vinaigrette.

Compound salads are made up from two or more ingredients and mixed together. For example, Russian salad is a mixture of vegetables (carrot, turnip, swede) cut into dice, garnished with peas, seasoned and bound with mayonnaise.

Dressings and sauces for salads

Vinaigrette and mayonnaise are used extensively for salads, but sour cream, tofu and yoghurt may also be used.

Types of oils

- olive
- corn
- sunflower
- peanut
- sesame
- safflower
- walnut
- soya

Types of vinegars

- cider
- red wine
- white wine
- malt
- herb
- lemon
- raspberry
- balsamic

Vinaigrettes with the addition of:

- garlic
- capers
- curry paste
- eggs
- blue cheese
- herbs

Seasonings

- English mustard
- French mustard
- Dijon mustard
- German mustard
- salt
- pepper
- spices
- herb salt

Herbs

- chervil
- tarragon
- thyme
- mint
- basil
- marjoram
- coriander
- fennel
- dill

Mayonnaise with the addition of:

- tomato ketchup
- horseradish
- lemon juice
- herbs
- capers
- gherkins
- curry powder

Also

- soured cream
- tofu
- yoghurt
- smetana
- crème fraîche
- quark

Oil-based sauces

These fall roughly into two categories, as follows.

1. Cold: mayonnaise and derivatives; vinaigrette and variations.
2. Hot: vinaigrette and variations; vinaigrettes used with some fish and vegetable dishes.

When preparing hot vinaigrettes, various flavoured oils and vinegars can be used to give a variety of tastes. Oils, such as olive, walnut, sesame seed, sunflower, grapeseed, peanut and safflower, can be flavoured by marinating herbs, for example basil, thyme, oregano, rosemary, garlic or onions, in them in one of two ways.

1. Place a bunch of the chosen herb/s into a bottle of oil, cork tightly and keep on a cool shelf.
2. Warm the oil with the herb/s for 15 to 20 minutes.

There is scope here for experimentation with various herbs, spices and vegetables, e.g. onion, garlic, shallots, so that a mise-en-place of several flavoured oils can be produced.

Red or white vinegars can be flavoured with herbs such as thyme, tarragon, dill, mint, rosemary, etc.

- Fruit vinegars include raspberry, strawberry, blackberry, peach, plum, apple, cherry.
- Floral vinegars, e.g. elderflower, rose.
- Sharp vinegars, e.g. chilli, garlic, horseradish.

When making vinaigrettes for use in hot dishes, there is obviously considerable room for experimentation, and the skill lies in the blending of the ingredients and flavours of both oils and vinegars to complement the dishes with which they are to be used and ensuring that they do not dominate.

For example, red mullet fillets or skate, lightly steamed, grilled or fried and lightly masked with a hot vinaigrette, is a basic recipe to which many variations can be applied, such as:

- A lightly cooked small brunoise of vegetables added.
- Finish with chopped fennel or dill.

Many vegetables simply cooked either by boiling or steaming can be given additional flavours by finishing with a light dribble of a suitably flavoured hot vinaigrette – for example:

- Sliced or diced beetroot, carrots, turnips, swedes.
- A mixture of cooked vegetables.
- Crisply cooked shredded cabbage.

Brown vegetable stock

	1 litre
onions ⎤	100 g
carrots ⎥ mirepoix	100 g
celery ⎥	100 g
leeks ⎦	100 g
sunflower oil	60 ml
tomatoes	50 g
mushroom trimmings	50 g
peppercorns	6
water	1 ½ litre
yeast extract	5 g

1. Fry the mirepoix in the oil until golden brown.
2. Drain and place in a suitable saucepan. Add all the other ingredients except the yeast extract and water.
3. Cover with the water, bring to the boil.
4. Add the yeast extract, simmer gently for approximately 1 hour. Then skim if necessary and use.

Fungi stock

White or brown fungi stock can be made by using white or brown vegetable stock recipe, adding 200–400 g mushrooms, stalks and trimmings (all well washed).

For white fungi stock, use white mushrooms; for brown, use open or field mushrooms.

 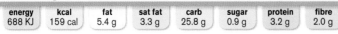

Anna potatoes

energy	kcal	fat	sat fat	carb	sugar	protein	fibre
688 KJ	159 cal	5.4 g	3.3 g	25.8 g	0.9 g	3.2 g	2.0 g

oil	
peeled potatoes	600 g
salt and pepper	
butter	25 g

1. Grease an anna mould using hot oil.
2. Trim the potatoes to an even cylindrical shape.
3. Cut into slices 2 mm thick.

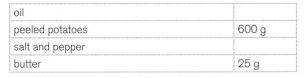

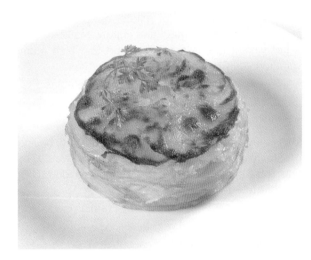

4. Place a layer of slices neatly overlapping in the bottom of the mould, season lightly with salt and pepper.
5. Continue arranging the slices of potato in layers, seasoning in between.
6. Add the butter to the top layer.
7. Cook in a hot oven (210–220°C) for ¾–1 hour, occasionally pressing the potatoes flat.
8. To serve, turn out of the mould and leave whole or cut into four portions.

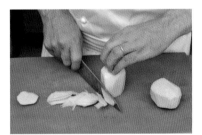

Finely slice the potatoes

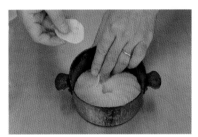

Layer the potato slices in the mould

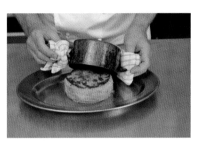

Carefully remove from the mould

 ## Maxim potatoes

energy	kcal	fat	sat fat	carb	sugar	protein	fibre
3456 KJ	822 cal	62.7 g	40.5 g	60.2 g	2.1 g	7.7 g	4.6 g

	4 portions	10 portions
large Desiree or Yukon Gold potatoes	4 (approx. 1400 g)	10 (approx. 3½ kg)
clarified butter	600 g	1½ kg
kosher salt		

1. Pre-heat the oven to 180–190°C.
2. Peel the potato and slice it into paper-thin rounds on a mandolin.
3. Toss the rounds with the clarified butter; they should be well coated.
4. Arrange them on a Silpat-lined baking sheet, overlapping the slices by half to form a solid sheet of potatoes, or lay them in overlapping circles in a large, heavy ovenproof skillet.
5. Sprinkle lightly with the salt.
6. Bake the potatoes for 45 to 50 minutes, or until they are crisp and golden brown. These can be made several hours ahead and left at room temperature.

5 Potato blinis

energy	kcal	fat	sat fat	carb	sugar	protein	fibre
1474 KJ	352 cal	21.7 g	11.1 g	28.1 g	1.6 g	13.1 g	1.9 g

	4 portions	10 portions
dried mash	500 g	1¼ kg
crème fraîche	125 g	300 g
flour	25 g	60 g
whole eggs	4	10
yolks	2	5
seasoning		

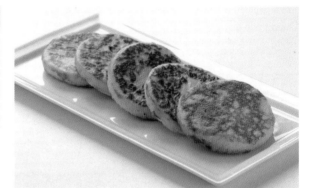

1. Mix the mash with the crème fraîche and the flour.
2. Separate the eggs and add the yolks to the mash.
3. Whip the egg whites to a snow, carefully fold in to the mash, check for seasoning and allow to rest for 1 hour.
4. Heat a little oil in a non-stick pan and place a small amount of mix in the pan (approx. 1 tbsp), turn over when it is golden brown.

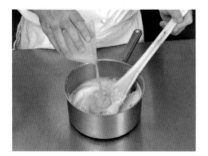

Combine the ingredients

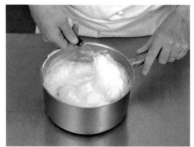

Whisk the mixture

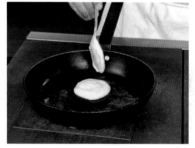

Drop enough mixture for one blini into the hot pan

6 Potato cakes with chives

energy	kcal	fat	sat fat	carb	sugar	protein	fibre
1181 KJ	282 cal	14.2 g	2.1 g	34.6 g	1.4 g	6.0 g	2.8 g

	4 portions	10 portions
large potatoes	4	10
egg yolks	2	5
butter	50 g	125 g
chives, chopped	50 g	125 g
salt and pepper		

1. Bake the potatoes in their jackets.
2. Halve and remove the potato from the skins.
3. Mash with the yolks and butter.
4. Mix in the chopped chives and season.
5. Mould into round cakes, 2 cm diameter.
6. Lightly flour and shallow-fry to a golden colour on both sides.

7 Irish potato cakes

	4 portions	10 portions
potatoes	250 g	650 g
head fresh garden cabbage, finely chopped	½	1
milk	90 ml	225 ml
bacon dripping or butter	50 g	125 g
salt and black pepper, freshly ground		
wholemeal flour	125 g	300 g
extra dripping or butter for frying		

1. Boil the potatoes in salted water until cooked. Drain, mash and leave to cool.

2. Place the cabbage in boiling salted water and cook for a few minutes. Drain and leave to cool.

3. Place the milk in a saucepan, add the bacon dripping and bring to the boil. Add the cooked potato and cabbage and blend together while the mixture heats through. Season with salt and pepper. Fold in the flour until the mixture comes away from the side of the saucepan.

4. Turn the mixture on to a cold surface and shape into cakes of approximately 5 cm diameter and 1 cm thick.

5. Fry in a little bacon dripping until brown and serve immediately.

8 Spicy potato cakes

	4 portions	10 portions
whole cumin seeds	¼ tsp	½ tsp
eggs	1	4
sweet potato, grated	300 g	1 kg
onion, grated	100 g	250 g
fresh coriander, chopped	40 g	100 g
fresh red chilli, diced	1 tsp	3 tsp
salt	¼ tsp	1 tsp
pepper	¼ tsp	1 tsp

1. In a small frying pan, toast the cumin seeds until just brown.

2. In a medium mixing bowl, whip the eggs, then mix in remaining ingredients, including the toasted cumin seeds.

3. Heat a large, heavy-bottomed skillet and oil lightly. Drop batter by spoonsful into the pan and cook slowly on each side until cakes are very golden, about 25 minutes.

9 Potatoes cooked with button onions and tomatoes

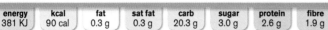

energy	kcal	fat	sat fat	carb	sugar	protein	fibre
381 KJ	90 cal	0.3 g	0.3 g	20.3 g	3.0 g	2.6 g	1.9 g

	4 portions	10 portions
potatoes, peeled	400 g	1¼ kg
button onions	100 g	250 g
garlic clove	1	2–3
vegetable stock	375 ml	1 litre
salt and pepper		
tomatoes, skinned, deseeded and diced	100 g	250 g

1. Trim and dice the potatoes into 2 cm pieces.

2. Add to the peeled onions, crushed garlic and stock.

3. Season and cook gently in a suitable pan in the oven or on the stove until the potatoes are just cooked.

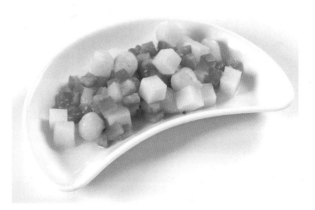

4. Add the tomatoes and cook for a few more minutes, then serve.

10 Potatoes Lyonnaise

energy	kcal	fat	sat fat	carb	sugar	protein	fibre
2714 KJ	648 cal	29.0 g	3.2 g	91.5 g	6.9 g	11.4 g	7.6 g *

	4 portions	10 portions
potatoes, sautéed	1 kg	2½ kg
onions, sautéed	275 g	650 g
parsley, chopped	12 g	30 g

1. Toss the sautéed potatoes and onions together in a frying pan.
2. Serve sprinkled with the chopped parsley.

Oil was used to sauté the potatoes and onions.

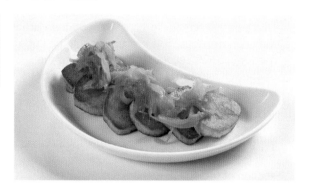

11 Rosemary Lyonnaise potatoes

	4 portions	10 portions
Desiree potatoes, sliced	600 g	1½ kg
shallots, sliced	200 g	500 g
garden rosemary, chopped	1 sprig	2 sprigs
duck fat	100 g	250 g
Parmesan, grated	40 g	100 g

1. Toss the sliced potato and onion together, and lightly season.

2. Place the fat in a deep ovenware dish and put into a preheated oven at 180°C.
3. Place the potatoes and onions in the fat and place into the oven.
4. Turn the potatoes after 10 minutes to colour evenly.
5. After another 20 minutes add the rosemary and turn the potatoes and onions.
6. Cook for a further 10 minutes.
7. Finish with the grated Parmesan and serve.

12 Potato gnocchi

energy	kcal	fat	sat fat	carb	sugar	protein	fibre
2288 KJ	540 cal	6.5 g	1.6 g	111.0 g	2.2 g	16.1 g	6.0 g

This recipe yields more gnocchi than are needed for a single recipe, but their versatility makes them an ideal item to have on hand. Use them as a garnish or serve them as a meal.

Part of what makes this a useful recipe is that the gnocchi freeze so well and they go directly from the freezer into boiling water so they're always at the ready.

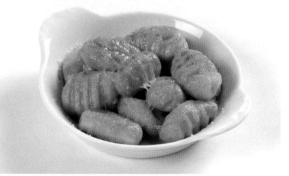

Potato gnocchi baked with cheese

	4 portions	10 portions
russet potatoes	1 kg	2½ kg
flour	350 g	875 g
egg yolks	4	10
Maldon salt to taste		

1. Pre-heat the oven to 180°C.
2. Bake the potatoes for 1 hour or until they are completely cooked.
3. Split the potatoes, scoop out the flesh and press

it through a potato ricer. Place the hot potatoes on a board or counter.

4. Make a well in the centre. Place one-third of the flour in the well, add the egg yolks, then add most of the flour and the salt.

5. Use a dough scraper to 'chop' the potatoes into the flour and eggs. This process should be done quickly (15–30 seconds) as overworking the dough will make the gnocchi heavy and sticky. Add more flour as necessary.

6. The resulting dough should be homogeneous and barely sticky on the outside. Shape the dough into a ball.

7. Roll the ball of dough lightly in flour. Pull off a section of the dough and roll it by hand on a lightly floured surface into a 'snake' about 1 cm thick. Cut into 1 cm pieces and, using your hand, roll each piece into a ball.

8. Roll the balls on a gnocchi paddle or over the back of a fork to create an oval shape with indentations. Test one gnocchi by placing it in a large pot of rapidly boiling, lightly salted water. It is cooked as soon as it floats to the surface.

9. Taste for seasoning and texture and add salt to the dough if necessary, or add a bit more flour if the gnocchi seem mushy.

10. Continue forming the remaining gnocchi, placing them on a lightly floured tray until ready to cook.

11. Place the gnocchi in the boiling water. Use a slotted spoon or skimmer to remove them to a bowl of ice water as they rise to the surface.

12. Once they have cooled (about 2 minutes) drain them briefly on paper towels or a kitchen towel. Lay them in a single layer on a parchment-lined baking sheet.

13. Store on a tray in the refrigerator if they will be used that day or place them in the freezer. Once they are frozen, they can be stored in well-sealed plastic bags and kept frozen for several weeks: cook/reheat them while they are still frozen.

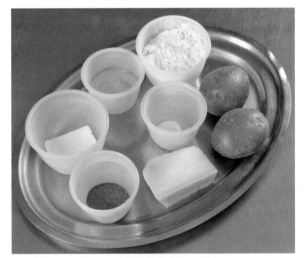

Ingredients

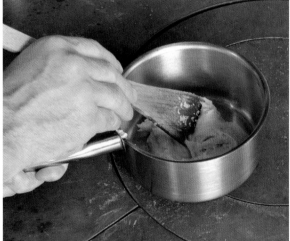

Mix the dough

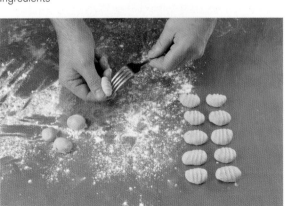

Shape the gnocchi

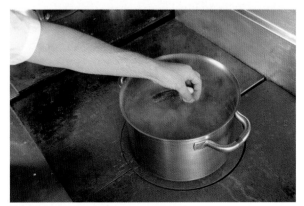

Put the gnocchi into the water to poach

13 Candied sweet potatoes

energy	kcal	fat	sat fat	carb	sugar	protein	fibre
641 KJ	151 cal	3.1 g	0.4 g	31.0 g	14.8 g	1.6 g	2.8 g

	4 portions	10 portions
oil or butter	1 tbsp	2½ tbsp
sweet potatoes, in 1 cm dice	400 g	1¼ kg
chopped onion	100 g	250 g
honey	2 tbsp	5 tbsp
cider vinegar	2 tbsp	5 tbsp
cinnamon	¼ tsp	½ tbsp
salt		

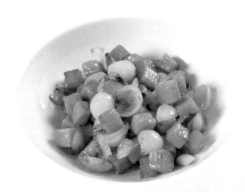

1. Heat the oil in a frying pan and add the sweet potatoes.
2. Cook for 10 minutes, stirring occasionally.
3. Add the onion and cook until brown.
4. Mix the honey, cider vinegar, cinnamon and salt in a bowl. Pour the honey mixture on to the potatoes, heat through, season and serve.

14 Sweet potato cakes

	4 portions	10 portions
sweet potatoes, peeled and cut into large chunks	400 g	1 kg
soy sauce	½ tsp	2 tsp
flour	40 g	100 g
salt	¼ tsp	1 tsp
sugar	¼ tsp	½ tsp
spring onion, chopped	1 tbsp	3 tbsp
fresh chilli, finely chopped (or more, to taste)	¼ tsp	½ tsp
lots of butter, for frying		

1. Steam the sweet potato until soft, then drain in a colander for an hour.
2. Mix all the ingredients together by hand: the mixture should be sticky, so if it's a little runny, add some flour. Avoid over-mixing as this will ultimately make the cakes chewy.
3. Dip your hands in water and shape walnut-sized balls with the potato cake mix, then flatten so you have round cakes around 5 cm in diameter and less than 1 cm thick.
4. Place on an oily surface.
5. Melt some butter in a nonstick pan. Using a fish slice, lift the cakes in to the pan and fry on moderate heat for about six minutes, turning as necessary, until you get a nice, brown crust.
6. Place between two sheets of kitchen towel, to soak up the excess butter. Serve hot.

15 Sweet potato and bacon Lyonnaise

	4 portions	10 portions
bacon	50 g	125 g
onion, chopped	200 g	500 g
sweet potatoes, peeled and cooked, sliced	650 g	1½ kg
salt	1 tsp	2 tsp

1. Cut the bacon into small dice. Place into a heavy frying pan with the onion and sauté until golden, or about 5 minutes.
2. Add the sliced sweet potatoes and season.
3. Cook uncovered over medium heat until the potatoes are hot through and acquire a golden crispy crust on the underside.
4. Serve immediately.

16 Vegetable soufflé

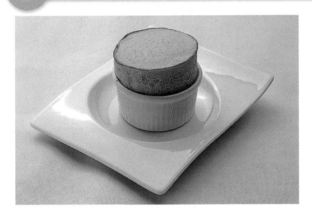

	4 portions	10 portions
eggs	3–4	7–10
seasoned vegetable purée, stiff	400 g	1 kg
double cream	2 tbsp	5 tbsp

1. Separate the eggs and stiffly beat the whites.
2. Mix the egg yolks and cream into the vegetable purée.
3. Fold in the beaten egg whites.
4. Prepare the soufflé moulds with butter and flour. Place the mixture into the moulds.
5. Bake in a hot oven at 220°C until set.

17 Aubergine soufflé

energy	kcal	fat	sat fat	carb	sugar	protein	fibre
1160 KJ	278 cal	18.5 g	9.9 g	13.9 g	7.7 g	15.2 g	4 g

	4 portions	10 portions
aubergines	2	5
thick béchamel sauce	250 ml	600 ml
grated Parmesan cheese	50 g	125 g
eggs, separated	3	7
salt and pepper		

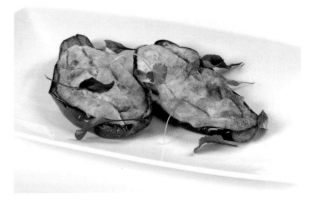

1. Cut the aubergines in halves.
2. Slash the flesh criss-cross and deep-fry for a few minutes.
3. Drain well, scoop out the flesh and finely chop.
4. Lay the skins in a buttered gratin dish.

5. Mix the aubergine flesh with an equal quantity of béchamel.

6. Heat this mixture through, then mix in the cheese and yolks, and season.

7. Fold in the stiffly beaten whites.

8. Fill the skins with this mixture, bake at 230°C for approximately 15 minutes and serve immediately.

> For extra lightness use 4 egg whites to 3 yolks (10 egg whites to 7 yolks for 10 portions).

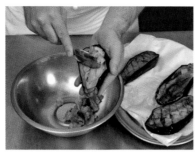
Scoop out the cooked flesh

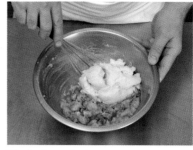
Mix the ingredients

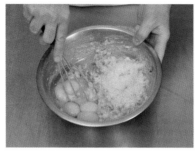
Whisk in the eggs

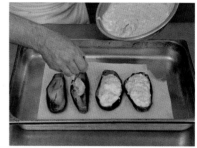
Fill the aubergine skins with the mixture

18 Cold mousses

A mousse is basically a purée of the bulk ingredient from which it takes its name, with the addition of a suitable non-dairy or cream sauce, cream and aspic jelly. The result should be a light creamy mixture, just sufficiently set to stand when removed from a mould.

> Care must be taken when mixing not to curdle the mixture as this will produce a 'bitty' appearance with small white grains of cream showing.
>
> The cream should only be half whipped as a rubbery texture will otherwise be obtained; also, if fresh cream is over-whipped the mixture will curdle.

Various types of mousse are used as part of other dishes as well as dishes on their own. A mould of a particular substance may be filled with a mousse of the same basic ingredient. Whole decorated chickens may have the breast reformed with a mousse such as ham, tomato or foie gras. Mousse may be piped to fill cornets of ham, borders for chicken suprêmes or cold egg dishes.

Although most recipes quote a lined mould for the mousse to be placed in when being served as an individual dish, mousses may often be poured into a glass bowl (or even smaller dishes for individual portions) to be decorated on top when set, then glazed. Although truffle is frequently quoted, other materials are now used for decoration.

> Convenience aspic jelly granules may be used for all mousse recipes.

19 Vegetable mousse

energy	kcal	fat	sat fat	carb	sugar	protein	fibre
839 KJ	203 cal	17.4 g	9.0 g	5.3 g	5.0 g	6.8 g	2.5 g

*

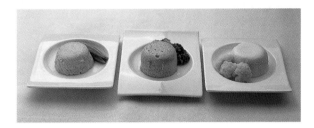

	4 portions	10 portions
eggs	3–4	7–10
seasoned vegetable purée	400 g	1 kg
double cream	2 tbsp	5 tbsp

> *i*
> Many vegetables are suitable for making a mousse – for example, asparagus, broccoli, carrot, cauliflower, aubergine, fennel, spinach. The mousse is usually shaped in a dariole or small timbale mould.
>
> The mousse may be served as the vegetable with a main course, as a garnish, or by itself as a light meal. When the mousse is served by itself, add an appropriate sauce, such as mushroom sauce with an asparagus mousse.

1. Thoroughly mix the eggs without over-beating.
2. Pass them through a fine strainer on to the cold vegetable purée. Add the cream and combine thoroughly.
3. Three-quarters fill the buttered moulds (this allows for expansion during cooking).
4. Place the moulds in a bain-marie of hot water and bake at 190°C until set.
5. Remove from the oven and allow to stand for 10 minutes before turning out.

Variations

Variations include the following.

- Use béchamel sauce in place of cream.
- Add extra ingredients, spices or herbs to the recipe. For example, add chopped garlic to an aubergine mousse; toasted pine nuts to spinach; chopped coriander to carrot; grated Parmesan cheese to broccoli.

* *Using carrots*

20 Tomato mousse

	4 portions	10 portions
vine plum tomatoes, chopped	10	25
seasoning		
sugar	2 tsp	3 tsp
Worcestershire sauce	2 tsp	3 tsp
gelatine leaves	2	5
chervil, chopped	½ tsp	1 tsp
basil, chopped	½ tsp	1 tsp
double cream	245 ml	650 ml

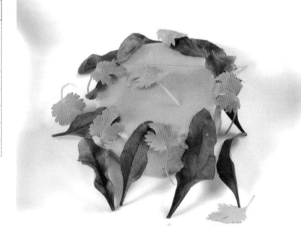

1. Quickly blitz the tomatoes with a large pinch of salt, ground pepper and the sugar. Push through a fine chinois and then reduce to 300 g in a thick-based saucepan over a moderate heat.
2. Add the Worcestershire sauce, and ground pepper to taste.

3. Soak the gelatine in cold water until soft.
4. Place the gelatine into the warm tomato reduction and mix until it has dissolved.
5. Chill over ice, stirring often.
6. Meanwhile, softly whip the cream until soft peaks are formed.

7. Once the tomato water thickens and begins to set, add the chopped herbs.
8. Gently fold in the whipped cream.
9. Place into ramekins and place in the fridge to allow to set.

21 Celery royale

	4 portions	10 portions
butter	25 g	75 g
celery, finely chopped	100 g	250 g
béchamel sauce, cold	2 tbsp	6 tbsp
egg	1	3
egg yolks	3	6
seasoning		

1. Cook the celery in the butter until soft.
2. Add the béchamel sauce and the beaten egg and egg yolks. Season.
3. Place in greased individual moulds or a dariole mould.
4. Place in a bain-marie in the oven at 180°C or a combination oven injected with steam for 25 to 30 minutes.

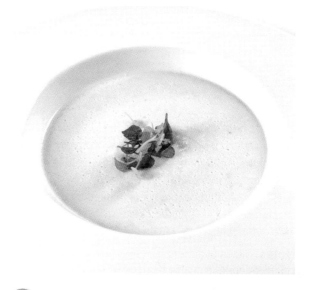

Variations

- Asparagus royale: use asparagus instead of celery.
- Leek royale: use leeks instead of celery.
- Green pea royale: use 100 g of pea purée instead of the celery, and white stock with a pinch of sugar instead of béchamel sauce.
- Tomato royale: as for green pea royale, using 200 g of tomato purée made with fresh tomatoes.
- Carrot royale: cook 75 g carrots in the butter and then purée them. Add 2 tbsp double cream to the béchamel sauce, with 1 egg and 2 egg yolks.

Royales are cut into various shapes and used as a garnish for soups, salads and other dishes.

A royale must be completely cold before shaping, to make it easy to handle.

22   Grilled vegetables

energy	kcal	fat	sat fat	carb	sugar	protein	fibre
308 KJ	73 cal	1.1 g	0.1 g	13.0 g	11.7 g	3.8 g	6.4 g

	4 portions
leeks	8
carrots	8
turnips	8
baby sweetcorn	8

Tender young vegetables can be cooked from raw and are best cooked on an under-fired grill or barbecue.

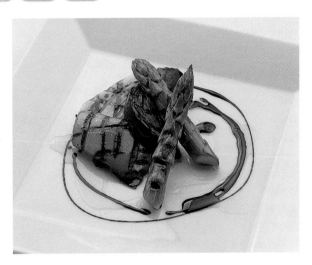

1. Wash, peel and trim the vegetables.
2. Dry well, brush with olive oil, season lightly.
3. Grill the vegetables with the tenderest last, e.g. turnips, carrots, leeks, sweetcorn.
4. Serve as a first course accompanied by a suitable sauce, e.g. spicy tomato sauce, or as a vegetable accompaniment to a main course.

Notes: Slices of aubergine, courgette and red and/or yellow peppers can also be used (discard the pith and seeds of the peppers).

Variation

If vegetables other than baby ones, e.g. carrot, turnip, parsnip, are grilled, then they first need to be cut into thickish slices and par-boiled until half-cooked, drained well, dried, then brushed with oil and grilled.

They can be served plain, sprinkled with chopped mixed herbs, or with an accompanying sauce.

23   *Baigan ka chokha* (Caviar of aubergine with spices and herbs)

	4 portions	10 portions
red onion	50 g	150 g
coriander leaves	20 g	60 g
mint leaves	20 g	60 g
ginger	10 g	30 g
green chilli	2	6
aubergines (large)	2	6
toasted cumin powder	10 g	30 g
lime juice	10 ml	30 ml
salt	½ tsp	1 tsp
olive oil	1 tbsp	3 tbsp

1. Chop the red onion into fine dice.
2. Wash and chop the herbs.
3. Scrape, wash and chop the ginger into fine dice and slice the chilli into thin roundels.

4. Roast the aubergines in a hot tandoor until charred. Remove, cook and skin.
5. Chop the aubergine flesh coarsely and store in the refrigerator until required.
6. Place the cold aubergine pulp in a mixing bowl. Add the spices, herbs, lime juice, olive oil and salt, and mix together.
7. Place back in the refrigerator for pulp to set, so it will be easy to handle with a spoon to form quenelles.
8. Use as an accompaniment to roasted lamb chops, for example.

This recipe was contributed by celebrity chef Atul Kochhar.

24 Bamboo shoots

energy	kcal	fat	sat fat	carb	sugar	protein	fibre
45 KJ	11 cal	0.2 g	0.1 g	0.7 g	0.7 g	1.5 g	1.7 g

 These are the shoots of young edible bamboo, stripped of the tough outer brown skin, so that the insides are eaten. They have a texture similar to celery and a flavour rather like that of globe artichokes. They are also sold preserved in brine.

Chopped bamboo shoots are used in a number of stir-fry dishes, meat and poultry casseroles and as a soup garnish. They can also be served hot with a hollandaise-type sauce or beurre blanc.

25 Bean sprouts

These are the tender young sprouts of the germinating soya or mung bean.

Rinse well and drain. The sprouts may be then stir-fried and served as a vegetable, mixed in with other ingredients in stir-fry dishes, used in omelettes and also served as a crisp salad item.

As bean sprouts are a highly perishable vegetable, it is best to select white, plump, crisp sprouts with a fresh appearance.

Bean sprouts are available all year round. It is essential that they are very thoroughly washed before being cooked.

26 Stir-fried bok choy

There are more than 20 varieties of bok choy available in Asia.

	4 portions	10 portions
baby bok choy	4 bunches	10 bunches
fresh ginger, grated	1 tsp	2½ tsp
soy sauce	2 tbsp	5 tbsp
sugar	1 tsp	2½ tsp
sesame oil	1 tsp	2½ tsp
vegetable oil	2 tbsp	2½ tbsp
water	1 tbsp	2½ tbsp

1. Wash the baby bok choy and drain. Separate the stalks and leaves.
2. Shred the bok choy coarsely.
3. Heat the vegetable oil in a wok. Add the ginger and stir-fry for about 30 seconds.
4. Add the bok choy. Quickly stir-fry for 1 minute.
5. Add the soy sauce, sugar and stir-fry for a further 1 minute.
6. Add the water. Simmer for 1 minute.
7. Stir in the sesame oil and serve.

27 Braised red cabbage with apples, red wine and juniper

energy	kcal	fat	sat fat	carb	sugar	protein	fibre
368 KJ	88 cal	5.8 g	0.6 g	8.2 g	7.8 g	1.3 g	3.3 g

	4 portions	10 portions
red cabbage, shredded	400 g	1¼ kg
vegetable oil	2 tbsp	5 tbsp
cooking apples, peeled, cored and diced	200 g	500 g
red wine	250 ml	600 ml
salt and pepper		
juniper berries	12	30

1. Blanch and refresh the cabbage.
2. Heat the oil in a casserole, add the cabbage and apples, and stir.
3. Add the wine, seasoning and juniper berries.
4. Bring to the boil, cover and braise for approximately 40–45 minutes until tender.
5. If any liquid remains when cooked, continue cooking uncovered to evaporate the liquid.

28 Cardoons

energy	kcal	fat	sat fat	carb	sugar	protein	fibre
34 KJ	8 cal	0.3 g	0.1 g	0.8 g	0.8 g	0.5 g	1.2 g

i Cardoons are a long plant, similar to celery, with an aroma and flavour like that of the globe artichoke.

Select cardoons with bright leaves, crisp stems and a fresh-looking appearance.

Remove the leaves, stalks and tough parts and cut into small pieces.

Cook in acidulated water for approximately 30–40 minutes.

Cardoons may be used as a plain vegetable, in other vegetable dishes or served raw as an appetiser.

29 Braised chicory

energy	kcal	fat	sat fat	carb	sugar	protein	fibre
476 KJ	114 cal	6.3 g	3.7 g	17.8 g	13.5 g	1.1 g	1.8 g

	4 portions	10 portions
fish or chicken stock	200 ml	500 ml
medium heads chicory	8	20
fresh lemon juice	3 tbsp	8 tbsp
caster sugar	3 tbsp	8 tbsp
sea salt and freshly ground black pepper		
butter	25 g	60 g

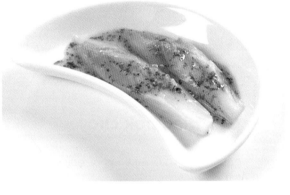

1. Have the stock ready and set aside.
2. Trim the chicory of any bruised outside leaves, then trim the ends and use a small, sharp knife to remove the bitter core at the base of each head.
3. Bring a pan of water to the boil and add the lemon juice, 1 tbsp of the sugar and salt to taste. Blanch the chicory for 8–10 minutes and drain well.
4. Drain all the liquid from the chicory and, in a large frying pan, heat the butter and brown the chicory on all sides, deglaze with a little stock and simmer for a few minutes, basting the chicory at all times.
5. Arrange the heads in a single layer on a platter, sprinkle with the remaining sugar, and season with salt and pepper. Leave to cool for about 10 minutes.

30 Christophene

energy	kcal	fat	sat fat	carb	sugar	protein	fibre
111 KJ	26 cal	0.2 g	0.0 g	5.6 g	4.7 g	1.1 g	1.7 g

i Christophene, also known as chow-chow, chayotte or vegetable pear, looks rather like a ridged green pear and is available in several varieties including white and green, spiny and smooth-skinned, rounded and ridged, or more or less pear-shaped. Christophenes usually weigh between 150–250 g, the inside flesh is firm and white with a flavour and texture resembling a combination of marrow and cucumber.

Peel the christophenes and remove the stones before cooking.

Cook by any method suitable for courgettes, or stuff and braise the christophenes.

31 Shallow-fried glazed fennel

	4 portions	10 portions
fennel bulbs	4	10
butter or margarine	25 g	62 g
sugar	1 tsp	2½ tsp
cider	275 ml	685 ml
cider vinegar	50 ml	125 ml

1. Trim the fennel bulbs and cut into quarters.
2. Cook the fennel in boiling water for approximately 10 minutes. Drain.

3. In a suitable pan, melt the butter and sugar and slightly caramelise the sugar. Brown the fennel in this butter and sugar mixture.
4. Add the cider and cider vinegar. Cover with a lid and cook for approximately 15 to 20 minutes until the fennel is tender.
5. Remove the fennel and reduce the cooking liquor to a glaze. Toss the cooked fennel in this glaze and serve.

32 Kohlrabi

energy	kcal	fat	sat fat	carb	sugar	protein	fibre
77 KJ	18 cal	0.2 g	0.0 g	3.1 g	3.0 g	1.2 g	1.9 g

i This is a stem that swells to a turnip shape above the ground. When grown under glass it is pale green in colour, when grown outdoors it is purplish.

Select kohlrabi with tops that are green, young and fresh. If the globes are too large they may be woody and tough.

Trim off the stems and leaves (these may be used for soups), peel thickly at the root end, thinly at top end, wash and cut into even-sized pieces.

Young kohlrabi can be cooked whole. Simmer in well-flavoured stock until tender.

Kohlrabi may be served with cream sauce, baked or stuffed, and added to casseroles (meat and vegetarian) and stews.

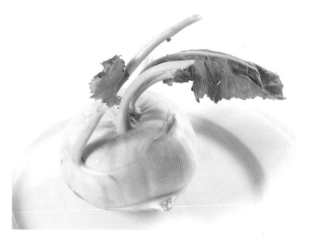

33 Mooli

energy	kcal	fat	sat fat	carb	sugar	protein	fibre
16 KJ	4 cal	0.0 g	0.0 g	0.7 g	0.7 g	0.2 g	0.0 g

i Mooli or white radish – or rettiche as it is sometimes known – is a parsnip-shaped member of the radish family and is available all year round. Mooli does not have a hot taste like radishes but is slightly bitter and is pleasant to eat cooked as a vegetable.

Mooli has a high water content, which can be reduced before cooking or serving raw by peeling and slicing, sprinkling with salt and leaving to stand for 30 minutes.

Otherwise, the preparation is to wash well and grate, shred or slice before adding to salads or cooking as a vegetable.

Mooli should have smooth flesh, white in appearance and be a regular shape.

 Mooli may be used as a substitute for turnips.

34 Wild mushrooms

Ceps, morels, chanterelles and oyster mushrooms are four of the most popular of the wide variety of wild mushrooms that may be gathered.

Ceps

> *i* Ceps are bun-shaped fungi with a smooth surface and a strong, distinctive flavour.

Dried ceps, if used, should be soaked in warm water for approximately 30 minutes before use. The soaking liquid should be used for cooking as it contains a good flavour.

Ceps hold a fair amount of water and need to be sweated gently in oil or butter and then drained, utilising the liquid.

Ceps may be used in soups, egg dishes (particularly omelettes), fish, meat, game and poultry dishes. They may also be: sautéed in oil or butter with garlic and parsley and served as a vegetable; stuffed with chopped ham, cheese, tomato and parsley; or sliced, passed through batter and deep-fried.

Morels

> *i* Morels appear in spring. They vary in colour from light to dark brown and have a meaty flavour.

Dried morels, if used, require soaking for 10 minutes, are squeezed dry and used as required.

Morels can be used in soups, egg dishes, meat, poultry and game dishes and as a vegetable, first course or as an accompaniment.

Chanterelles

> *i* Chanterelles are common, trumpet-shaped and frilly. They are generally bright yellow with a delicate flavour, slightly resembling apricots, and are obtainable in summer and autumn. There are many varieties.

Dried chanterelles, if used, require about 25 minutes' soaking in warm water before cooking.

Because of their pleated gills, chanterelles must be washed carefully under running cold water then dried well. As they have a rubbery texture they require lengthy gentle cooking in butter or oil.

They can be served with egg, chicken or veal dishes.

Oyster mushrooms

> *i* Oyster mushrooms are ear shaped, grey or greyish brown in colour, and have an excellent flavour.

Oyster mushrooms can be tough in texture and therefore need careful cooking. Cook in butter or oil with parsley and garlic, or flour, egg and breadcrumbs, then deep-fry.

35 Okra

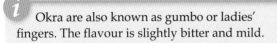

energy	kcal	fat	sat fat	carb	sugar	protein	fibre
65 KJ	16 cal	0.5 g	0.2 g	1.5 g	1.3 g	1.4 g	2.0 g

> *i* Okra are also known as gumbo or ladies' fingers. The flavour is slightly bitter and mild.

Select pods that are firm, bright green and fresh looking.

Cut off the conical cap at the stalk end, scrape the skin lightly, using a small knife, to remove any surface fuzz and the tips, then wash well.

Okra can be served as a plain vegetable, tossed in butter or with tomato sauce, may be prepared in a similar fashion to a ratatouille. Okra are also used in soups, stews, curries, pilaff rice and fried as fritters.

> Okra contain a high proportion of sticky glue-like carbohydrate which, when they are used in stews, gives body to the dish.

36 Confit onions

	4 portions	10 portions
duck fat or olive oil	750 ml	3 kg
button onions	24	12
fresh bay leaf	1	3
garlic clove, split	1	3
sprig of thyme	1	3

1. Place all the ingredients into a medium-sized saucepan, heat gently to approx. 65°C and cook for 45 minutes to 1 hour until the onions are tender.
2. Do not allow the oil to reach a high temperature as the onions will deep-fry.

37 Palm hearts

i Palm hearts are the tender young shoots or buds of palm trees and are generally available tinned or bottled in brine. Fresh palm hearts have a bitter flavour and need to be blanched before being used.

Palm hearts can be boiled, steamed or braised and are served hot or cold, usually cut in halves lengthwise.

When hot they are accompanied by a hollandaise-type sauce or *beurre blanc*, when cold by mayonnaise or a herb-flavoured vinaigrette.

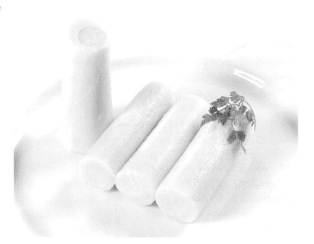

38 Parsnip and vanilla purée

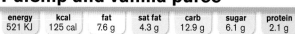

energy	kcal	fat	sat fat	carb	sugar	protein	fibre
521 KJ	125 cal	7.6 g	4.3 g	12.9 g	6.1 g	2.1 g	4.6 g

	4 portions	10 portions
parsnips, peeled and stalks removed	400 g	1 kg
butter	30 g	75 g
vanilla pod, split	½	1
seasoning		
milk, to aid purée		

1. Place the parsnips, butter and vanilla in a vacuum packing bag or pouch and steam until soft. Remove the pod and scrape out the seeds, add the rest of the ingredients and blitz, adding milk if necessary.
2. Pass through a fine drum sieve and season.

39 Braised-roast salsify

energy	kcal	fat	sat fat	carb	sugar	protein	fibre
598 KJ	145 cal	11.6 g	7.1 g	14.3 g	3.4 g	2.6 g	4.0 g

	4 portions	10 portions
fish or chicken stock	200 ml	500 ml
salsify	500 g	1¼ kg
cold water	700 ml	1¾ l
milk	100 ml	250 ml
lemons, juice of	1	3
rock salt	1 tbsp	3 tbsp
butter	50 g	125 g
fresh bouquet garni	1	2
sea salt and ground white pepper		

1. Have the stock ready and set aside.
2. Wash the salsify well, then peel, top and tail. Place immediately into a saucepan with the water, milk, lemon juice and rock salt.
3. Bring to the boil, then remove from the heat and leave the salsify to cool.
4. Drain, then cut into 4 cm batons or thick julienne strips. Preheat the oven to 180°C.
5. Heat the butter in a large, ovenproof frying pan or shallow, cast-iron casserole. Add the salsify batons and fry gently until they start to colour a little and caramelise.
6. Pour in the stock to just cover the salsify. Stir, add the bouquet garni and cook, uncovered, in the oven for 12–14 minutes until the liquid has evaporated and the salsify has become nicely glazed. Check the seasoning and serve.

40 Salsify fritters

Mix 400 g cooked salsify in 2 tablespoons olive oil, salt, pepper, chopped parsley and lemon juice, and leave for 30–45 minutes.

Dip in a light batter, deep-fry to a golden brown and serve.

(Increase the proportions 2½ times for 10 portions.)

41 Salsify with onion, tomato and garlic

energy	kcal	fat	sat fat	carb	sugar	protein	fibre	
558 KJ	135 cal	10.7 g	6.5 g	13.2 g	4.1 g	2.1 g	3.8 g	*

	4 portions	10 portions
salsify	400 g	1¼ kg
margarine, oil or butter	50 g	125 g
onions, chopped	50 g	125 g
clove of garlic, crushed and chopped	1	2–3
tomatoes, skinned, deseeded and diced	100 g	250 g
tomato purée	25 g	60 g
white stock	250 ml	600 ml
seasoning		
parsley, chopped		

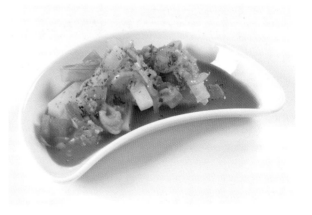

1. Wash and peel the salsify, cut into 5 cm lengths. Place immediately into acidulated water to prevent discoloration.
2. Place salsify into a boiling blanc or acidulated water with a little oil and simmer until tender, approximately 10–40 minutes. Drain well.

3. Melt the margarine, oil or butter, add the onion and garlic. Sweat without colour.
4. Add the tomatoes, and tomato purée, cook for 5 minutes.
5. Moisten with white stock, correct seasoning.
6. Place the cooked and well-drained salsify into the tomato sauce.

7. Serve in a suitable dish, sprinkled with chopped parsley.

If oil is used instead of butter: 636 kJ, 151 kcal, 12.9 g fat of which 1.3 g saturated, 12.9 g carbohydrate of which 3.7 g sugars, 2.0 g protein, 3.8 g fibre.

42 Scorzonera (salsify)

energy	kcal	fat	sat fat	carb	sugar	protein	fibre
99 KJ	23 cal	0.4 g	0.0 g	8.6 g	1.4 g	1.1 g	3.5 g

i Scorzonera, also known as black-skinned salsify or oyster plant, has a white flesh when skinned, with a slight flavour of asparagus and oysters.

Select salsify with fresh-looking leaves at the top.

Wash well, boil or steam in the skin, then peel using a potato peeler and immediately place in a blanc to prevent discoloration.

Cut into suitable-length pieces and serve plain, with butter, with cream or as for any cauliflower recipe.

If peeling salsify raw, immediately place into cold water and lemon juice and cook in a blanc or in water with ascorbic acid (vitamin C) to prevent discoloration.

Salsify requires approximately 20–30 minutes' cooking; test by pressing a piece between the fingers – if cooked, it will crush easily.

i A blanc is a traditional cooking liquor of water with a little flour, lemon juice and salt. It keeps the vegetables white. The modern method is to keep and cook the vegetables in water with ascorbic acid – this is more efficient.

43 Leaf spinach with pine nuts and garlic

energy	kcal	fat	sat fat	carb	sugar	protein	fibre
614 KJ	149 cal	12.5 g	1.1 g	3.0 g	2.8 g	6.0 g	3.4 g

	4 portions	10 portions
spinach	1 kg	2½ kg
pine nuts	50 g	125 g
oil or butter	1 tbsp	2–3 tbsp
garlic clove, chopped	1	2–3
salt and pepper		

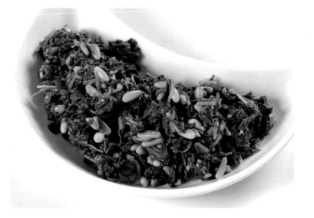

1. Cook the spinach for 2–3 minutes and drain well.
2. Lightly brown the pine nuts in oil, add garlic and sweat for 2 minutes.
3. Add coarsely chopped spinach and heat through over a medium heat.
4. Correct seasoning and serve.

44 Squash

energy	kcal	fat	sat fat	carb	sugar	protein	fibre
155 KJ	36 cal	0.1 g	0.0 g	8.3 g	4.5 g	1.1 g	1.6 g

i There are many different varieties of squash, which is a relative of the pumpkin. Squash should be firm with a blemish-free skin; summer squash should have a more yielding skin than winter squash, which are allowed to harden before harvesting.

The most usual variety sold is the custard squash, which is best when eaten young.

Custard squash can be cooked in similar ways to courgettes – sliced and lightly boiled, stewed or fried with the skins on and served with butter.

Winter squash have the skin removed before cooking and can then be cooked like marrow, e.g. stuffed.

45 Baby sweetcorn

energy	kcal	fat	sat fat	carb	sugar	protein	fibre
96 KJ	23 cal	0.4 g	0.0 g	2.0 g	1.4 g	2.9 g	1.5 g

i These are cobs of corn that are harvested when very young. They are used widely in oriental cookery and are available from December to March.

Always select cobs that look fresh and are undamaged.
1. Remove the corns from their protective husks.
2. Cook for a few minutes in unsalted water.
3. Serve whole or cut in slices and coated with butter or margarine.

Unlike fully grown sweetcorn, baby corn are not removed from the cob before eating – when cooked the vegetable is tender enough to eat whole.

Baby sweetcorns are used in stir-fry dishes, e.g. with chicken, crab or prawns, and may also be served cold with vinaigrette.

Baby corn looks attractive when served as one of a selection of plated vegetables.

46 Vegetable broth

	4 portions	10 portions
medium-sized carrots	2	5
small parsnip	1	3
small turnip	1	3
medium-sized onion	1	3
large celery stalks	2	5
large leek	1	3
butter	25 g	75 g
vegetable stock	1 litre	2½ litres
pearl barley	1 tbsp	2½ tbsp
salt and pepper		

1. Cut the carrots, parsnip and turnip into dice. Chop the onions and celery. Cut the leek into fine shreds.
2. Melt the butter in a saucepan, add the vegetables and cover the pan.
3. Fry gently, without browning, for 5 or 6 minutes, shaking the pan frequently.
4. Pour in the stock, add the barley and salt and pepper to taste.
5. Bring to the boil and then reduce the heat, cover the pan and simmer gently for around 1¼ hours, stirring occasionally, until the barley is soft.
6. Ladle into 4 warm soup bowls and serve hot.

47 Japanese broth

	4 portions	10 portions
dashi kombu	115–130 square cm	280–300 square cm
cold, filtered water	350 ml	1 litre
packets (usually 5 g) of dried bonito flakes	1 or 2	3 to 5

i Dashi kombu is a type of seaweed called kelp, used to make dashi. Bonito flakes for dashi are also known as katsuo boshi.

1. Pour the water over the kelp in a stock pot. Cover and steep for 30 minutes.
2. Turn on the heat to medium, achieve a temperature of 80 to 81°C degrees or until the bubbles just begin to move from the base of the pan. Avoid boiling the broth, as this might result in a bitter flavour.
3. Remove the kelp, which will have doubled in size; some deposits will be left behind but this is fine.
4. Sprinkle the bonito flakes over the broth. Allow to steep for 3 to 4 minutes. During this time many of the flakes should sink.
5. Line a fine strainer with a couple layers of muslin, and place over a large bowl or storage container. Strain the broth, then discard the bonito flakes.

48 *Sop bobor* (spinach and coconut soup)

	4 portions	10 portions
onions, finely chopped	25 g	60 g
vegetable oil	75 ml	150 ml
garlic, chopped	12 g	30 g
lesser galangal, peeled and finely chopped	12 g	40 g
salam leaf	1	2½–3
lemon grass stalk, crushed	1	2½–3
coriander powder	3 g (½ tsp)	10 g (1½ tsp)
brown sugar	12 g	25 g
chicken stock	500 ml	1¼ litres
coconut milk	250 ml	600 ml
spinach leaves	100 g	250 g
coconut flesh, diced	100 g	250 g
salt and pepper		
Garnish		
spinach leaves, finely chopped	50 g	125 g
coconut flesh, diced	50 g	125 g

1. Sauté the onions in the oil, add the garlic and lesser galangal. Sweat for 2–3 minutes without colour.
2. Add the salam leaf, lemon grass, coriander powder and brown sugar. Sauté for a further 2–3 minutes.
3. Cover with chicken stock, add the coconut milk, bring to the boil, stir frequently.
4. Add the chopped spinach leaves and diced coconut flesh. Season with salt and pepper. Reduce the heat, simmer for 15 minutes.
5. Remove the salam leaf and lemon grass.
6. Purée the soup in a liquidiser.
7. Serve in individual soup bowls, garnished with finely shredded spinach and diced coconut flesh.

If fresh coconut flesh is not available, use dried coconut flakes soaked in water for 10 minutes.

 Lesser galangal *(kencur)* is a rhizome that originated in India and is used sparingly. It has a hot, strong flavour. Fresh *kencur* can be found in Asian food stores, and can also be purchased in a powdered form *(kaempferia galanga)*.

Wood fungus *(jamur kuping)* may be added to this recipe. It is also called cloud ear fungus, because it swells to a curled shape when soaked in water. Sold in dried form and greyish black in colour, it turns brown and translucent when soaked.

49 Borscht

energy	kcal	fat	sat fat	carb	sugar	protein	fibre
428 KJ	102 cal	2.4 g	0.8 g	11.1 g	10.1 g	9.5 g	2.9 g

	4 portions	10 portions
Stock		
duck (half-roasted)	1 × 2 kg	2 × 2 kg
boiling beef, e.g. topside, thin flank (blanched and refreshed)	200 g	500 g
beef stock	2 litres	5 litres
beetroot juice	250 ml	600 ml
onion	50 g	125 g
carrots	50 g	125 g
celery	50 g	125 g
leek	50 g	125 g
bouquet garni		
Garnish		
carrot	50 g	125 g
leek	50 g	125 g
cabbage	50 g	125 g
beetroot	50 g	125 g
cooked duck, diced	50 g	125 g
cooked beef, diced	50 g	125 g
Accompaniments		
beetroot juice		
sour cream		
small duck patties		

i This is an unclarified broth of eastern European origin, mainly from Russia and Poland.

1. Make a good brown stock with the stock ingredients: allow to simmer for 2–3 hours and reduce by half.
2. Strain through a fine strainer or double muslin, skim well and correct the seasoning.
3. Prepare the vegetables for the garnish, cutting them into a fine julienne or paysanne.
4. Add the garnish of vegetables, diced duck and beef to the soup. Serve with the accompaniments.

Accompaniments

To make beetroot juice, grate raw peeled beetroot and squeeze firmly.

Duck patties can be made as small as possible from any type of paste, e.g. short or puff, and the filling should be a well-flavoured and seasoned duck mixture with, for example, sweated chopped onion and cabbage.

50 Roasted plum tomato and olive soup

energy	kcal	fat	sat fat	carb	sugar	protein	fibre
873 KJ	208 cal	10.7 g	2.6 g	22.9 g	9.4 g	6.6 g	2.9 g

	4 portions	10 portions
plum tomatoes	400 g	1½ kg
small onions	1	2
cloves of garlic	1	2
sprigs of basil	2	4
tomato purée	2 tbsp	4 tbsp
olive oil	25 g	50 g
black and green olives	50 g	100 g
balsamic vinegar	1 tsp	3 tsp
water	500 ml	1½ litres
salt and pepper		
sugar	10 g	25 g
croutes	2	3
sundried tomato paste	1 tbsp	3 tbsp
Parmesan	25 g	75 g
black olives	2	5
chopped parsley	25 g	50 g

1. Roughly chop the plum tomatoes, onion, garlic and basil.
2. Place into a roasting tray with tomato purée and a few drops of olive oil. Roast at 204°C for 10 minutes.
3. Remove from the oven and put into a saucepan. Add water.
4. Simmer for 20 minutes, stirring occasionally.
5. Liquidise for 2–3 minutes with olives. Pass through a conical sieve.
6. Check the consistency of the soup, add seasoning, a pinch of sugar and a few drops of balsamic vinegar.
7. Slice the dinner rolls into rounds and lightly toast both sides.
8. Spread with sundried tomato paste and Parmesan.
9. When the soup is required, bring to the boil. Put into soup cups and top with croutes and a slice of black olive and chopped parsley.

51   Watercress and beetroot soup

energy	kcal	fat	sat fat	carb	sugar	protein	fibre
2822 KJ	681.2 cal	53.4 g	32.8 g	42.3 g	9.8 g	10.3 g	8.0 g

	4 portions	10 portions
Beetroot		
large beetroots	2	5
water for cooking		
white wine vinegar	150 ml	375 ml
water	100 ml	250 ml
sugar	150 ml	375 ml
bay leaf	1	2
Watercress soup		
onions	160 g	400 g
leeks	175 g	430 g
butter (for the onions and leeks)	125 g	300 g
potatoes, diced small	750 g	1.8 kg
water	1.8 litres	4.5 litres
salt	15 g	30 g
pepper to taste		
spinach	125 g	300 g
watercress	600 g	1½ kg
butter (for the spinach and watercress)	125 g	300 g

For the watercress soup

1. Sweat the onion and leek without colour in the butter. Cook until very tender.
2. Add the potatoes and bring quickly to the boil with the water. Season with salt and pepper and allow to cool (blast chill).
3. Separately sweat the spinach and watercress in the butter until wilted. Transfer to a suitable container and add ice (to help preserve the colour).
4. When both are cool, liquidise each mix separately and pass through a chinois.
5. Add the potato purée to the watercress purée until the correct consistency and flavour has been achieved.
6. Correct seasoning.
7. Meanwhile place a small amount of the drained beetroot in each serving bowl and top with the hot soup.

For the beetroot

1. Place the beetroot in a pan and cover with the water. Bring to the boil.
2. Turn down to a simmer until cooked (about 1½ hours).
3. While the beetroot is cooking, place the vinegar, water and sugar in a separate pan and bring to the boil.
4. Boil this for 5 minutes, then take off the heat.
5. Once the beetroot is cooked, drain the liquid and peel the beetroot while it is still warm, then cut into dice.
6. Add the bay leaf to the vinegar/water/sugar mixture, and pour over the diced beetroot. Reserve for at least 2 hours before using.

The beetroot for this dish is best left overnight to develop the flavour.

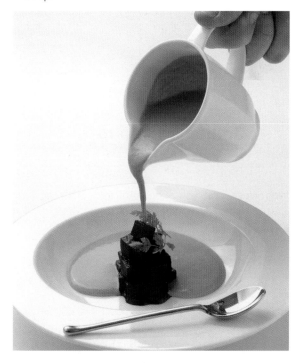

52   Blackberry soup

	4 portions	10 portions
fresh blackberries	450 g	1.2 kg
sugar	120 g	275 g
water	420 ml	1 litre
natural yoghurt	500 ml	1.2 litres
lemon, juiced and zest finely grated	1	2
natural yoghurt to serve	100 ml	250 ml
berries and mint to garnish		

1. Place all the ingredients except the yoghurt into a food processor and mix to a purée.
2. Strain into a clean bowl and add the yoghurt. Mix well and pour into serving bowls.
3. Garnish with a small spoonful of yoghurt, half a blackberry and mint.

53   Melon soup

	4 portions	10 portions
cantaloupe melon, peeled and seeded	250 g	650 g
watermelon, peeled and seeded	270 g	800 g
honeydew melon, peeled and seeded	200 g	600 g
sugar	80 g	200 g
dry sherry	20 ml	60 ml
lime, juiced and zest finely grated	1	3
melon salad (mixture of ¼ inch dice of watermelon, cantaloupe and honeydew)	200 g	600 g

1. Place all the ingredients, except the salad, into a food processor and mix to a purée.
2. Strain into a clean bowl and mix well.
3. Pour into serving bowls. Garnish with a small spoonful of melon salad.

54   Chilled fruit soup

	4 portions	10 portions
fresh orange juice	150 ml	450 ml
cranberry juice	150 ml	450 ml
honeydew melon, peeled and seeded	200 g	500 g
dried apricots	80 g	200 g
strawberries, washed and hulled	150 g	450 g
small banana	1	3
natural yoghurt	200 ml	600 ml
sugar	80 g	200 g
lime, juiced and zest finely grated	1	3
strawberries and mint to garnish		

1. Place all the ingredients into a food processor and mix to a purée.
2. Strain into a clean bowl and mix well.
3. Pour into serving bowls. Garnish with a half strawberry and mint.

Chilled fruit gazpacho soup

	4 portions	10 portions
orange	1	3
lime	1	3
honeydew melon, peeled and seeded	200 g	600 g
blueberries	80 g	200 g
sugar	80 g	200 g
honey	1 tbsp	3 tbsp
dark rum	2 tbsp	6 tbsp
strawberries, washed and hulled	150 g	450 g
raspberries	150 g	450 g
lime, juiced and zest finely grated	1	3
orange, juice of	1	3
sour cream	250 ml	650 ml
coriander, chopped	1 tsp	3 tsp
strawberry halves and mint to garnish		

1. Place the fruit, sugar, honey, rum and juices together into a food processor, and pulse into a chunky purée.
2. Mix in the sour cream, but retain a little for the garnish, and add cinnamon to taste.
3. Pour into serving bowls. Garnish with a half strawberry, a little of the sour cream, a pinch of cinnamon and mint.

Lightly jellied tomato and tea consommé

	100 shot glasses
tomatoes, chopped	50
sundried tomatoes (no oil)	30
chervil	1 bunch
water	3 litres
jasmine tea	1 tbsp or 3 jasmine tea bags
gelatine	6 leaves
spring onions, finely sliced and black fungus for garnish	

1. Mix tomatoes, dried tomatoes, chervil and water in a pan.
2. Bring to a gentle simmer but do not boil.
3. Gently simmer for 10 minutes, then remove from heat.
4. Add the jasmine tea and allow to infuse for 20 minutes. Season.
5. Strain through a fine sieve and then through a coffee filter.
6. Skim and allow sediment to settle.
7. Remove the consommé leaving the sediment (similar to clarifying butter).
8. Reheat the oiled, soaked leaf gelatine, garnish with finely sliced spring onions and chopped black fungus.
9. Allow to set, place into liqueur glasses and finish each glass with tomato concassée. Serve as a canapé.

57 Basic vinaigrette

	Makes approx. ¼ litre
wholegrain mustard	1 tsp
sherry vinegar	25 ml
grapeseed/corn oil	50 ml
light olive oil	125 ml
seasoning	

1. Place the mustard, vinegar and corn/grapeseed oil into a large bowl and whisk to an emulsion.
2. Slowly add the olive oil, about 50 ml at a time, bringing to an emulsion at each stage. Add seasoning.
3. Pour into a jar or bottle and store in the fridge until ready to use. If the mix separates during storage, simply shake the bottle or jar to re-emulsify.

Variations

	Additions per 250 ml of basic vinaigrette
Basil vinaigrette	1 tsp chopped basil
Chilli vinaigrette	½ tsp chopped red chillies
Herb vinaigrette	1 tsp chopped herbs (e.g. chervil, tarragon, basil and parsley)
Honey vinaigrette	2 tsp honey
Pesto vinaigrette	2 tsp pesto
Tomato vinaigrette	1 tbsp tomato ketchup and 50 g tomato concassée

58 Balsamic dressing

	Makes approx. 250 ml
balsamic vinegar	50 ml
grapeseed/corn oil	50 ml
light olive oil	125 ml
seasoning	

1. Place the vinegar and corn/grapeseed oil in a large bowl and whisk to an emulsion.
2. Slowly add the olive oil, about 50 ml at a time, bringing to an emulsion at each stage. Season.
3. Pour into a jar or bottle and store in the fridge until ready to use. If the mix separates during storage, simply shake the bottle or jar to re-emulsify.

59 Beetroot dressing

beetroot, cooked, peeled	400 g
white wine vinegar	40 g
corn oil	125 g
seasoning	

1. Blitz the cooked and peeled beetroot in a liquidiser with the white wine vinegar for 1 minute.
2. Pass through a fine chinois into a bowl.
3. Whisk in the oil and season to taste.
4. Refrigerate.

Variations on mayonnaise

	Additions to 250 ml mayonnaise
Basil mayonnaise	1 tbsp chopped basil
Ginger mayonnaise	1 tbsp finely grated fresh ginger
Green sauce	3 tbsp spinach purée 2 tsp chopped mixed herbs (parsley, chervil, tarragon)
Honey-flavoured mayonnaise	1 tbsp honey
Honey and ginger mayonnaise	1 tbsp finely grated fresh ginger 1 tbsp honey

Garlic-flavoured mayonnaise

	4 portions	10 portions
egg yolks	2	5
vinegar or lemon or lime juice	2 tsp	5 tsp
salt, ground white pepper		
mustard	⅛ tsp	⅜ tsp
cloves of garlic (juice or chopped)	2	5
olive oil or vegetable oil	250 ml	625 ml
boiling water	1 tsp	2 tsp

1. Place the yolks, vinegar or juice, seasoning and garlic in a bowl and mix well.
2. Gradually pour on the oil very slowly, whisking continuously.
3. Add the boiling water, whisking well.
4. Correct the seasoning.

Other suggested additions:
- tomato ketchup
- anchovy essence
- tomato and anchovy essence
- horseradish, finely grated.

Fresh tomato sauce (raw) or coulis

	4 portions	10 portions
tomatoes, skinned and pips removed	400 g	1¼ kg
vinegar	½ tbsp	1½ tbsp
oil	3 tbsp	8 tbsp
salt and mill pepper		
chopped parsley and tarragon	1 tbsp	3 tbsp

1. Squeeze the tomatoes to remove excess juice then liquidise the flesh.
2. Place in a bowl and gradually whisk in the vinegar and oil.
3. Season and mix in the herbs.

Note: Other herbs (e.g. basil, oregano) may be used in place of tarragon.

63   Plum sauce

	Makes approx. 700 ml
preserved plums, mashed	20
onion, minced	1 tbsp
ginger, minced	1 tsp
red chilli, minced	1 tsp
clove of garlic, minced	1
water	450 ml
lime, zest	1
lime juice to taste	
brown sugar to taste	

1. Combine all the ingredients in a saucepan.
2. Bring to the boil, stirring constantly, and then simmer a few minutes to blend the flavours.
3. Reduce to sauce consistency and season as required with lime juice and sugar.
4. Allow to cool, then chill.

This sauce tastes best if it is refrigerated, covered, overnight to allow the seasonings to mellow.

64   *Cervelle de canut*

sour cream	200 g
cider vinegar	5 g
walnut oil	2 g
fine herbs, chopped (chervil and parsley)	10 g
shallots, washed, finely chopped	50 g
seasoning	

i   This is a sauce based on sour cream. The name translates as 'silk workers' brains'.

Take a small container of the sour cream and fold in the shallots, herbs, cider vinegar, walnut oil and seasoning. Just make sure there is enough seasoning and the flavour is light and tasty.

65   Sauce maltaise

	Makes approx. 600 ml
water	8–9 tbsp
vinegar	2 tbsp
cracked pepper	pinch
fine salt	pinch
egg yolks	5
butter, melted and warm	500 g
blood oranges	2
grated blood orange zest	big pinch

1. Place 4 tablespoons of the water, and the vinegar, cracked pepper and fine salt, into a saucepan and reduce by two-thirds.
2. Place the saucepan over a double boiler; add 1 tablespoon water and the egg yolks; gradually whisk in the butter, a little at a time, interspersing it with 3 to 4 tablespoons more water, to make a light sauce.
3. Once the sauce is nicely thickened, blend in the juice of 2 blood oranges with a big pinch of grated zest.

Sauce bavaroise

	Makes approx. 600 ml
water	8–9 tbsp
vinegar	2 tbsp
cracked pepper	pinch
fine salt	pinch
egg yolks	5
butter, melted and warm	500 g
picked thyme leaves, chopped	1 tsp
horseradish cream	2 tbsp

1. Place 4 tablespoons of the water, and the vinegar, cracked pepper and fine salt, into a saucepan and reduce by two-thirds.
2. Place the saucepan over a double boiler; add 1 tbsp water and the egg yolks; gradually whisk in the butter, a little at a time, interspersing it with 3 to 4 tablespoons more water, to make a light sauce.
3. Once the sauce is nicely thickened, blend in the chopped thyme and the horseradish cream.

 ## Fig and apple chutney

cooking apple, peeled and cut into 2.5 cm dice	1
onion, diced	25 g
dried fig, chopped	50 g
white wine vinegar	25 ml
English mustard	⅓ tbsp
cayenne pepper	pinch
clove garlic	½
sultanas	50 g
sugar	10 g

1. Combine all the ingredients in a heavy saucepan.
2. Bring to the boil then lower the heat and simmer for 2 hours until thick.
3. Add a splash of water if the mixture dries out before the 2 hours are up. Leave to cool, then briefly liquidise the mixture until it is the consistency of jam. Store in the refrigerator.

 ## Apricot chutney

red wine vinegar	250 g
demerara sugar	250 g
ginger, cut into fine brunoise	30 g
diced onion	125 g
nutmeg	0.1 g
saffron	0.1 g
vanilla pod	½
tomato concasse	250 g
dried apricots, cut into sixths	500 g
lemon juice	2 g
lemon zest	6 g
Szechuan pepper	5 turns of the mill
black pepper	10 turns of the mill
Muscatel vinegar	20 g

1. Make a thick syrup with the red wine vinegar and the sugar.
2. Add the ginger, onion, nutmeg, saffron, vanilla and concasse. Reduce to a thick syrup. Add the apricots and reduce again.
3. Allow to cool. Once cold, add the rest of the ingredients.

69 Peach and saffron summer chutney

diced shallots	1¼ kg
olive oil	large splash
mixed spice	15 tsp
chillies, diced	10
garlic cloves, finely grated	10
saffron strands	5 tsp
sea salt	5 tsp
caster sugar	1½ kg
cider vinegar	1¾ litre
peaches, cut into chunks	6 kg

1. Sweat the shallots in a touch of oil with the mixed spice, chilli, finely grated garlic and saffron strands. Add the salt and gently cook until the shallots are slightly soft.
2. When the onions are soft, add the sugar and the cider vinegar and cook this down to a caramel colour; this will take approx. 30–40 minutes.
3. When the onions have a caramel colour, add the peaches and gently cook down for approx. 1 hour until the chutney has become nice and thick. Now check the seasoning and chill.
4. Store in vacuum pack bags or kilner jars.

Use the best peaches you can find for this recipe, and good quality olive oil.

70 Red onion confit/marmalade

red onions, sliced	1 kg
butter	50 g
soft brown sugar	50 g
red wine vinegar	250 ml
blackcurrant cordial or red wine (optional)	60 ml

1. Slowly sauté the onions in the butter in a thick-bottomed pan.
2. Cook thoroughly but with little or no colour.
3. Add the other ingredients and reduce slowly until slightly thick.
4. Season lightly with salt and mill pepper.
5. When cold, store in covered jars or basins in the refrigerator.

Note: Can be served as a garnish/accompaniment to many dishes hot or cold.

71 Aubergine raita

energy	kcal	fat	sat fat	carb	sugar	protein	fibre
1008 KJ	240 cal	11.6 g	6.8 g	20.8 g	20.6 g	15.1 g	14.0 g

	4 portions	10 portions
aubergines (approx. 150 g each)	1	3
yoghurt	1 litre	2½ litres
pinch of salt		
piece of ginger, finely chopped	1	2½
cumin seeds	1 tsp	2½ tsp
fenugreek	1 tsp	2½ tsp
ghee or sunflower oil	1 tbsp	2½ tbsp

3. In a small saucepan or wok, fry the ginger, cumin and fenugreek for a minute in the ghee or oil and add to the raita.
4. When the aubergine is cooked, cool in water for a few minutes, then cut in half, scrape the flesh of the skin and cut it in very small pieces or, better, blend it roughly then add to the raita.
5. Cool in the refrigerator for half an hour before serving.

1. Prick the skin of the aubergine and bake in the oven at 200°C until soft.
2. While the aubergine is cooking, whisk the yoghurt with 100 ml of water and the salt in a large salad bowl.

There are many types of raita and they are a very popular side dish in India. They are made of yoghurt, water, spices and some kind of vegetable or fruit. A very refreshing dish in hot weather.

72 Vegetable crisps

Vegetable crisps may be made from the following vegetables: parsnips, beetroot (golden is ideal), carrots, mooli, root ginger, potato, courgette, aubergine, sweet potato.

1. Peel and slice the vegetables very thinly (wash and dry the potatoes) using a mandolin.
2. Deep-fry in deep hot oil at 185°C until crisp.
3. Drain well on kitchen paper and use as a garnish.

Vegetable crisps may be used as a garnish. They are fatty, so only use a few.

73 Falafel

This is a popular Middle Eastern dish.

As a main dish it is served as a sandwich, stuffed in pitta bread with lettuce, tomatoes and tahini or couscous. As an appetiser, it is served as a salad or with hummus and tahini.

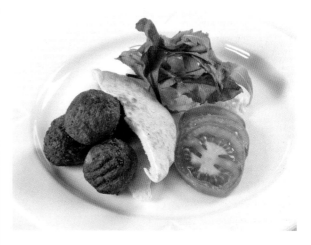

	4 portions	10 portions
sunflower oil	2 tbsp	5 tbsp
onion, finely chopped	1	2
garlic cloves	1	2
dried chickpeas, soaked, cooked in boiling water and drained	200 g	500 g
ground cumin	1 tsp	2½ tsp
ground coriander	1 tsp	2½ tsp
parsley, chopped	1 tbsp	2½ tbsp
mixed herbs	1 tsp	2½ tsp
egg, beaten	1	3

1. Heat a tablespoon of oil in a suitable pan. Fry the onion and garlic until soft.
2. Place the chickpeas and ground spices into a food processor and mix to a purée.
3. Stir in the chopped onion and garlic. Add the parsley and mixed herbs. Season.
4. Add the beaten egg. Mix well.
5. Mould into balls evenly, then flatten into patties.
6. Heat the remaining oil in a suitable pan. Fry the falafels carefully on both sides for approx. 3 minutes until golden brown and firm.

Tomato and olive tapenade

Tomatoes	
cherry tomatoes, halved	210 g
basil, crushed	12 g
white wine vinegar	1 drop
garlic, crushed	15 g
gold olive oil	15 g
fine salt	pinch (0.5 g)
black pepper	0.1 g
Tapenade	
black olives, pitted	280 g
lemon zest	30 g
anchovy fillets (optional)	11 g
thyme	1 g
olive oil	10 g
garlic	4 g

1. Mix the tomatoes and all the associated ingredients together in a bowl and marinade for two hours before use.
2. Make the tapenade by blending all the ingredients in a Robo Coupe until they form a paste. Chill until required.

Use as a garnish for soups and cold meats, or as a filling for tartlets or spring rolls.

Gribeche

egg, hard-boiled, finely grated	100 g
capers, chopped	40 g
shallot, finely diced	20 g
Muscatel vinegar	5 g
salt	4 g
parsley, chopped	4 g
crème fraîche	50 g

Combine all the ingredients. Store until required.

Serve on toast as an appetiser or canapé.

 Garlic and cream cheese on rosemary crouton

Garlic and cream cheese	
goats' cheese (*fromage de chevre*)	490 g
garlic	8 g
double cream	750 g
seasoning	
Rosemary croutons	
olive oil	100 ml
sprig of rosemary	
baguette, thinly sliced	1

3. Place the mix into the mixer and beat with the paddle attachment.
4. When the cheese is soft, add the cream a little at a time.
5. When all the cream has been added, season to taste.

Rosemary croutons

1. Pour the oil into a non-stick tray.
2. Rub the rosemary all over the bottom of the tray with the oil.
3. Add the slices of baguette. Cook at 180°C for 8 minutes.

Serve together as an appetiser.

Garlic and cream cheese

1. Chop the goats' cheese into small pieces.
2. Purée the garlic and add it to the cheese.

77 Vegetarian terrine

	4 portions	10 portions
fresh washed spinach	300 g	750 g
salt and pepper		
ground allspice	1 tsp	2½ tsp
chopped chives	25 g	60 g
carrots ⎫ washed and	400 g	1 kg
celeriac ⎭ peeled	400 g	1 kg
choux pastry	375 ml	1 litre
double cream or crème fraîche	190 ml	475 ml

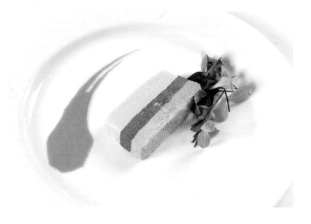

1. Cook, refresh and drain the spinach well, purée in food processor and season with salt, pepper, allspice and chopped chives.
2. Cut carrots and celeriac into even pieces, cook and purée separately.
3. To each purée add 125 ml of choux pastry and 60 ml of double cream (× 2½ for 10 portions). Mix well.
4. Take a large well-greased loaf tin, preferably aluminium foil (disposable).
5. Layer carrot purée over the base. Next layer with celeriac and finish with the spinach.
6. Cover with foil. Cook in a bain-marie in the oven at 180°C for approximately 1¼ hours.
7. Remove from oven, cool and serve cold, sliced with a suitable sauce, e.g. green peppercorn and paprika (see below).

> Drain and dry out the puréed vegetables to remove excess moisture, and make sure the choux pastry is not too wet.

Green peppercorn and paprika sauce

	4 portions	10 portions
plum tomatoes	200 g	500 g
green peppercorns, crushed	25 g	60 g
paprika	12 g	25 g
double cream	250 ml	600 ml
lemon, juice of	½	1–2

1. Purée the plum tomatoes, place in a suitable pan with the peppercorns and bring to the boil. Simmer for 5 minutes.
2. Add paprika, simmer for a further 5 minutes.
3. Finish with cream, bring back to boil.
4. Add lemon juice, pass through a fine strainer, cool and serve chilled.

This sauce may be used to accompany the vegetarian terrine.

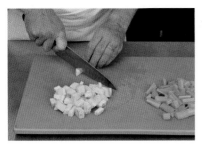

Chop the vegetables

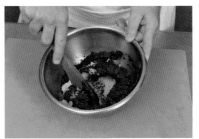

Mix together the ingredients for each layer

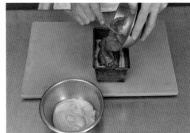

Layer the mixtures into the mould

78 Tian of green and white asparagus

	4 portions	10 portions
garlic	10 g	25 g
thyme	½ tsp	1 tsp
black pepper	pinch	10 g
gelatine sheets	1	3
green asparagus (medium)	400 g	1 kg
white asparagus (medium)	400 g	1 kg
salt	pinch	½ tsp
shallots	100 g	250 g
chives, chopped	1 tbsp	2 tbsp
extra virgin olive oil	20 ml	50 ml
sundried tomatoes in oil	30 g	75 g

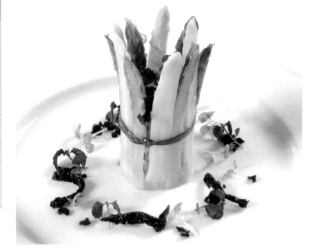

To make the jelly

1. Bring 500 ml of water to the boil in a pan. Add a touch of garlic, thyme and black pepper.
2. Melt the gelatine in warm water and add to the bouillon.
3. Pass through a fine sieve and leave to cool.

To make the tian

4. Trim and peel the asparagus.
5. Cook the colours separately in salted water infused with thyme for approx. 4–5 mins. Cool down immediately in iced water.
6. Trim each length of asparagus to exactly 8 cm long. (Keep the trimmings.)
7. Slice the trimmings of asparagus and sauté with the shallots and remaining garlic, leave to cool.
8. Using a metal ring (approx. 7 cm in diameter) place the spears of asparagus around the inside of the ring in alternate colours. Use the sautéed mixture to fill the centre of the ring and pack tightly.
9. Pour the jelly over the top of the mixture inside the metal ring and place in the refrigerator to set.

To make the sauce

10. Finely chop the chives and add to the olive oil. Cut the tomatoes into a fine julienne and add to the mixture. Season well.

To plate

11. Heat the metal ring of asparagus very quickly with a flame torch to loosen the edges. Place in the centre of a plate and carefully spoon the dressing in a circle around the edge.

79 Light fluffy omelette

For each omelette
2–3 egg yolks
salt and pepper
2–3 egg whites
25 g butter or margarine

1. Beat the yolks with salt and pepper.
2. Half beat the whites, fold the yolks into the whites.
3. Heat the butter or margarine in the omelette pan and pour in the mixture; cook, stirring with a fork, until nearly set.
4. Fold the omelette in half, finish cooking in the oven until set.
5. Serve on individual plates immediately.

Soft-boiled eggs with mushroom duxelle and cheese sauce

energy	kcal	fat	sat fat	carb	sugar	protein	fibre
1629 KJ	392.2 cal	30.6 g	14.7 g	16.2 g	2.2 g	14.0 g	0.7 g

	4 portions	10 portions
eggs	4	10
short pastry	100 g	250 g
Duxelle		
shallots	25 g	60 g
mushrooms, chopped	100 g	250 g
butter or margarine	50 g	125 g
salt and pepper		
mornay sauce (cheese sauce)	125 ml	600 ml
grated Parmesan cheese	25 g	60 g

1. Soft boil the eggs for 5–6 minutes then remove and place in a basin of cold water to cool. Shell. Retain in cold water.
2. Line individual tartlet moulds with short pastry and bake blind.
3. Prepare the mushroom duxelle and season.
4. Place tartlet cases in individual serving dishes and fill with the duxelle.
5. Reheat the eggs in simmering salted water, drain. Place the reheated eggs in the tartlet cases.
6. Mask with mornay sauce, sprinkle with grated Parmesan cheese and gratinate. Serve immediately.

 Ratatouille pancakes with a cheese sauce

energy	kcal	fat	sat fat	carb	sugar	protein	fibre
2398 KJ	571 cal	35.8 g	6.5 g	46.1 g	19.0 g	19.6 g	6.5 g

	4 portions	10 portions
Pancake batter		
flour	100 g	250 g
skimmed milk	250 ml	625 ml
egg	1	2–3
pinch of salt		
sunflower margarine, melted	10 g	25 g
Ratatouille		
courgettes	200 g	500 g
aubergines	200 g	500 g
red pepper	1	2–3
green pepper	1	2–3
tomatoes	100 g	250 g
yellow pepper	1	2–3
onion, chopped	50 g	125 g
clove garlic, chopped	1	2
sunflower oil	4 tbsp	10 tbsp
tin plum tomatoes	400 g	1¼ kg
tomato purée	50 g	125 g

Cheese sauce		
skimmed milk	500 ml	1¼ litres
sunflower oil	50 g	125 g
flour	50 g	125 g
onion, studded with clove	1	2–3
Parmesan, grated	25 g	60 g
egg yolk	1	2–3
seasoning		

1. Prepare and make the pancakes.
2. Prepare the ratatouille and cheese sauce.
3. Season with salt and cayenne pepper.
4. Fill the pancakes with the ratatouille, roll up and serve on individual plates or on a service dish, coated with cheese sauce and sprinkled with grated Parmesan. Finish by gratinating under the salamander.

82 Vegetable, bean and saffron risotto

energy	kcal	fat	sat fat	carb	sugar	protein	fibre
2017 KJ	485 cal	35.8 g	8.6 g	4.5 g	34.8 g	5.6 g	4.5 g

	4 portions	10 portions
vegetable stock	185 ml	1 litre
saffron	5 g	12 g
sunflower margarine	50 g	125 g
onion, chopped	25 g	60 g
celery	50 g	125 g
short-grain rice	100 g	250 g
small cauliflower	1	2–3
sunflower oil	4 tbsp	10 tbsp
large aubergine	1	2–3
cooked haricot beans	100 g	250 g
cooked peas	50 g	125 g
cooked French beans	50 g	125 g
tomato sauce made with sunflower margarine and vegetable stock	250 ml	600 ml
grated Parmesan cheese	25 g	60 g

1. Infuse the vegetable stock with the saffron for approximately 5 minutes by simmering gently, while maintaining the quality of stock.
2. Melt the margarine, add the onion and celery and cook without colour for 2–3 minutes. Add the rice.
3. Cook for a further 2–3 minutes. Add the infused stock and season lightly. Cover with a lid and simmer on the side of the stove.
4. While rice is cooking prepare the rest of the vegetables. Cut the cauliflower into small florets, wash, blanch and refresh, quickly fry in the sunflower oil in a sauté pan. Add the aubergines cut into ½ cm dice and fry with the cauliflower. Add the cooked haricot beans, peas and French beans.
5. Stir all the vegetables together and bind with tomato sauce.
6. When the risotto is cooked, serve in a suitable dish. Make a well in the centre. Fill the centre with the vegetables and haricot beans in tomato sauce.
7. Sprinkle the edge of the risotto with grated Parmesan cheese to serve.

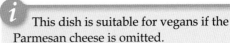

i This dish is suitable for vegans if the Parmesan cheese is omitted.

83 Vegetable olives (vegetable pancakes)

energy	kcal	fat	sat fat	carb	sugar	protein	fibre
2321 KJ	554 cal	29.5 g	10.2 g	48.4 g	24.3 g	26.7 g	6.7 g

	4 portions	10 portions
mushrooms	100 g	250 g
carrots	100 g	250 g
onions	100 g	250 g
leeks	100 g	250 g
capsicums	100 g	250 g
aubergine	100 g	250 g
basil leaves, bunch		
crêpes (pancakes)	8 × 15 cm	20 × 15 cm
tomato sauce	1.2 litre	3 litre
béchamel	250 ml	600 ml
mozzarella cheese	150 g	375 g
seasoning		

1. Cut the vegetables into a paysanne and sweat.
2. Place a basil leaf on a crêpe, add the vegetable mixture and roll up.
3. Place in an earthenware dish on a little tomato sauce.
4. Cover completely with the remaining tomato sauce, cover with foil and bake to heat thoroughly at 150°C for approximately 15 minutes.
5. Remove from the oven, remove the foil, coat the centre with a little béchamel, top with cheese and grill.
6. Sprinkle with chopped basil and serve with Italian garlic bread or French bread.

This recipe was contributed by Gary Thompson and Neil Yule.

84 Aubergine stir-fry, Japanese style

	4 portions	10 portions
aubergines, sliced into ½ cm thick pieces	2	5
miso (soy bean paste)	1 tbsp	3 tbsp
mirin	½ tsp	1½ tsp
sugar to taste		
oil	½ tsp	
garlic, chopped	½ tsp	1 tsp
onion, sliced	½	1
green peppers, thinly sliced	1	2
carrot, cut into julienne	25 g	50 g
spring onion, sliced	10 g	20 g
salt to taste		

1. Soak the auberinges in a bowl of water for 10 minutes and drain. Dry with paper towels.
2. Mix the miso, mirin, and sugar in a small bowl and set aside.
3. Heat the oil in a medium skillet and fry the garlic and onion until fragrant.
4. Add the aubergines and cook on a medium heat until softened.
5. Add the green peppers and stir-fry until softened. Turn down the heat to low.
6. Stir in the carrot and spring onion, then add the miso mixture.
7. Stir quickly together and season to taste.

85 Thai-style potato curry

energy	kcal	fat	sat fat	carb	sugar	protein	fibre
1687 KJ	401 cal	14.2 g	1.9 g	63.9 g	20.7 g	8.4 g	7.6 g

	4 portions	10 portions
potatoes	1 kg	2½ kg
onion	50 g	125 g
sunflower oil	50 ml	125 ml
small piece of fresh ginger root		
fresh lemon grass stick, smashed to extract flavour	1	2
fresh green chillies, chopped and seeds removed	2	5
coconut milk	210 ml	525 ml
dry mango powder (if not available, the juice of 2 limes or lemons)	1 tbsp	2½ tbsp
plum tomatoes, peeled and chopped into 1 cm dice	12	30

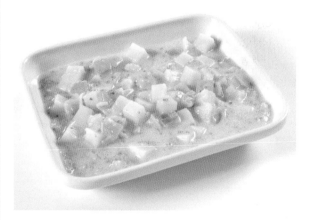

1. Peel and wash the potatoes and cut them into dice. Chop the onion finely and fry in sunflower oil on medium heat until golden brown.
2. Add the grated ginger, the lemon grass, chopped finely, and the chopped chillies, and fry for another 2 minutes, stirring constantly, then add the potatoes, the coconut milk, the mango powder or lemon/lime juice, the tomatoes and, if needed, water to cover.
3. Bring to the boil then lower the heat and leave to simmer for 35 minutes on a low heat, stirring occasionally. Serve with freshly cooked rice.

Variation

The potatoes can be replaced with 400 g of soaked butter beans, cooked for 1 hour in water, to make a Thai-style butter bean curry. Cooked green lentils and spinach can be added at the end of the cooking process; serve immediately on a bed of brown rice.

86 Stuffed vegetables

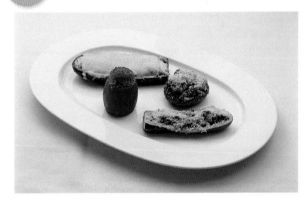

Certain vegetables can be stuffed and served as a first course, as a vegetable course and as an accompaniment to a main course.

The majority of vegetables used for this purpose are the bland, gourd types, such as aubergines, courgette and cucumbers, in which case the stuffing should be delicately flavoured so as not to overpower the vegetable.

Below are some of the more popular types of vegetable used for this purpose and the usual type of stuffing in each case. There is, however, considerable scope for variation and experimentation in any of the stuffings.

Artichoke bottoms

Use duxelle stuffing; serve with a cordon of thin demi-glace or jus-lié flavoured with tomato.

Aubergine

The cooked chopped flesh is mixed with one of the following to make the stuffing:

- Cooked chopped onion, sliced tomatoes and chopped parsley
- Duxelle, sprinkled with fresh breadcrumbs, grated cheese – and gratinated
- Cooked chopped onion, garlic, tomato concassée, parsley, breadcrumbs – and gratinated
- Diced or minced cooked mutton, cooked chopped onion, tomato concassée, cooked rice and chopped parsley.

Serve with a cordon of tomato sauce or coulis.

Mushrooms and ceps

Use duxelle stuffing.

For stuffed ceps, forest style, use equal quantities of duxelle stuffing and sausagemeat (or omit the meat for a vegetarian version).

Stuffed cabbage

Use veal stuffing and serve with pilaff rice.

Cucumber

This can be prepared in two ways.

1. Peeled, cut into 2 cm pieces, the centres hollowed out with a parisienne spoon and then boiled, steamed or cooked in butter.
2. The peeled whole cucumber is cut in halves lengthwise, the seed pocket scooped out and the cucumber cooked by boiling, steaming or in butter.

Suitable stuffings can be made from a base of duxelle, pilaff rice or chicken forcemeat, or any combination of these.

To stuff the cucumber pieces, pipe the stuffing from a piping bag and complete the cooking in the oven. When the whole cucumber is stuffed, rejoin the two halves, wrap in pig's caul and muslin and braise.

Lettuce

Stuff with two parts chicken forcemeat and one part duxelle, and braise. For a vegetarian version, stuff with duxelle only.

Turnips

Peel the turnips, remove the centre almost to the root and blanch the turnips.

Cook and purée the scooped-out centre and mix with an equal quantity of potato purée.

Refill the cavities and gently cook the turnips in butter in the oven, basting frequently.

Turnips may also be stuffed with cooked spinach, chicory or rice.

Pimentos

Stuff with pilaff rice, varied if required with other ingredients, e.g. mushrooms, tomatoes or duxelle.

Use duxelle stuffing with garlic and diced ham. Serve with a cordon of demi-glace flavoured with tomato.

Use chopped hard-boiled egg bound with thick béchamel, grated cheese and gratinated. Serve with a cordon of light tomato sauce.

Use scrambled egg, mushrooms and diced ham, sprinkled with breadcrumbs fried in butter.

Use risotto with tomato concassée. Coat with thin tomato sauce.

Use cooked tomato concassée, chopped onion, garlic and parsley, bound with fresh breadcrumbs – gratinate. May be served hot or cold.

Use pilaff rice in which has been cooked dice of tomato and red pimento. Cook gently in oven and sprinkle with chopped parsley.

Baked christophenes with onion and cheese filling (*cristophene au gratin*)

87

	4 portions	10 portions
large christophenes	2	5
butter	75 g	180 g
onions, finely chopped	150 g	375 g
Parmesan cheese, freshly grated	8 tbsp	20 tbsp
salt	1 tsp	2½ tsp
freshly ground black pepper		

A christophene is a type of squash.

1. Wash the christophenes under cold running water, drain, and cut them lengthwise into halves. Drop them into enough lightly salted boiling water to cover them completely and cook briskly for about 30 minutes, or until they are tender and show only slight resistance when pierced with the point of a small, sharp knife.
2. Drain the christophenes and, when they are cool enough to handle, remove and discard the seed and scoop out the pulp from each half with a small spoon to make boat-like shells about ½ cm thick. Set the shells aside on paper towels to drain completely. Chop the scooped-out pulp coarsely.
3. Preheat the oven to 180°C. In a heavy 25 to 30 cm skillet, melt four-fifths of the butter over a moderate heat. When the foam begins to subside, drop in the onions and, stirring frequently, cook for about 5 minutes, until they are soft and transparent but not brown.
4. Add the chopped pulp, ¾ of the cheese, the salt and some pepper.
5. Cook briskly until most of the liquid in the pan has evaporated and the mixture is thick enough to hold its shape lightly in the spoon.
6. Fill the christophene shells with the onion mixture, patting it in firmly. Arrange the shells side by side in a shallow baking dish large enough to hold them comfortably. Dot the tops with the remaining butter in ½ cm pieces.
7. Sprinkle the squash with the remaining cheese and bake in the middle of the oven for about 20 minutes, or until the tops are a delicate golden brown. Serve at once.

88 Galette of aubergines with tomatoes and mozzarella

energy	kcal	fat	sat fat	carb	sugar	protein	fibre
940 KJ	224 cal	9.6 g	6.2 g	20.7 g	17.0 g	15.0 g	3.4 g

	4 portions	10 portions
aubergines	400 g	1 kg
onions, finely chopped	100 g	250 g
garlic, crushed and chopped	2	5
vegetable oil		
low-fat yoghurt	500 ml	1¼ ltr
cornflour	2 tsp	5 tsp
coriander, finely chopped	1 tsp	2½ tsp
sugar	1 tsp	2½ tsp
plum tomatoes	400 g	1 kg
buffala mozzarella	150 g	375 g
seasoning		
coriander, to garnish		

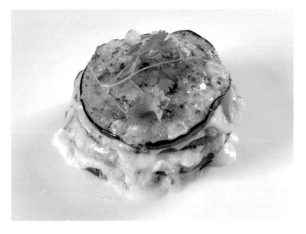

1. Slice the aubergines thinly. Place on a tray and sprinkle with salt. Leave for 1 hour.
2. Dry the aubergines in a cloth. Quickly fry in oil until golden brown on both sides. Remove from pan, drain well.
3. Sweat the finely chopped onion and garlic in oil without colour.
4. Mix together the yoghurt, cornflour, coriander and sugar, add to the onion and garlic. Bring to the boil and season lightly. Remove from heat.
5. Blanch and peel the tomatoes, chop into ½ cm slices.
6. Arrange 4 large slices of aubergine on a greased baking sheet. Spread the yoghurt mixture on each slice, and top with tomato and mozzarella. Continue to build layers of aubergine, tomato and mozzarella. Finish with a layer of yoghurt mixture.
7. Bake in a hot oven (220°C) for 20 minutes until golden brown. Serve immediately, garnish with coriander.

89 Gratin of nuts with a tomato and red wine sauce

	4 portions	10 portions
onion, finely chopped	100 g	250 g
green pepper, in brunoise	50 g	125 g
celery, in brunoise	50 g	125 g
butter or margarine	25 g	60 g
garlic cloves	2	5
cooked fresh or canned chestnuts *or*	200 g	500 g
dried chestnuts (well soaked then cooked in vegetable stock	75 g	180 g
cashew nuts	200 g	500 g
walnuts	50 g	125 g
Cheddar cheese	100 g	250 g
red wine	60 ml	150 ml
brandy	60 ml	150 ml
paprika	10 g	25 g
thyme (dried)	5 g	12 g
eggs	1	2–3

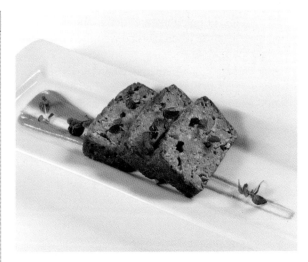

1. Sweat the onion, green pepper and celery in the butter or margarine without colour.
2. Add the crushed and chopped garlic, continue to sweat for 1 minute.
3. Add the finely chopped nuts and grated Cheddar cheese, mix well.
4. Add the red wine, brandy and herbs, season well and bind with an egg.
5. Place mixture into a well-greased and silicone paper-lined 400 g loaf tin.
6. Cover with aluminium foil and bake at 190°C for approximately 45 minutes. (Alternatively, bake in a bain-marie in the oven.)
7. When cooked, turn out and carefully portion into individual plates on to a red wine and tomato sauce with basil (see below). Decorate with fresh basil and a little tomato concassée.

Tomato and red wine sauce flavoured with basil

	4 portions	10 portions
fresh tomato coulis	125 ml	300 ml
red wine	125 ml	300 ml
sprigs chopped basil	2	5
natural yoghurt or single cream	60 ml	150 ml
seasoning		

1. Bring the tomato coulis to the boil, add the red wine and chopped basil. Simmer for 2 minutes.
2. Finish with natural yoghurt or single cream, and correct seasoning and consistency. Pass through a fine strainer if necessary before use.

90 Parsnip and cheese roulade with mixed herbs

	4 portions	10 portions
Roulade		
butter or margarine	40 g	100 g
plain flour	25 g	62 g
milk	275 ml	700 ml
egg yolks	3	8
egg whites	3	8
Parmesan cheese, grated	100 g	250 g
chopped mixed herbs (basil, chervil, parsley)	1 tbsp	2½ tbsp
salt and white pepper to season		
hazelnuts or almonds, chopped and roasted		
Herb mix layer		
butter or margarine	40 g	100 g
onions, finely chopped	200 g	500 g
mixed chopped herbs (parsley, chervil, basil)	2 tbsp	5 tbsp
white breadcrumbs	75 g	200 g
seasoning		
Filling		
parsnips	350 g	875 g
butter or margarine	25 g	62 g
double cream or crème fraîche	2 tbsp	5 tbsp
grated nutmeg		

1. Make the herb mix by melting the butter or margarine in a suitable pan. Sweat the chopped onions in the butter without colour.

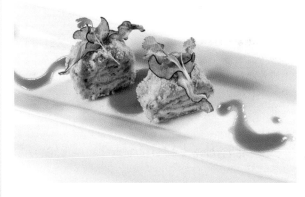

2. Add the mixed herbs, breadcrumbs and seasoning. Stir well and place on a Swiss roll tin lined with parchment paper (use a 30 cm × 20 cm tin for 4 portions).
3. Prepare the roulade. Make a béchamel sauce with the butter, flour and milk. Cook for approximately 10 minutes, then add the egg yolks, mixing well. Add the Parmesan and mixed herbs. Season lightly with salt and white pepper.
4. Beat the egg whites to full peak. Add a spoonful of the white into the cheese sauce mixture, then carefully fold in the remainder of the egg whites.
5. Carefully and evenly spread the mixture on top of the herb mix in the Swiss roll tin.
6. Bake in a preheated oven for approximately 20 minutes at 200°C.

7. Cook the parsnips by steaming or boiling. Once cooked, purée them. Add the butter, cream or crème fraîche, and nutmeg.

8. Lay a sheet of baking parchment on a table. Sprinkle with the chopped nuts.

9. When baked, turn the roulade out onto the nuts. Peel off the base paper.

10. Spread the creamed parsnips all over the roulade, on top of the herb mix layer.

11. Roll up the roulade carefully and sprinkle with Parmesan.

12. Serve sliced with a hot fresh tomato coulis.

91 Tofu and vegetable flan with walnut sauce

energy	kcal	fat	sat fat	carb	sugar	protein	fibre
2359 KJ	568 cal	45.8 g	9.3 g	25.8 g	5.6 g	15 g	2.5 g

	4 portions	10 portions
shortcrust pastry	150 g	375 g
sunflower oil	4 tbsp	10 tbsp
carrots, diced	50 g	125 g
mushrooms, sliced	50 g	125 g
celery, diced	50 g	125 g
broccoli florets, blanched and refreshed	100 g	250 g
fresh chopped basil	3 g	7½ g
chopped dill weed	3 g	7½ g
skimmed milk	125 ml	300 ml
egg	1	2–3
tofu	200 g	500 g
seasoning		

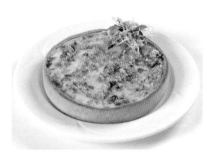

1. Line 18 cm flan ring(s) with shortcrust pastry and bake blind for approximately 8 minutes in a preheated oven at 180°C.

2. Heat the sunflower oil in a sauté pan, add the carrots, mushrooms and celery, gently cook for 5 minutes without colouring.

3. Add the broccoli, cover and cook gently until just crisp, stirring frequently and adding a little water if the mixture begins to dry.

4. Sprinkle over the herbs. Cook for 1 minute. Drain vegetables and allow to cool.

5. Warm the milk to blood heat. Whisk the egg and tofu in a basin, add seasoning then gradually incorporate milk. Whisk well.

6. Fill the flan case with the drained vegetables and add the tofu and milk mixture.

7. Bake for 20 minutes approximately at 180°C. Serve with walnut sauce (see below).

Walnut sauce

	4 portions	10 portions
onion, finely chopped	100 g	250 g
garlic clove, chopped	1	2–3
walnut oil	50 g	125 g
brown sugar	10 g	25 g
curry powder	25 g	60 g
lemon, grated zest and juice	1	2–3
peanut butter	25 g	60 g
soy sauce	1 tsp	2–3 tsp
tomato purée	25 g	60 g
vegetable stock	375 ml	900 ml
seasoning		
walnuts, very finely chopped	100 g	250 g
arrowroot	10 g	25 g

1. Fry the onion and garlic in the walnut oil, add the sugar and cook to a golden-brown colour.

2. Add the curry powder, cook for 2 minutes.

3. Add zest and juice of lemon, peanut butter, soy sauce and tomato purée. Mix well.

4. Add vegetable stock, bring to boil, simmer for 2 minutes, season.

5. Add chopped walnuts.

6. Dilute the arrowroot with a little water and gradually stir into sauce. Bring back to the boil stirring continuously. Simmer for 5 minutes.

7. Correct seasoning and consistency.

Vegetable gougère (filled choux ring)

choux pastry (see page 325)	4 portions	10 portions
water	250 ml	625 ml
sunflower margarine	100 g	250 g
strong flour	125 g	300 g
eggs (medium)	4	10
Gruyère cheese, diced	75 g	180 g
seasoning		

1. Make the choux pastry, cool and add the finely diced Gruyère cheese.
2. With a 1 cm plain tube, pipe individual rings approximately 8 cm in diameter on to a very lightly greased baking sheet.

3. Brush lightly with eggwash and relax for approximately 15 minutes.
4. Bake in a preheated oven at 190°C for 20 to 30 minutes.
5. When cooked, place on individual plates. Fill the centre with a suitable filling.

Possible fillings:
- Ratatouille
- Stir-fry vegetables
- Cauliflower cheese
- Button mushrooms in a tomato and garlic sauce
- Leaf spinach with chopped onions in a béchamel sauce
- Button mushrooms and sweetcorn in a béchamel yoghurt sauce.

93 Spinach, ricotta and artichoke filo bake with cranberries

energy	kcal	fat	sat fat	carb	sugar	protein	fibre
2191 KJ	523 cal	25.2 g	12.9 g	51.2 g	14.7 g	24.3 g	7.5 g

	4 portions	10 portions
spinach	400 g	1 kg
ricotta	500 g	1¼ kg
tinned artichokes, drained	200 g	500 g
filo pastry	275 g	700 g
frozen cranberries	500 g	1¼ kg
butter	25 g	60 g
olive oil	1 tbsp	2–3 tbsp
onion, sliced	100 g	250 g
salt, freshly ground black pepper		
chopped fresh parsley to taste		

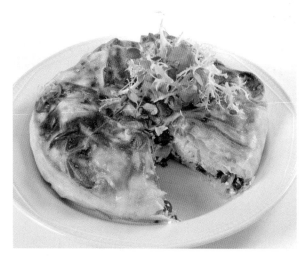

1. Cook, refresh and drain the spinach, then chop finely.
2. Break down the ricotta and mix with the spinach.
3. Sauté the onion in the olive oil without colour. Add to the ricotta and spinach with the chopped parsley. Season to taste.
4. Line a lightly buttered flan dish with 3 layers of filo pastry, leaving overhang.
5. Fill with spinach mixture and press drained artichokes evenly around the dish.

6. Top with cranberries.
7. Gather in the overhanging filo pastry, adding more layers to cover centre.
8. Russe up pastry, brush with butter and bake at 180°C for 35 minutes approximately.

This recipe was contributed by Gary Thompson.

94 Ravioli stuffed with spinach and cumin served with lemon sauce

	4 portions	10 portions
pasta dough	200 g	500 g
Filling		
butter	25 g	75 g
garlic cloves, crushed	1	3
cumin seeds	1 tsp	2½ tsp
salt, pepper, nutmeg		
spinach, chopped	250 g	625 g
ricotta	100 g	250 g
Parmesan, grated	1 tbsp	2½ tbsp
olive oil	1 tbsp	2½ tbsp
Lemon sauce		
unsalted butter	175 g	500 g
garlic, crushed	1	2
vegetable stock	100 ml	250 ml
lemon zest and juice	1	2
parsley, chopped	1 tbsp	2 tbsp

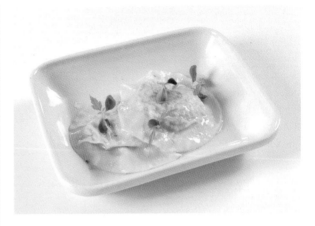

1. Prepare the ravioli filling: heat the butter in a suitable pan with the garlic and cumin seeds.
2. Add the spices to taste, heat for 30 seconds.
3. Add the spinach and cook over a low heat for 3–4 minutes.
4. Place filling in a bowl, and allow to cool.
5. Add the ricotta and Parmesan. Mix well. Season with salt, pepper and nutmeg.
6. Roll out the pasta dough and prepare the ravioli. The sheets of ravioli should be rolled out on a lightly dusted surface of semolina. Brush the dough with water, place on pieces of filling in rows 5 cm apart. Cover with a second sheet and cut into squares with a pasta wheel or sharp knife. Press down the edges well to seal the dough. Place the ravioli squares on a tray dusted with semolina.
7. Cook the ravioli in boiling salted water for 2–3 minutes, remove and drain well on a cloth.
8. Place ravioli onto plates, drizzle with olive oil, keep warm.

9. For the sauce, melt the butter with the garlic in a pan, add the stock, bring to the boil. Simmer for 5 minutes.
10. Add the lemon juice and zest. Season.
11. Pour sauce over ravioli, serve garnished with julienne of zest of lemon and flat parsley. Alternatively, garnish with basil leaves and add a little chopped basil to the lemon sauce.

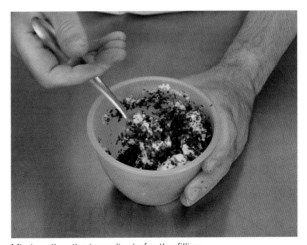

Mix together the ingredients for the filling

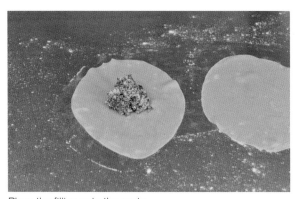

Place the filling onto the pasta

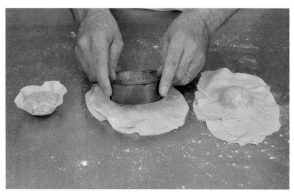

Trim the ravioli

95 Tagliatelle Arrabiata

energy	kcal	fat	sat fat	carb	sugar	protein	fibre
988 KJ	233 cal	4.0 g	0.4 g	44.3 g	7.4 g	7.9 g	2.9 g

	4 portions	10 portions
dried tagliatelle	200 g	500 g
olive oil	1 tbsp	2½ tbsp
onion, peeled and finely chopped	25 g	60 g
garlic cloves, peeled and finely chopped	2	4
red chilli, finely chopped	1	2
white wine	100 ml	250 ml
tomato purée	30 g	75 g
pomodorino cherry tomatoes	400 g	1 kg
salt and freshly ground black pepper		

1. Half fill a large saucepan with water. Season with salt and bring to the boil.
2. Cook the tagliatelle in the salted water as per the packet instructions.
3. In a medium saucepan, heat the oil.
4. Sauté the onion for 2 minutes, to soften. Stir in the garlic and chilli.
5. Pour in the wine, bring to the boil and cook off for 2 minutes.
6. Stir in the tomato purée and tomatoes, and bring the mixture to simmering point.
7. Simmer for 8–10 minutes. Season.
8. Drain the pasta and stir it into the sauce.

96 Textured vegetable protein lasagne

	4 portions	10 portions
textured vegetable protein (TVP)	100 g	250 g
cold water	280 ml	700 ml
carrots, finely diced	75 g	180 g
celery, finely diced	75 g	180 g
mushrooms, finely diced	75 g	180 g
courgettes, finely diced	75 g	180 g
parsnips, finely diced	75 g	180 g
onion, finely chopped	50 g	125 g
vegetable oil	2 tsp	5 tbsp
plum tomatoes, chopped	400 g	1 kilo
fresh oregano, chopped	1 tsp	2½ tsp
lasagne sheets, cooked	8–10	20–25
cheese sauce	600 ml	1½ litres
cheddar or Parmesan, grated		

1. Soak the TVP in cold water for 10 minutes, then drain.
2. Sweat the vegetables in the oil until tender without colour.
3. Add the tomatoes and oregano and simmer for 10 minutes. Season.
4. Lightly grease a suitable dish. Arrange the lasagne sheets in the dish, with the vegetable mix and cheese sauce. Finish with the cheese sauce.
5. Sprinkle with cheddar cheese or Parmesan and finish in an oven at 180°C for 20 minutes, until brown.

97 Vegetable curry using textured vegetable protein

	4 portions	10 portions
textured vegetable protein (TVP) chunks	100 g	250 g
vegetable stock	500 ml	1¼ litres
onion, finely chopped	50 g	125 g
garlic, crushed and chopped	2	5
vegetable oil	2 tbsp	5 tbsp
curry powder	1 tbsp	2½ tbsp
garam masala	¼ tsp	¾ tsp
fresh ginger, grated	½ tsp	1¼ tsp
cooking apple, peeled and finely chopped	75 g	180 g
carrots, cut into ½ cm dice	50 g	125 g
celery, cut into ½ cm dice	50 g	125 g
mushrooms, sliced	100 g	250 g
plum tomatoes (canned are suitable in their juice)	400 g	1 kg
tomato purée	2 tsp	5 tsp
water or vegetable stock	280 ml	700 ml

1. Soak the TVP in the vegetable stock for 10 minutes. Drain.
2. Fry the onion and garlic in the vegetable oil until cooked and slightly coloured.
3. Add the TVP, curry powder, garam masala and ginger. Stir well.
4. Add the apple, carrot, celery, mushrooms, chopped tomatoes and tomato purée. Simmer for 2 minutes.
5. Add the water or vegetable stock. Simmer for approx. 15–20 minutes.

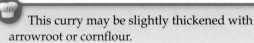 This curry may be slightly thickened with arrowroot or cornflour.

98 Tomato and lentil dahl with roasted almonds

	4 portions	10 portions
vegetable oil	2 tbsp	5 tbsp
butter or margarine	25 g	60 g
onions, finely chopped	50 g	125 g
carrots, finely chopped	1	2
garlic cloves	3	7
cumin seeds, crushed and chopped	2 tsp	5 tsp
yellow mustard seeds	2 tsp	5 tsp
grated root ginger	1 tsp	2½ tsp
ground turmeric	2 tsp	5 tsp
chilli powder	1 tsp	2½ tsp
garam masala	1 tsp	2½ tsp
red lentils	200 g	500 g
water	400 ml	1 litre
coconut milk	400 ml	1 litre
tomatoes, peeled, deseeded and finely diced	5	12
seasoning		
lime juice	2 limes	5 limes
coriander, fresh, chopped	4 tbsp	10 tbsp
almonds, flaked	50 g	125 g

1. Heat the oil and butter in a suitable saucepan. Add the onion and sweat for 5 minutes without colour. Add the carrot, garlic, cumin and mustard seeds, and ginger. Cook for a further five minutes.
2. Stir in the ground turmeric, chilli powder and garam masala and cook for 1 minute. Stir well.
3. Add the lentils, water, coconut milk and tomatoes. Season and bring to the boil. Simmer for approximately 45 minutes, stirring occasionally.
4. Stir in the lime juice and fresh coriander. Cook for a further 15 minutes until the lentils are tender.
5. Serve sprinkled with coriander and flaked almonds.

99 Honey-roasted vegetables with cracked wheat

energy	kcal	fat	sat fat	carb	sugar	protein	fibre
2166 KJ	517 cal	13.4 g	1.8 g	92.4 g	25.8 g	11.4 g	6.1 g

	4 portions	10 portions
sweet potatoes, peeled	2	5
onions, red	2	5
red peppers	1	3
yellow peppers	1	3
courgettes	2	5
olive oil	2 tbsp	5 tbsp
clear honey	2 tbsp	5 tbsp
salt and black pepper		
cinnamon stick	1	3
Cracked wheat		
cracked bulgar wheat	250 g	625 g
olive oil	2 tbsp	5 tbsp
lemon zest, grated	1	3
ground cumin	3 tsp	8 tsp
garlic, crushed and chopped	2	5

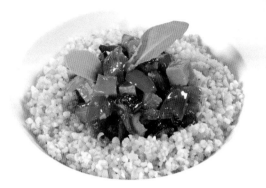

1. Prepare the vegetables. Cut the sweet potatoes into 2 cm dice and cut the red onions into wedges to match the sweet potato size. Deseed the peppers and cut into 2 cm squares. Cut the courgettes into 1 cm slices.
2. Place the vegetables in a roasting tin. Sprinkle with oil and add 1 tablespoon of honey.
3. Season with salt and black pepper and add the cinnamon stick. Roast in oven at 200°C for approximately 12–15 minutes. The vegetables should not be over-cooked, they should remain crisp.
4. Drizzle with the remaining honey, then place back in the oven for a few minutes.
5. Soak the cracked wheat in boiling water for a few minutes, then drain.
6. In a suitable pan, heat the oil, add the grated lemon zest, sweat for 2 minutes. Add the cumin and garlic and fry for 30 seconds.
7. Stir in the cracked wheat and fry for 1–2 minutes. Season.
8. Place the cracked wheat in a serving dish with the roasted vegetables in the centre.

100 Bulgur wheat and lentil pilaff

	4 portions	10 portions
green lentils	100 g	250 g
bulgur wheat	100 g	250 g
coriander, ground	1 tsp	2½ tsp
cinnamon, ground	1 tsp	2½ tsp
olive oil	1 tbsp	2½ tbsp
streaky bacon, finely chopped	200 g	500 g
onion, finely chopped	50 g	125 g
garlic clove, finely chopped	1	3
cumin seeds	1 tsp	2½ tsp
salt and pepper		
parsley, finely chopped	2 tbsp	5 tbsp

1. Soak the lentils in cold water for 1 hour. Soak the bulgur wheat in boiling water for 15–20 minutes. Drain both.
2. Place the lentils in a saucepan with the coriander and cinnamon and approximately half of the water – enough to cover the lentils. Bring to the boil and simmer until the lentils are cooked and the liquid has been absorbed.
3. Heat the olive oil in a pan and fry the bacon until crisp. Remove and drain.
4. Add the onion and garlic to the pan. Add a little more oil if required and sweat for approximately 10 minutes until the onion is slightly brown.
5. Stir in the cumin seeds and cook for 1 minute. Return the bacon to the pan.
6. Stir the drained bulgur wheat into the cooked lentils, then add the mixture to the frying pan. Season with salt and pepper, stir in the parsley and serve.

In this chapter you have learned to:

1. produce starters, main courses, accompaniments and garnishes suitable for vegetarians.

2. prepare vegetables to accompany meat and fish.

3. understand vegetables and their cooking.

5 Meat

This chapter covers Unit 305: Advanced Skills and Techniques in Producing Meat Dishes.

In this chapter you will learn to:

1. Prepare meat, cuts, joints and associated products
2. Produce starters, main courses, accompaniments and garnishes.

Composition

Meat is a natural and therefore not a uniform product, varying in quality from carcass to carcass, while flavour, texture and appearance are determined by the type of animal and the way it has been fed. There is no reason to think that flavour is obtained only in meat that possesses a proportion of fat, although fat does give a characteristic flavour to meat and helps to keep it moist during roasting. Neither is the colour of meat any guide to quality. Consumers are inclined to choose light-coloured meat – bright red beef, for example – because they think that it will be fresher than an alternative dark-red piece. Freshly butchered beef is bright red because the pigment in the tissues, myoglobin, has been chemically affected by the oxygen in the air. After several hours, the colour changes to dark red or brown as the pigment is further oxidised to become metamyoglobin. The colour of fat can vary from almost pure white in lamb, to bright yellow in beef. Colour depends on the feed, on the breed and, to a certain extent, on the time of year.

Tenderness and quality

The most useful guide to tenderness and quality is a knowledge of the cuts of meat and their location on the carcass. The various cuts are described under their respective headings, but in principle:

- The leanest and tenderest cuts – the 'prime' cuts – come from the hindquarters.
- The 'coarse' cuts, or meat from the neck, legs and forequarters, those parts of the animal that have had plenty of muscular exercise and where fibres have become hardened, provide meat for braising and stewing.

Many consider these coarse cuts to have more flavour, although they require slow cooking to make them tender. The meat from young animals is generally more tender and since tenderness is a prime factor, animals may be injected before slaughter with an enzyme, such as papin, which softens the fibres and muscles. This merely speeds up a natural and more satisfactory process: meat contains its own proteolytic enzymes, which gradually break down the protein cell walls as the carcass ages; that is why meat is hung for 10–20 days in controlled conditions of temperature and humidity before being offered for sale. Meat that is aged longer becomes more expensive as the cost of refrigeration is high and the meat itself shrinks because of evaporation and the trimming of the outside hardened edges.

Carcass electrical stimulation

Electrical stimulation is widely used to improve the tenderness of beef and lamb; it may also be used on other meats. Electrical stimulation causes the muscle in the carcass to contract violently. The muscle converts to meat more quickly, the pH level drops faster and rigor mortis sets in sooner than in an unstimulated carcass.

This technique may improve the appearance and colour of meat as well as the tenderness. It protects against cold shortening. The quality characteristics of the meat (such as bright red muscle colour, muscle firmness and marbling) develop more quickly. Beef that is electrically stimulated does not need to be aged for as long as other beef.

Cooking

Meat is an extremely versatile product that can be cooked in a multitude of ways, and matched with practically any vegetable, fruit and herb. The cut (shin, steak, brisket), the method of heating (roasting, braising, grilling), and the time and temperature all affect the way the meat will taste. Raw meat is difficult to chew because the muscle fibre contains an elastic protein (collagen), which is softened only by mincing – as in steak tartare – or by cooking. When you cook meat, the protein gradually coagulates as the internal temperature increases. At 69°C coagulation is complete, the protein begins to harden and further cooking makes the meat tougher.

Time and temperature

Since tenderness combined with flavour is the aim in meat cookery, much depends on the ratio of time and temperature. In principle, slow cooking retains the juices and produces a more tender result than does fast cooking at high temperatures. There are, of course, occasions when high temperatures are essential: for instance, you need to grill a steak under a hot flame for a very limited time in order to obtain a crisp, brown surface and a pink, juicy interior – using a low temperature would not give you the desired result.

But in potentially tough cuts such as breast or where there is a quantity of connective tissue (neck of lamb), a slow rate of cooking converts the tissues to gelatine and helps to make the meat more tender. Meat containing bone will take longer to cook because bone is a poor conductor of heat. Tough or coarse cuts of meat should be cooked by braising, pot roasting or stewing.

Marinating and searing

Marinating in a suitable marinade, such as wine and wine vinegar, helps to tenderise the meat and imparts an additional flavour. *Searing* meat in hot fat or in a hot oven before roasting or stewing helps to produce a crisp exterior by coagulating the protein but does not, as is widely supposed, seal in the juices. However, if the external temperature is too high and cooking prolonged, rapid evaporation and contraction of the meat will cause considerable loss of juices and fat. Salt sprinkled on meat before cooking will also hasten loss of moisture since salt is hygroscopic and absorbs water.

Elastin and collagen

To take this one step further, when fibrous proteins are heated they contract and squeeze out the associated water. For example, when a steak is cooked the proteins contract, therefore squeezing out all the water/juices. If the heat is increased or continues, the steak will then become dry and, consequently, the eating quality will be impaired. Cuts of meat also contain *elastin* and *collagen*: elastin (the muscle group associated with tendons and arteries) is extremely stretchy and further cooking adds to its strength; collagen (the main muscle proteins, which amount to the highest proportion of mass in the muscle) is rather tough and chewy. Meat that has a higher proportion of both, usually from the major and highly worked muscle groups, would not be suitable for prime cooking. However, these cuts of meat may be cooked for longer at the correct temperature (braising), dissolving the collagen as it is water soluble, forming gelatine and offering a tasty joint of meat.

Prime cuts

Prime cuts, such as beef fillets, have little collagen in their make-up (approximately 3 per cent) and do not require long cooking to tenderise the joint. Although most chefs would adopt a high temperature for a short period on the prime cuts, this does not always yield a perfect result. Due to the lack of fat and collagen in such cuts of meat, high heat will render the muscle fibres dry and, consequently, the eating quality is impaired. A lower temperature and longer in the oven will produce a gradual heat, therefore there is less extreme coagulation in the tissues and less fluid will have been squeezed out in the process.

To put this theory into simple terms – traditionally, when cooking meat, a fillet steak (for example) would be sealed in hot oil (180°C to 200°C or even hotter) and then the heat would be reduced slightly to finish the cooking. The process that takes place is one of (to put it scientifically) 'thermal energy' or molecular conduction: the first layer of molecules heating the next, and so on, until the desired degree of cooking is achieved at the core (rare, medium, etc.). To achieve a core temperature of 55°C to 60°C, 25 per cent of the meat would be overcooked. Therefore, if the temperature was to be reduced to a constant 59°C (just before the protein collapses) and the meat cooked for longer, adopting the molecular conduction theory, more than 95 per cent of the meat would be perfectly cooked.

The *Maillard* reaction

When cooking meats at low temperatures there is one obvious flaw: the meat will not be exposed to the high cooking temperatures that develop that beautiful roasted flavour. This chemical reaction of browning is called the *Maillard* reaction and is an extremely complicated chain of reactions that involves carbons, proteins, sulphurs, etc. One thing we do know about this reaction is that at 140°C and above, you will start to release the wonderful roasted meat flavours. Therefore, when slow-cooking meats they will need to be started very quickly on a hot pan on the stove to initiate this Maillard reaction in the meat and give the meat a roasted flavour. In some cases you will need to quickly return the meat to the pan to re-caramelise the outside; alternatively, if the joint is dense and large, remove from the low oven and increase the temperature to 190 to 200°C. When the oven is up to temperature, return the joint to it for a short while to crisp up the outside. The density of the meat and size of the joint will ensure that there will be very little secondary cooking or residual heat left to cook through to the core.

Basting and braising

The collagen that makes up connective tissue requires long cooking at moderate temperature to render it supple in the mouth and to be converted into gelatine (a form of secondary/internal basting). When basting, care should be taken not to destroy the secondary basting properties of the collagen as at temperatures above 88°C the collagen will dissolve rapidly into the braising medium, impairing the eating quality. As cooking methods and understanding of meats develop, we now know more about the effect that heat has on the make-up of meat. Therefore, the traditional braising method of bringing the casserole to a simmer and placing it in the oven at 140°C could, in theory, render the structure of the meat dry due to the fact that at 88°C collagen rapidly dissolves into the cooking medium, yielding a beautifully gelatinous and well-flavoured sauce, and making the eating quality of the meat dry and tough.

To modernise the braising approach the cooking medium would need to be at between 80°C and 85°C; this is best controlled on the top of the stove. Alternatively, set your oven at 90°C (approximately), checking the cooking medium once in a while.

Pay constant attention

All the techniques above, which are used to slow-cook prime, secondary and highly worked muscle groups, are very controlled and accurate, and rely on constant attention to ensure that they are not rapidly cooking, and that they are in fact actually cooking, if cooking at low temperatures. The general rule of thumb is: the more collagen, the higher the temperature needed to enable the collagen to dissolve, forming gelatine that will then in turn baste the meat and offer a perfectly braised and moist piece of meat.

When slow-cooking prime joints, the rule of thumb is to reduce the temperature of cooking as, in some cases, shrinkage can occur from 59°C ranging up to 65°C for sirloin of beef.

Sirloin of beef obviously has more collagen than fillet (it is essentially a worked muscle group) and is generally cooked on a high heat, either roasted or pan-fried. To adopt the above method, you can render the sirloin extremely tender, full of moisture, with a roasted outer and the flavoursome roasted meat taste that is craved. An average sirloin joint for roasting can weigh from 2 to 5 kg whole off the bone. The method is to seal the meat on the outside, as you would normally, place into a pre-heated oven at 180°C, cook at 180°C for 10 minutes, then reduce the temperature to 64°C (the oven door will need to be open at this stage). Once the oven has come down to 64°C, close the door and cook for a further 1 hour 50 minutes. This will give you an extremely tender piece of sirloin.

Degree of cooking

This is not a sure-fire rule to find out how well cooked the meat is, but it can certainly help those who do not cook meat on a regular basis. First, open the hand you do not write with, with your palm facing towards you, then using little pressure touch your thumb with your little finger; next, with the first finger of your strongest hand touch the muscle under the thumb – this is the feeling you should look for when you require well-done meat. Follow this technique through the fingers, as follows, according to the degree of cooking you require:

- Little finger – well done – 72–78°C
- Next finger – medium to well – 64–70°C
- Middle finger – medium – 60–64°C
- Forefinger – rare to medium – 58–59°C.

Use of a heat probe will ensure greater accuracy.

Carving

- Before cooking: remove any bones, sinew or gristle from meat joints that may hinder carving; tie securely to retain shape; remove wishbones from poultry.
- When cooked: if to be served hot, allow to rest for 15 minutes before carving; if served cold, ideally cook on the same day as required to keep meat or poultry moist and succulent, and to eliminate the need for refrigeration.
- Keep carving knives sharp and use sharpening steel frequently to keep a good edge on the blade, ensuring that the blade is wiped clean after each use of the steel.
- When carving joints of meat, carve across the grain, with the exception of saddle of lamb or mutton.

Preservation

Salting

Meat can be pickled in brine; this method of preservation may be applied to silverside, brisket and ox tongues. Salting is used in the production of bacon, before the sides of pork are smoked, and for hams.

Chilling

This means that meat is kept at a temperature just above freezing point in a controlled atmosphere. Chilled meat cannot be kept in the usual type of cold room for more than a few days, sufficient time for the meat to hang, enabling it to become tender.

Freezing

Small carcasses, such as lamb and mutton, can be frozen; their quality is not affected by freezing. They can be kept frozen until required and then thawed out before being used. Some beef is frozen, but it is inferior in quality to chilled beef.

Canning

Large quantities of meat are canned; corned beef is worth mentioning here since it has a very high protein content. Pork is used for tinned luncheon meat.

Types of meat

Beef

The cuts of beef vary considerably, from the very tender fillet steak to the tough brisket or the shin, and there is a greater variety of cuts in beef than in any other type of meat. While their names may vary, there are 14 primary cuts from a side of beef, each one composed of muscle, fat, bone and connective tissue. The least developed muscles, usually from the inner areas, can be roasted or grilled, while leaner and more sinewy meat is cut from the more highly developed external muscles. Exceptions are rib and loin cuts, which come from external but basically immobile muscles.

Knowing where the cuts come from helps to designate the cooking method.

Fillet

Taken from the back of the animal, this is the tenderest part, cut from the centre of the sirloin. It is usually cut into steaks and can be fried or grilled.

Sirloin

A boneless steak, which is more tender than rump, but not as tender as fillet. It is suitable for grilling or frying.

Rump

A good-quality cut, though it is less tender than fillet or sirloin. It is suitable for grilling or frying.

Rib

Sold on the bone or unboned and rolled, it is suitable for roasting.

Topside

A lean, tender cut from the hindquarters, it is suitable for braising or pot roasting.

Silverside

Taken from the hindquarters, this is a cut from the round. It can be pot roasted, used for traditional boiled beef or cured for Bresaola (see recipe 40).

Flank

A boneless cut from the mid-to-hindquarters; suitable for braising or stewing.

Skirt

A boneless rather gristly cut. It is usually stewed or made into mince.

Brisket

A cut from the fore end of the animal, below the shoulder. Quite a fatty joint, it is sold on or off the bone or salted. It is suitable for slow roasting.

Lamb and mutton

Lamb is the meat from a sheep under a year old; above that age the animal is called a 'hogget', and its meat becomes mutton. The demand for lamb in preference to mutton is partly due to the fact that the lamb carcass provides smaller cuts of more tender meat. Mutton needs to be well ripened by long hanging before cooking and, as it is usually fatty, needs a good deal of trimming as well.

Good-quality lamb should have a fine, white fat, with pink flesh where freshly cut; in mutton the flesh is a deeper colour. Lamb has a very thin, parchment-like covering on the carcass, known as the 'fell', which is usually left on roasts to help them maintain their shape during cooking. It should, however, be removed from chops. The flesh of a younger lamb is usually more tender. A good way to judge age is through weight – especially with legs of lamb: the highest quality weighs about 2.3 kg and never more than 4 kg. Smaller chops are also more tender and, therefore, more expensive.

Mutton remains less popular than lamb, but a number of organisations are trying to promote it as a less expensive and more cost-effective meat than lamb.

Best end
A small joint sold with bone. It is suitable for roasting.

Cutlets
Best end of neck divided between the bones. They can be grilled or sautéed.

Loin chop
This contains part of the back bone and is suitable for grilling, frying or braising.

Chump chop
Cut from between leg and loin, it is grilled or fried.

Leg
A tender cut, often divided into fillet and shank. It is sold on the bone for roasting or boned for casseroles.

Shoulder
Sold on the bone, it has quite a lot of fat. It can be roasted whole or boned and rolled, or cut up for kebabs or casseroles.

Breast
A cut that contains quite a lot of fat. It is usually sold boned for stuffing and slow roasting.

Scrag end
Bony and fatty, it is usually used for stews.

Riblets
Breast meat on the bone that has been separated between the ribs. It is usually cooked in liquid.

Neck fillets
Used for stews and braising (e.g. hot pots).

Pork

Pork is the culinary name for meat from the farmed domestic pig. For the majority of the pork market pigs are slaughtered when they are 5 to10 months old (usually 6 months).

- The lean flesh of pork is usually pale pink. The fat should be white, firm and not excessive and the bones small, fine and pink.
- The skin/rind will depend on the breed.
- Suckling pigs weigh 5–9 kg and are roasted whole.
- Boars are wild or uncastrated male pigs.

Fillet
A boneless cut of lean meat from the hindquarters. It is suitable for grilling or frying.

Loin
A lean joint that sometimes includes the kidney. It is suitable for roasting.

Loin chop
Taken from the hind loin, it is suitable for grilling or frying.

Chump
Available on or off the bone from the hind loin, it is suitable for roasting.

Leg
The hind leg, usually roasted.

Shoulder
A tender fore end cut that is available boned or on the bone. It is used for casseroles and kebabs.

Spare rib
Taken from the fore end of the animal, it is sold whole or as spare rib chops. It is suitable for roasting, grilling or frying.

Belly

This generally yields bacon, but is sometimes sold fresh and used in sausage-making; otherwise it is grilled or baked.

Hock

A small bony cut from the hindquarters. It is stewed or used for soups.

Ribs

Rib bones taken from the underside; they are used for barbecuing.

Restrictions on pork

Pork is a banned meat in some cultures and religions (e.g. Muslims and Jews).

Some consider pig meat to be unclean and will not eat it. Certainly in some hotter climates it used to be considered a health hazard and this has become part of their culture.

However some nations have long held pork in esteem as a tender, prime meat.

Veal

Veal is the meat from dairy calves, usually slaughtered at 3 months of age. Today this meat is in short supply – due to more efficient dairy production from fewer animals – and expensive, with ethical values now playing a part in the buying market.

Unlike beef, veal can be judged by the colour of the meat. The whiter it is, the greater proportion of the calf's diet has been milk and the more likely the meat is to be tender with a delicate flavour.

Fillet

A boneless cut from the hindquarters. Sometimes sold for roasting but more often sliced into escalopes.

Loin

A cut from the back of the animal that is available on the bone or boned and rolled. It can be roasted.

Veal chops

These are taken from the loin and have the bone in them. They may be grilled or fried.

Best end

A cut that is suitable for roasting, braising or stewing.

Leg

A prime cut that is usually roasted.

Knuckle

This is the end of the leg. It is a bony cut and is used for boiling and stewing (e.g. osso bucco).

Shoulder

This can be boned and rolled for roasting, but is usually cut up for stews and pies.

Use of bones in cooking

Meat bones are useful for giving flavour to soups and stocks, especially beef ones with plenty of marrow. Veal bones are gelatinous and help to enrich and thicken soups and sauces. Fat can be rendered down for frying, or used as an ingredient when suet or lard is called for.

Offal and other edible parts of the carcass

Offal is the name given to the edible parts taken from the inside of a carcass of meat: liver, kidneys, heart and sweetbreads. Tripe, brains, tongue, head and oxtail are also sometimes included under this term.

Fresh offal (unfrozen) should be purchased as required and can be refrigerated under hygienic conditions at a temperature of 1–4°C, at a relative humidity of 90 per cent for up to seven days. Frozen offal must be kept in a deep freeze and defrosted in a refrigerator as required.

Liver

Liver is a good source of protein and iron, and also contains vitamins A and D. It is low in fat.

Quality points:
- Liver should look fresh, moist and smooth, with a pleasant colour and no unpleasant smell.
- Liver should not be dry or contain an excessive number of tubes.

Calf's liver

Is considered the best in terms of tenderness and flavour. It is also the most expensive.

Lamb's liver

Is mild in flavour, light in colour and tender. Sheep's liver, being from an older animal, is firmer in substance, deeper in colour and has a stronger flavour.

Ox or beef liver

Is the cheapest and, if taken from an older animal, can be coarse in texture and strong in flavour. It is usually braised.

Pig's liver

Has a strong, full flavour and is used mainly for pâté recipes.

Kidneys

The nutritional value of kidneys is similar to that of liver.

Quality points:

- Suet – the saturated fat in which kidneys are encased – should be left on otherwise the kidneys will dry out. The suet should be removed when kidneys are being prepared for cooking; the butcher will remove it before delivery.
- Both suet and kidneys should be moist and have no unpleasant smell.

Lamb's kidneys

Are light in colour, delicate in flavour and ideal for grilling and frying.

Sheep's kidneys

Are darker in colour and stronger in flavour.

Calf's kidneys

Are light in colour, delicate in flavour and used in a variety of dishes.

Ox kidney

Is dark in colour, strong in flavour, and is either braised or used in pies and puddings (mixed with beef).

Pig's kidneys

Are smooth, long and flat and have a strong flavour.

Sweetbreads

Sweetbreads are the pancreas and thymus glands, known as heart breads and neck. The heart bread is round, plump and of better quality than the neck bread, which is long and uneven in shape. Calf's heart bread, considered the best, weighs up to 600 g, lamb's heart bread up to 100 g.

Sweetbreads are an easily digested source of protein, which makes them valuable for use in invalid diets.

Quality points:

- Heart and neck breads should be fleshy and of good size.
- They should be creamy white in colour and have no unpleasant smell.

Tongues

Ox tongues, lamb and sheep tongues are those most used in cooking. Ox tongues are usually salted then soaked before being cooked.

Quality points:

- Tongues must be fresh and have no unpleasant smell.
- There should not be an excess of waste at the root end.

Oxtail

Oxtails usually weigh 1½–2 kg; they should be lean with not too much fat. There should be no sign of stickiness and no unpleasant smell.

Preparing a saddle of lamb

The saddle may be divided as follows.

Remove skin, starting from head to tail and from breast to back, and split down the centre of the back bone to produce two loins. Each loin can be roasted whole, boned and stuffed, or cut into loin and chump chops.

Preparing saddle for roasting (see recipe 11):

1. Skin and remove the kidney.
2. Trim the excess fat and sinew.
3. Cut off the flaps, leaving about 15 cm each side so as to meet in the middle under the saddle.
4. Remove the aitch, or pelvic bone.
5. Score neatly and tie with string.
6. For presentation the tail may be left on, protected with paper and tied back.
7. The saddle can also be completely boned, stuffed and tied.

1 Stock-reduced base sauce

	Makes 4 litres
veal bones, chopped	4 kg
calves' feet, split lengthways	2
carrots	400 g
onions	200 g
celery	100 g
tomatoes, quartered	1 kg
mushrooms, chopped	200 g
large bouquet garni	1
unpeeled cloves of garlic (optional)	4

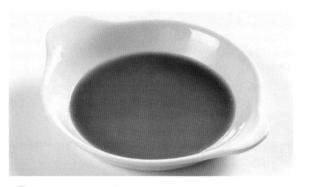

1. Brown the bones and calves' feet in a roasting tray in the oven.
2. Place the browned bones in a stock pot, cover with cold water and bring to simmering point.
3. Using the same roasting tray and the fat from the bones, brown off the carrots, onions and celery.
4. Drain off the fat, add the vegetables to the stock and deglaze the tray.
5. Add the remainder of the ingredients, simmer gently for 4–5 hours. Skim frequently.
6. Strain the stock into a clean pan and reduce until a light consistency is achieved.

i Most establishments have stopped using traditional espagnole and demi-glace as the basis for brown sauces. Instead rich, well-flavoured brown stocks of veal, chicken, etc., are reduced until the lightest form of natural thickening from the ingredients is achieved.

No flour is used in the thickening process and consequently a lighter-textured sauce is produced.

Take care when reducing this type of sauce so that the end product is not too strong or bitter.

2 Lamb jus (meat base)

	Makes 2 litres
thyme	bunch
bay leaves, fresh	4
garlic	2 bulbs
red wine	1 litre
lamb bones	20 kg
veal bones	10 kg
white onions, peeled	6
large carrots, peeled	8
celery sticks	7
leeks	4
tomato purée	6 tbsp

1. Pre-heat the oven to 175°C. Place the herbs, garlic and the wine in a large, deep container. Place all the bones onto a roasting rack on top of the container of herbs and wine, and roast in the oven for 50–60 minutes. When the bones are completely roasted and have taken on a dark golden-brown appearance, remove from oven.
2. Place all the ingredients in a large pot and cover with cold water. Put the pot onto the heat and bring to the simmer; immediately skim all fat that rises to the surface.
3. Turn the heat off and allow the bones and vegetables to sink. Once this has happened, turn the heat back on and bring to just under a simmer, making as little movement as possible to create more of an infusion than a stock.

4. Skim continuously. Leave to simmer (infuse) for 12 hours then pass through a fine sieve into a clean pan and reduce down rapidly, until you have about 1.5 litres remaining.

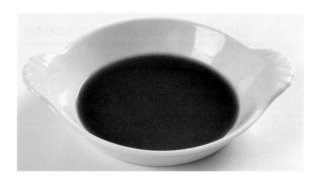

3 Sauce Colbert

	Makes approx. 650 ml
water	8–9 tbsp
vinegar	2 tbsp
cracked pepper	pinch
fine salt	pinch
white wine	100 g
egg yolks	5
butter, melted and warm	500 g
reduced brown stock or meat glaze, warmed	30 g

1. Place 4 tablespoons of water, the vinegar, cracked pepper and fine salt in a saucepan and reduce by two-thirds.

2. In a separate pan, reduce the white wine to 20 g by boiling it over a moderate heat.

3. Place the saucepan over a double boiler. Add 1 tablespoon of water and the egg yolks. Gradually whisk in the butter, a little at a time, interspersing it with 3 to 4 tablespoons more water, to make a light sauce.

4. Once the sauce is nicely thickened, whisk in the reduced white wine, and then blend in the reduced stock until rich and smooth.

4 Serving of cold cooked meats

Roast the meats and allow them to cool quickly, directly from the oven either at ambient temperature or by blast chilling. In this way the meat is cool and succulent for eating.

Cold cooked meat should be sliced as near to serving time as possible, and arranged neatly on a dish. Finely diced or chopped aspic may be placed around the edge. It may be decorated with a bunch of picked watercress or presented in the piece with 3 or 4 slices cut.

Whole joints, particularly ribs of beef, are often placed on a buffet table. They should either be boned or have any bones that may hinder carving removed before being cooked. They should be trimmed if necessary, strings removed and, after glazing with aspic jelly or brushing with oil, dressed on a dish garnished with watercress; lettuce leaves and fancy-cut pieces of tomato may also be used to garnish the dish.

Fillet of beef Wellington and roast suckling pig are popular cold buffet dishes.

5 Pâtés and terrines

Pâtés and terrines are similar, the difference being the actual cooking and the receptacle in which they are cooked.

The filling consists of a forcemeat, prepared from the required meat, poultry or game, well seasoned with herbs, spices and any other garnish that may be relevant.

1. To make a pâté en croute, line a raised pie mould with pie pastry (recipe 6), then with thin slices of larding bacon.

2. Add the forcemeat with the garnish in between layers until the mould is full, the last layer being forcemeat.

3. Cover the top with larding bacon and pie pastry, neatly decorated.

4. Make one or more holes, 1 cm, in the top and insert short, oiled, stiff-paper funnels to enable steam to escape during cooking.

5. Egg wash the top 2–3 times and bake for 1¼–1½ hours at 190°C.

6. When cold, fill the pie through the holes in the top with a well-flavoured aspic jelly or a flavour to suit the pie.

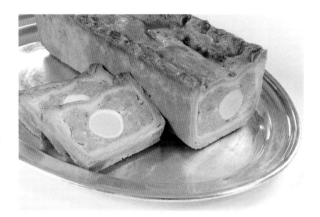

6   Pie pastry

	4 portions	10 portions
flour	400 g	1¼ kg
salt		
butter or margarine	100 g	250 g
lard	100 g	250 g
egg	1	2–3
water	125 ml	300 ml

1. Sieve the flour and salt.
2. Rub in the fat.
3. Add beaten egg and water.
4. Mix well and allow to rest before using.

7   Quenelles using a panada

Quenelles are said to originate from Lyon in France. The word quenelle comes from the German *knodel* (dumpling).

Quenelles may be made with meat such as veal, or with chicken or fish.

	4 portions	10 portions
veal, chicken or fish fillets	100 g	250 g
unsalted butter	100 g	250 g
eggs	2	6
egg whites	1	2
milk	100 ml	250 ml
flour	120 g	300 g
seasoning		
nutmeg		
stock or water		

There are three important steps in preparing quenelles – making the panada, mixing the forcemeat and packing.

1. Bring the milk to the boil in a suitable saucepan. Add a quarter of the butter and the sieved flour, and beat vigorously until the mixture is thickened. Stir continuously until the panada is dried out. Allow the panada to cool.

2. Place the mixture in a basin over ice and add the egg whites. Mix well. Add the cooled panada and mix well.

3. Add the whole eggs and then the softened butter. Mix well and allow to cool.

4. Shape into a quenelle shape with two large spoons. Allow two quenelles per portion.

5. Bring the stock or water to the boil. Place the quenelles in the cooking liquor. Poach for approximately 10–15 minutes. When cooked, remove from the cooking liquor and drain.

6. Serve on suitable plates masked with an appropriate sauce such as prawn, lobster, crab, vermouth, supreme, white wine, rosé or mustard.

8 Quenelles using mousseline

Quenelles have a delicate consistency and subtle taste of meat or fish. This recipe may be made from meat, chicken or fish mousseline.

	4 portions	10 portions
veal, chicken or fish (e.g. pike, sole)	500 g	1¼ kg
egg whites	2	5
double cream	400 ml	1 litre
seasoning		
stock		

1. Purée the veal, chicken or fish in a food processor. Pass through a sieve.
2. Place the mixture in a bowl of ice and beat in the egg whites.
3. Gradually add the double cream. Season.
4. Mould the quenelles using two large spoons and gently poach in stock until cooked, approximately 10–15 minutes depending on the size. Shape into quenelles using two large tablespoons or serving spoons.
5. Serve with an appropriate sauce such as suprême sauce or white wine and mustard sauce. Fish quenelles may be served with prawn, lobster (see page 242) or white wine sauce.

9 Pojarski

A pojarski may be made from any white meat, e.g. veal, pork, chicken, pheasant or fish (pike, sole, salmon, bream, monkfish, cod, etc.).

	4 portions	10 portions
meat or fish	500 g	1¼ kg
butter	120 g	300 g
white breadcrumbs soaked in milk	120 g	300 g
seasoning		
eggs, beaten	1	2
vegetable oil for frying		

1. Mince or purée the meat in a food processor. Season. Add butter and mix well.
2. Add the breadcrumbs. Squeeze out excess milk and add the beaten egg.
3. Divide the mixture into equal portions. Shape into cutlets on breadcrumbs mixed with a little flour.
4. Shallow fry the cutlets in hot oil until cooked and coloured on both sides.
5. Serve on suitable plates with a suitable sauce such as prawn, lobster (see page 242), crab, suprême, white wine, mushroom or fresh tomato coulis.

Accompaniments

The pojarski may be garnished with asparagus, mushrooms or tomatoes.

They may be served on a bed of buttered or creamed spinach, creamed parsnip or buttered Jerusalem artichokes.

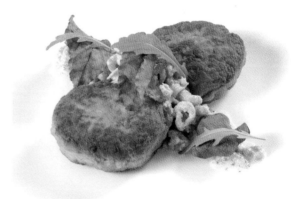

Pojarski made with pike

10 Pot roast chump of lamb with root vegetables

energy	kcal	fat	sat fat	carb	sugar	protein	fibre
3231 KJ	781 cal	66.1 g	37.7 g	24.4 g	16.7 g	23.7 g	6.3 g

*

	4 portions	10 portions
beef dripping	100 g	250 g
lamb chump, trimmed and boned	400 g	1 kg
small whole onions, peeled	400 g	1 kg
small carrots, peeled	400 g	1 kg
celery sticks, cut in three	400 g	1 kg
swede, peeled and cut into chunks	200 g	500 g
field mushrooms	100 g	250 g
hot stock	275 ml	700 ml
clarified butter	200 ml	500 ml
bay leaves	1	3
sprig of thyme		
butter	25 g	60 g
flour	25 g	60 g
seasoning		

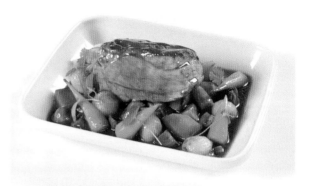

1. Pre-heat the oven to 140°C.
2. Melt the dripping in a thick cooking pot, and when it's hot put in the lamb and sear and brown it all over, then transfer it to a plate. Next, lightly brown the onions, carrots, celery and swede, and remove them temporarily to the plate.
3. Empty all the fat from the pot, then replace the lamb chump and arrange the vegetables and mushrooms around the meat. Add the hot stock, clarified butter, bay leaves and thyme, and a little salt and pepper. Cover with foil and a tightly fitting lid and, as soon as you hear simmering, place in the centre of the oven and leave for about 15 minutes.

4. When ready, place the meat and vegetables on a warmed serving dish, then skim off the fat. Bring the liquid to the boil and boil briskly until reduced slightly. Mix the butter and flour to a paste, then add this to the liquid and whisk until the sauce thickens. Serve with the meat and some sharp English mustard.

This method of cookery traps in flavour, keeps the meat moist and makes a sauce while doing so. The root vegetables in this will give the meat flavour, which makes them a suitable garnish with the lamb.

* Contains beef dripping, butter and clarified butter.

11 Slow-cooked saddle of lamb, braised cabbage and chocolate

energy	kcal	fat	sat fat	carb	sugar	protein	fibre
2677 KJ	641 cal	33.6 g	4.7 g	40.9 g	35.5 g	45.8 g	6.3 g

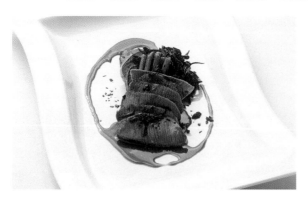

For the lamb

1. Crush the garlic and mix with the oil and thyme. Place the trimmed lamb loin in the oil and allow to infuse overnight.
2. Preheat the oven to 59°C. When ready to cook, drain off the oil and seal in a hot pan until all sides are golden (this should take no more than 1½ minutes). Then wrap in cling film and place in the preheated oven for a minimum of 35 minutes (the lamb will start to overcook after 60 minutes, so be mindful of this).

For the cabbage

1. Slice and sweat the red onions in a pan and put to one side.
2. Slice the red cabbage and add to the red onions in a pan along with the red wine, cinnamon, cassis and brown sugar.
3. Cover with tin foil and put in the oven at 150°C; check after 1 hour.
4. When cooked, strain off the liquor, reduce to a glaze and finish with the redcurrant jelly.
5. Mix the glaze into the cabbage and chill.

For the sauce

1. Remove the lamb from the oven and take off the cling film.
2. Heat a little oil in a non-stick pan and place the lamb saddles in for a short period, just to re-seal. This should take no more than 1 minute. Allow to rest for 2 minutes.
3. Meanwhile, reheat the lamb jus, and add the sherry vinegar (to taste) and the peas.

	4 portions	10 portions
Lamb		
garlic cloves	2	5
oil	50 ml	125 ml
sprig of thyme		
long saddle (boned, sinew and fat removed – eye of loin)	1	2
Cabbage		
red onions	2	5
head of red cabbage	½	1
red wine	500 ml	1¼ litres
stick cinnamon	½	1
cassis	150 ml	375 ml
brown sugar	50 g	125 g
redcurrant jelly	1 tbsp	2 tbsp
Sauce		
lamb jus	200 ml	500 ml
sherry vinegar	5 ml	12 ml
cooked peas	200 g	500 g
To finish		
good-quality dark chocolate, chopped into small pieces	75 g	200 g
cooked green beans	200 g	500 g
portion of sautéed potatoes		

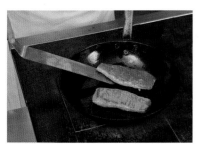

Seal the meat in a hot pan

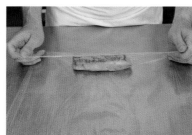

Wrap the meat in cling film

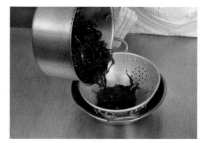

Strain the liquor from the cabbage

To finish

1. Place a mound of cabbage in the centre of the plate and top with buttered green beans.
2. Carve the lamb into equal portions and divide between the plates.
3. Pour over the sauce and finish with a sprinkling of chocolate around the plate and side orders of sautéed potatoes.

> The method of cookery here – slow-cooking at low temperature – permits you to use saddle of lamb instead of best end, giving you the same results in terms of tenderness and a deeper flavour from the lamb.

12 Slow-roast leg of lamb with minted couscous and buttered peas

	Up to 10 portions
Leg of lamb	
leg of lamb	1 (1.8–2 kg)
olive oil	3 tbsp
seasoning	
garlic cloves	4
rosemary	2 sprigs
butter	40 g
brown stock	300 ml
white wine	200 ml
Couscous	
light chicken stock	400 ml
olive oil	50 ml
salt	
cayenne pepper	
couscous	200 g
mint leaves, cut into julienne	3
lemon	½
Garnish	
fresh peas	400 g
butter	50 g
seasoning	

Slow-roast leg of lamb

1. Preheat the oven to 200°C.
2. Rub the leg of lamb with a little oil, salt and pepper.
3. Peel 3 cloves of garlic and cut in half lengthways. Make six incisions in the leg of lamb and insert a piece of garlic and a small piece of rosemary into each one.
4. Break up the rest of the garlic without peeling.
5. Place the lamb and the rest of the oil in a hot roasting tray that is on a medium heat. Sear over a medium heat until golden on all sides. Add the butter and remaining garlic and continue to heat until foaming.

6. Turn the oven down to 190°C. Place the lamb in the oven and cook for 15 minutes at this temperature.
7. Turn down the oven to 85°C and cook for a further 1 hour and 10 minutes.
8. Remove the lamb. Allow to rest and keep warm.
9. Meanwhile, return the roasting tray to the stove and scrape the tray with a spatula to lift the roasting sugars.
10. Add the stock and wine, bring to the boil, skim and reduce by half. Any juices that have run from the leg of lamb can be added to the roasting tray. Pass the sauce through a fine sieve and retain for serving.

Minted couscous

1. Bring the stock, oil, salt and cayenne pepper to the boil.
2. Place the couscous in a bowl and pour over the liquid. Cover tightly with cling film and leave for 5 minutes.
3. Remove the cling film and add a little more oil to help free the grains.
4. Add the mint into the mix and allow to infuse.
5. Finish with the squeezed lemon and check the seasoning.

To serve

1. Bring a pan of water to the boil. Add the peas and cook for 3 minutes until just cooked but still retaining their vibrant green colour.
2. Drain. Season and add a knob of butter. Toss well.
3. Place in a hot serving dish; the peas can be served communally.
4. Carve the lamb. Serve with a mound of couscous and a sauce boat of the fine roast gravy.

13 Slow-cooked shoulder of lamb with *boulangère* potatoes

	Up to 10 portions
Shoulder of lamb	
shoulder of lamb	1 (1.8–2 kg)
olive oil	3 tbsp
seasoning	
garlic cloves	4
rosemary	2 sprigs
butter	40 g
Boulangère potatoes	
butter	180 g
onions, sliced	2
bay leaves	2
paprika	1 tsp
russet or maris piper potatoes, peeled	1½ kg
lamb or chicken stock (amount depends on size of cooking dish)	400 ml
seasoning	
ground black pepper	

Shoulder of lamb

1. Preheat the oven to 200°C. Rub the shoulder of lamb with a little oil, salt and pepper.
2. Peel the garlic and cut in half lengthways. Make eight incisions in the shoulder of lamb and insert a piece of garlic and a small piece of rosemary into each one.
3. Place the lamb and the rest of the oil in a hot roasting tray. Sear the meat over a medium heat until golden on all sides. Add the butter and continue to heat until foaming.
4. Place in the oven and cook on 200°C for 20 minutes, then turn down the oven to 85°C and cook for a further 1 hour and 30 minutes.
5. Remove the lamb from the roasting tray. Continue to boil and add any juices that have run from the leg of lamb. When reduced by half, whisk in a knob of butter, then pass the sauce through a fine sieve. Serve with the lamb and vegetables.

Boulangère potatoes

1. Preheat oven to 180°C. Melt 60 g of butter in a sauté pan over a medium heat.
2. Add the onions, bay leaves and paprika. Sauté until translucent. Season lightly with salt and pepper. Remove onions and cool.
3. Slice the potatoes and place flat side down in a buttered and seasoned baking dish.
4. Top this with a thin layer of the onions. Repeat the layers until the potato and onion are depleted.
5. Pour in enough stock to cover the potatoes and onions two-thirds of the way up the dish.
6. Cover the top layer of potatoes with the remaining butter and mill some freshly ground pepper over the top.

To cook and finish

1. Once the potatoes are cooked (approx 50 minutes), check with the tip of a small knife. Turn down the oven to 140°C. Place the golden shoulder of lamb on a cooling wire suitable for the oven and place on top of the *boulangère* potatoes: this will allow excess juice from the meat to baste the potatoes.
2. Place in the oven and cook for 30 minutes.
3. Remove the lamb and allow to rest.
4. Turn the oven up to 200°C, allowing the potatoes to develop a golden top: this will take 10 minutes.
5. Meanwhile, when the lamb is well rested, carve, lay on the plates and serve with roast root vegetables, with the *boulangère* in the centre of the table.

Slow-cooked best end of lamb with lentils

	4 portions	10 portions
lamb stock	300 ml	1 litre
baby onions, cooked	200 g	500 g
tomato concasse	100 g	250 g
puy lentils, soaked overnight	50 g	120 g
bouquet garni		
small onion, peeled and halved	1	3
small carrot, peeled	1	3
sherry vinegar	30 ml	75 ml
butter	40 g	100 g
Savoy cabbage, cut into fine strips	100 g	240 g
whole best ends of lamb (8 bones each)	2	5
lemon thyme and parsley, chopped	2 tbsp	5 tbsp
olive oil	50 ml	120 ml
garlic mashed potato	350 g	1 kg
seasoning		

1. Have the lamb stock, cooked baby onions and tomato concasse ready. Boil the lamb stock until reduced by two-thirds. Set aside.
2. Drain the lentils, then place in a saucepan with the bouquet garni, onion and carrot. Cover with fresh water, bring to the boil, then turn down to a simmer and cook for about 15–20 minutes until just tender. Drain, remove the bouquet garni, onion and carrot, then set aside.
3. At this point, sprinkle the lentils with a little sherry vinegar while warm, allowing the flavour to go into the lentils.
4. In a small pan, melt half the butter and sweat the cabbage for 2 minutes or until just wilted, stirring occasionally. Mix with the lentils and set aside.
5. Preheat the oven to 70°C. Mix together the herbs and roll the best end in the herbs on the meat side.
6. Heat the oil in an ovenproof pan and brown the meat on all sides. Slow roast in the oven for 35–40 minutes.
7. Meanwhile, add the baby onions and tomato concasse to the sauce. Reheat the garlic mashed potato. Reheat the lentils and cabbage with a little butter and keep warm.
8. Once the lamb is cooked, place the cabbage and lentils in the centre of the plate. Carve the lamb (4 cutlets each) and arrange over the cabbage mixture.
9. Bring the sauce to the boil, correct the seasoning and pour over the lamb dish to serve.

Slow-braised and roast belly of lamb with cauliflower risotto and balsamic jelly

15

	4 portions	10 portions
Belly of lamb		
lamb breast (belly) (250–300 g each)	1–2	4
vegetable oil	15 ml	50 ml
braising stock	200 ml	1 litre
cloves of garlic	1	3
sprig of thyme	1	
bay leaf	1	1
large cut mirepoix	200 g	500 g
Balsamic jelly		
balsamic vinegar (not aged)	100 ml	250 ml
mombazilliac wine (or other white wine)	50 ml	125 ml
apple juice	50 ml	125 ml
agar agar, powdered	1 g	2.5 g
Cauliflower risotto		
chicken stock	500 ml	1200 ml
vegetable oil	15 ml	50 ml
shallots, finely chopped	1	2
clove of garlic, split	½	½
carnaroli rice	110 g	250 g
white wine	1 tbsp	4 tbsp
butter	30 g	75 g
Parmesan cheese, grated	20 g	50 g
cauliflower florets, roasted	150 g	400 g
chives, chopped	1 tsp	2 tsp
seasoning		
To finish		
spinach, washed	75 g	200 g
baby carrots, peeled, cooked	5	12
lamb jus	75 ml	200 ml

Slow-braised lamb belly

1. Trim the excess fat from the bellies.
2. Seal quickly in hot oil.
3. Place the braising stock, garlic, thyme, bay leaf and mirepoix into a pan. Bring to the boil.
4. Place the bellies into the liquid and cook for 1½ hours (depending on size and thickness).
5. When cooked, drain off the liquid and retain. Place between two trays and press, with a little weight on top to assist pressing.

6. When cold, place on a board and cut into the portion size required.

Balsamic jelly

1. Reduce the vinegar by half.
2. Combine the mombazilliac wine and apple juice and reduce by half.
3. Mix the two reductions together and allow to cool.
4. Add the agar agar, mixing well.
5. Return to the boil, whisking for 1 minute.
6. Pour into a shallow container and allow to set at room temperature.
7. Store in the fridge until ready.

Cauliflower risotto

1. In a saucepan, bring 1 litre of the chicken stock to a simmer.
2. In a separate, heavy pan, heat the vegetable oil over a medium heat and sweat the shallots and garlic for 3 minutes without allowing them to colour. Add the rice and sweat for a further 2 minutes, again without colouring.
3. Pour in the wine and simmer until it has reduced to a glaze.
4. Begin adding the stock in small stages of about 50–75 ml. Bring the risotto to the boil each time, allowing the stock to evaporate while stirring continuously. Each process of adding and simmering will take approximately 3 minutes.
5. Repeat several times until the rice is cooked but not chalky to the bite: in total it should take about 20–22 minutes from the first addition of chicken stock.
6. Add the butter, Parmesan and cauliflower florets and work to an emulsion. Add the chives and correct the seasoning and consistency: if too thick, add a little more stock; if too wet, reduce the liquid a little. The risotto is then ready to serve.

To complete the dish

1. Prepare the lamb bellies as above. Start cooking the risotto. When halfway through the cooking process, take the retained cooking liquor from the lamb and heat it in a separate pan. Place the lamb bellies carefully into the liquor.

2. Bring to a simmer and take off the heat, allowing the bellies to slowly heat through.
3. Meanwhile, finish the risotto and heat the vegetable garnish in a little butter.
4. Cut the jelly into even dice and place into the lamb jus. Gently heat through: the jelly will melt at 83°C, so be mindful not to simmer or boil the jus.

5. Arrange the vegetables on the plate. Remove the lamb from the liquor and drain. Place the risotto on the plate with the vegetables; top with the drained lamb and sauce.

Stuffed saddle of lamb with apricot farce

energy	kcal	fat	sat fat	carb	sugar	protein	fibre
4086 KJ	983 cal	70.2 g	27.8 g	40.8 g	19.6 g	49.2 g	8.0 g

*

	4 portions	10 portions
Lamb		
saddle, boned	1	2
best lamb mince	250 g	625 g
dried apricots, chopped	100 g	250 g
chives, chopped	1 tsp	2 tsp
seasoning		
pig's caul/crepinette	200 g	500 g
oil	50 ml	125 ml
lamb jus	200 ml	500 ml
Fondant potato		
medium potatoes, preferably Maris Pipers	4	10
vegetable oil	50 ml	125 ml
garlic cloves, split	2	5
butter	150 g	375 g
water or white stock	100 ml	250 ml
seasoning		
Roast vegetables		
butter	50 g	125 g
oil	50 ml	125 ml
medium carrots, peeled and cut into 4	2	5
medium parsnips, peeled and cut into 4	2	5
leeks, trimmed of green and root, cut into 10 cm lengths	2	5

(best lamb mince, dried apricots, chives, seasoning = farce)

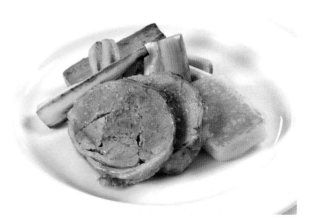

4. Open up the crepinette onto the board and lay the lamb inside. Tightly double-wrap the lamb with crepinette and tie in four equal sections (tie tightly, but not overtight, as during cooking the lamb will expand and either burst from the wrap or split the string).
5. Heat the oil in a thick-bottomed pan and seal the lamb saddle all over until golden. Place in the oven for 20 minutes on 180°C, then reduce the temperature to 65°C for a further 45 minutes.
6. Check if cooked by inserting a probe in the centre, which should read 55–59°C.

For the lamb

1. Preheat the oven to 180°C.
2. With the lamb on the chopping board, fat side down, bat out the fat flanks either side.
3. Mix all the farce ingredients and place in the lamb's centre cavity. Wrap over the fat flanks, encasing the farce and creating a tight cylinder shape.

For the fondant potato

1. Preheat the oven to 170°C.
2. Peel the potatoes and cut into slabs approximately 4 cm thick.
3. Using a round pastry cutter, cut the slabs of potato into 5 cm rounds and trim off the sharp edges.
4. In an ovenproof saucepan, heat the vegetable oil over a medium-high heat.

5. Add the potatoes and garlic, brown the potatoes on one side, taking care not to scorch them. Turn the potatoes over when golden brown and add the butter, water and seasoning.
6. Bring to a simmer, then transfer to the oven for 12–15 minutes or until the centre of the potatoes is soft. Remove from the oven and leave to soak up the butter for about 1 hour.
7. If the liquid in the pan has evaporated and only butter is left as the cooking medium, top up the pan with hot liquid and bring back to an emulsion.

To finish

1. Start to cook the fondant potatoes (see above).
2. Start to cook the lamb (see above).
3. Meanwhile, place the butter and oil for the vegetables in a thick pan, and heat and cook the vegetables until golden on the stove.

4. Drain into colander and keep warm.
5. Remove the lamb from the oven when ready and allow to rest for 10 minutes.
6. Remove the string and place on a carving board.
7. Meanwhile, arrange the fondants and roast vegetables on the plate. Slice the lamb into four equal pieces and place neatly over the vegetables.
8. Finish the dish by coating the lamb and around with lamb jus.

Variation

Omit the dried apricots for mint and peas, then substitute the roast vegetables and potato for a light couscous salad and wilted greens.

Tripe was used for pig's caul, for this analysis.

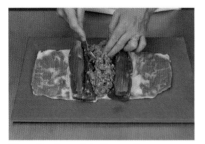
Place the farce into the cavity

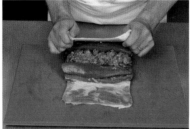
Wrap over the flanks

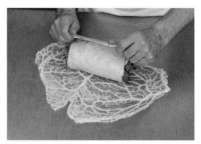
Wrap in crepinette

17 Lamb and rice stuffing

medium onion, finely chopped	1
ghee or butter	1 tbsp
salt	2 tsp
black pepper	1 tsp
cinnamon or mixed spices	1 tsp
rice, washed and drained	200 g
lamb shoulder, finely chopped	500 g
water	350 ml

1. Sauté the onions in the ghee until soft.
2. Mix the onions and ghee, salt, pepper and cinnamon into the rice.
3. Add the meat and water. Mix well.

This stuffing can be used in stuffed and baked vegetables, or shaped and cooked separately

18 Changezie champen

	4 portions
lamb chops or cutlets	8
Marinade	
garlic paste	20 g
green chilli paste	10 g
toasted fennel seeds	5 g
mace powder	¼ tsp
cardamom powder	½ tsp
double cream	250 ml
crushed black pepper	½ tsp
salt	½ tsp
roasted gram flour	30 g
vegetable oil	50 ml
sesame seeds	30 g

1. Mix all the spices and pastes in double cream to form a marinade.
2. Stir in the roasted gram flour and vegetable oil and leave the marinade for 30 minutes at room temperature.
3. Add the lamb chops to the marinade and leave it to rest at room temperature for 1½ hours.
4. Skewer the lamb chops and cook for 15 minutes in a moderately hot tandoor.
5. Remove and rest the chops for 5 minutes, baste with oil.
6. Roll the chops over sesame seeds on the edges and cook again for another 5 minutes.
7. Remove, baste with butter and sprinkle on crushed black pepper and lemon juice.
8. Serve with mint chutney and sliced onions.

> *i* In the tandoor, the intense heat chars the meat. Alternatively, chops can also be cooked on a hot grill or in an oven, although this will sacrifice the barbeque flavour.

This recipe was contributed by Atul Kochhar.

19 Palak lamb

> *i* This is a medium-spiced dish from the Punjab.

	4 portions	10 portions
vegetable ghee or oil	62 ml	155 ml
cumin seeds	1 tsp	2½ tsp
onion, finely chopped	50 g	125 g
fresh ginger, finely chopped	12 g	30 g
garlic clove, crushed	1	3
shoulder loin or leg of lamb, cut into 2½ cm dice	400 g	1 kg
hot curry paste	2 tsp	5 tsp
natural yoghurt	125 ml	312 ml
salt, to taste		
tomato purée	25 g	62 g
spinach, chopped	200 g	500 g
coriander lemon for garnish		

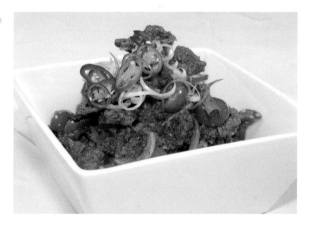

1. Heat the ghee or oil in a suitable frying pan.
2. Add the cumin seeds and fry for 1 minute.
3. Add the onion and fry until golden brown.
4. Add the ginger and garlic and stir-fry until all is brown.
5. Add the lamb and simmer for 15–20 minutes.
6. Add the curry paste, yoghurt and salt.
7. Cook for 5 minutes. Add water if necessary to prevent sticking.
8. Stir in the tomato purée and spinach. Cover and simmer for 10–15 minutes, until the lamb is tender.
9. Serve garnished with coriander leaves.

Rendang kambang kot baru (lamb in spicy coconut sauce)

	4 portions	10 portions
peanut oil	35 ml	125 ml
shallots	25 g	60 g
garlic clove, finely chopped	1	2½
candlenuts or brazils or macadamia nuts, ground	50 g	125 g
turmeric powder	5 g (1 tsp)	12 g (2½ tsp)
coriander powder	5 g (1 tsp)	12 g (2½ tsp)
lemon grass stalk, finely chopped	1	2–3
loin chops	4 × 150 g	10 × 150 g
white cabbage leaves, blanched	4	10
spicy coconut sauce (see recipe 21)	500 ml	1¼ litres

1. Place the peanut oil, shallots, garlic and ground nuts in a basin. Sprinkle with turmeric and coriander. Add the lemon grass and season. Mix to a thick paste. Add oil until a spreadable mixture is obtained.
2. Spread mixture on to the lamb, marinate for 2 hours in a refrigerator.
3. Quickly fry the lamb on both sides for 1 minute.
4. Wrap each chop in a blanched cabbage leaf.
5. Place the lamb in a suitable pan for braising, cover with hot spicy coconut sauce. Place a lid on the pan and braise in a moderate oven (180°C) for approximately 10 minutes.
6. Serve with stir-fry vegetables, flavoured with turmeric.

 Saus rendang (spicy coconut sauce)

	Makes 500 ml
peanut oil	35 ml
shallots, finely chopped	50 g
ginger, finely chopped	12 g
garlic clove, finely chopped	1
greater galangal, peeled and finely chopped	12 g
candlenuts, brazil nuts or macadamia nuts	25 g
lemon grass stalk, chopped	1
kaffir lime leaves	4
turmeric powder	2 g
coriander powder	2 g (½ tsp)
red chilli juice	375 ml
coconut milk	250 ml
salt	

i Greater galangal is less aromatic and pungent than lesser galangal. It is always used fresh in Indonesia. If unavailable, use fresh ginger but double the amount.

1. In a saucepan, heat the peanut oil and sauté the shallots, ginger, garlic and greater galangal for approximately 5 minutes, until they are a light-brown colour.
2. Add the nuts, lemon grass, lime leaves, turmeric and coriander. Continue to sauté for a further 2 minutes.
3. Add the chilli juice and coconut milk and season. Bring to the boil and simmer for approximately 6–10 minutes, stirring continuously.
4. Remove the lime leaves.
5. Liquidise and pass through a strainer, use as required.

22 Lamb faggots with mint

	4 portions	10 portions
Lamb mousse		
lamb fillet	100 g	500 g
salt		
whipping cream	100 g	500 g
Lamb faggot mix		
onion, finely diced	200 g	1 kg
cumin powder	2 g	5 g
lamb sweetbreads, cooked	250 g	700 g
butter		
confit lamb breast (belly)	250 g	700 g
lamb jus	50 ml	130 ml
mint, chopped	10 g	25 g
seasoning		

Lamb mousse

1. Place the fillet in the blender with a pinch of salt.
2. Blend for 1 minute and then add another pinch of salt and slowly add the cream.
3. When all the cream is incorporated, take out of the blender and store in a bowl.

Lamb faggots

1. Sweat the onion until soft and add the cumin.
2. Cook out for about 2 minutes, then chill.
3. Chop the sweetbreads until very small.
4. Roast in butter until golden brown.
5. Pick the confit belly, ensuring no fat remains.
6. Combine all the ingredients together and season.
7. Test the mix.
8. Create 25 g balls of the mixture. Wrap each ball in cling film and steam for 8 minutes.
9. Take out of the cling film and roast in a pan with a little butter and deglaze with a little vinegar.
10. Add some jus and butter and reduce until it coats the faggots and becomes sticky.

23 Mutton cawl

	4 portions	10 portions
mutton, cubed	500 g	1.4 kg
smoked bacon, cubed	500 g	1.4 kg
onions, coarsely chopped	2	5
carrots, chopped	4	10
parsnips, chopped	2	5
small swede, chopped	1	2
vegetable stock	500 ml	1½ litres
peppercorns	12	30
cloves	4	10
bay leaf	1	2
sprig of thyme	1	2
potatoes, peeled and cubed	500 g	1.2 kg
leeks, sliced	4	10
salt and pepper to season		

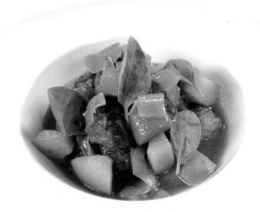

1. Brown the mutton and bacon well in a large pan.
2. Pour off the excess fat, then add all the vegetables, except the potatoes and leeks. Add the stock, peppercorns, thyme, cloves and bay leaf and simmer for about 3 hours.
3. Add the potatoes and leeks. Bring back to the boil, then simmer for another 30 minutes.

24 Mutton and turnip pie

	4 portions	10 portions
neck fillet of mutton, cut into rough 2 cm pieces	500 g	1.4 kg
plain flour for dusting		
vegetable oil		
large onions, peeled, finely chopped	1	3
rosemary, sprig		
chicken or lamb stock	1 litre	2 litres
salt and freshly ground black pepper		
turnips, peeled, cut into rough 2–3 cm chunks	400 g	1 kg
puff pastry, rolled to about 1 cm thick	250 g	800 g
egg, beaten	1	1

1. Pre-heat the oven to 200°C.
2. Season the pieces of mutton and dust generously with about 1 tbsp of flour.
3. Heat the vegetable oil in a heavy-bottomed saucepan and fry the pieces of mutton and onions for 3–4 minutes, without colouring them too much.
4. Add the rosemary and stock, bring to the boil and simmer gently for about 1½–2 hours, until the mutton is soft and tender.
5. Add the turnips. Cover with a lid and add a little boiled water if necessary. Simmer for about 15 minutes, until the turnips are cooked. Remove from the heat and leave to cool.
6. Meanwhile, cut the pastry a little larger than the pie dish (or dishes, if you are making individual pies).
7. When the mutton mixture has cooled, transfer it to the pie dish.
8. Brush the edges of the pastry with some egg and lay the pastry on the dish, pressing the edges onto the rim.
9. Cut a slit of about 2–3 cm in the centre to let the steam out, or for a larger pie use a pie funnel.
10. Bake the pie for 40–45 minutes until golden.

25 Leg of mutton

	10–15 portions
leg of mutton	1
white chicken stock	5 litres
white wine	
bouquet garni	
onions	2
carrots	2
celery, stick	¼
button mushrooms	200 g
leeks	2
cream	400 ml
capers, washed	60 g
seasoning	
Garnish	
carrots, cut into julienne	200 g
celeriac, cut into julienne	200 g
celery, cut into julienne	200 g
new potatoes, cooked, sliced	500 g

1. Take the leg of mutton and soak in water.
2. Place the leg in a pan and cover with white chicken stock and white wine with a bouquet garni. Bring to the boil, skim and simmer for 30 minutes.
3. Peel, wash and cut the vegetables into large dice and place into the pot with the leg of mutton. Cook for a further 2 hours until the leg is totally cooked through and tender (exact cooking time will depend on size).
4. Remove the leg and reduce the resulting liquor so it becomes much richer in texture and taste.
5. Pass the liquor through a fine sieve; pour in the double cream. Bring back to the boil and simmer for a few minutes only. Then add the capers. Season to taste.
6. Slice the leg and pour the sauce over the top. Garnish with new potatoes and the celery, carrot and celeriac.

26 Lambs' kidneys with juniper and wild mushrooms

energy	kcal	fat	sat fat	carb	sugar	protein	fibre
821 KJ	193.9 cal	3.5 g	1.1 g	18.0 g	1.2 g	23.7 g	0.4 g

	4 portions	10 portions
English lambs' kidneys	12	30
shallots, chopped	25 g	60 g
juniper berries, crushed	12	30
gin, marinated with the berries for one day	60 ml	150 ml
English white wine	125 ml	300 ml
strong lamb stock	½ litre	1¼ litre
selected wild mushrooms	50 g	125 g
oil and butter, to sauté large potatoes	2	5

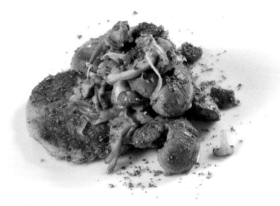

1. Remove the fat and thin film of tissue covering the kidneys.
2. Season well and sauté in a hot pan, keeping them pink. Remove and keep warm.
3. Add the shallots and some crushed juniper berries to the pan, flambé with a little gin, pour in the white wine and reduce well. Add the lamb stock and reduce by half. Pass and finish with butter.
4. Prepare the mushrooms and sauté in hot oil, adding butter to maintain their earthy flavour, then keep warm.
5. Finely shred the potatoes into matchsticks on a mandolin, dry in a clean cloth, season and cook in butter as a fine potato cake.
6. To serve, place the potato cake in the centre of a serving dish, slice the kidneys and arrange attractively in a circle on the potato. Garnish the kidneys with the wild mushrooms, cordon the dish with the sauce and serve immediately.

27 Lambs' liver flavoured with lavender and sage, served with sherry sauce

energy	kcal	fat	sat fat	carb	sugar	protein	fibre
2123 KJ	509 cal	38.62 g	13.3 g	17.6 g	15.6 g	24.0 g	2.0 g

	4 portions	10 portions
lamb's liver	400 g	1 kg
milk	250 ml	625 ml
honey	50 g	125 g
sage (chopped) bunch	1	2
lavender, bunch	1	2
garlic cloves	2	4
sesame oil	25 ml	50 ml
Sauce		
baby onions	200 g	500 g
garlic clove, crushed	1	1
sesame oil	25 ml	50 ml
sherry	50 ml	125 ml
veal stock	250 ml	625 ml
unsalted butter	50 g	125 g

1. Remove skin and arteries from the liver, and place on one side.
2. Mix the milk, honey and half the chopped sage, with the lavender and uncrushed garlic cloves.
3. Place the liver in the milk mixture and leave for 24 hours.
4. For the sauce, peel the baby onions, blanch them, then refresh.
5. Sauté the crushed garlic in sesame oil with the baby onions. Add the sherry and reduce by half.
6. Add the veal stock and reduce this by two-thirds. Take off heat and cool slightly.
7. Whisk in the unsalted butter and season.
8. Heat sesame oil for the liver, remove the liver from the marinade and drain. Season liver with salt, pepper, remaining sage and any remaining lavender.
9. Sauté liver lightly until pink.
10. To serve, pour the sauce onto the plate, place the liver on top. Garnish with the onions from the sauce. Finish with sprigs of lavender.

28 Roast wing rib with Yorkshire pudding

energy	kcal	fat	sat fat	carb	sugar	protein	fibre
3185 KJ	758 cal	31.04 g	13.0 g	31.6 g	4.5 g	90.0 g	1.6 g

	10 portions
Beef	
piece wing rib of beef	1 × 2 kg
beef dripping	25 g
Yorkshire pudding	
eggs	2
milk	200 ml
ice cold water	100 ml
plain flour	110 g
Gravy	
carrots ⎫ mirepoix	50 g
onion ⎭	50 g
red wine	200 ml
plain flour	30 g
beef stock	300 ml
prepared English mustard or horseradish sauce, to serve	

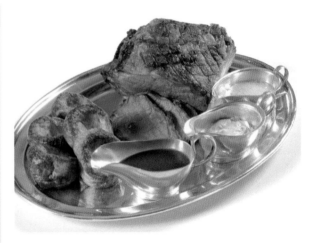

For the Yorkshire pudding

1. Place the eggs, milk and water in a bowl and combine well with a whisk.
2. Gradually add the flour to avoids lumps, and whisk to a smooth batter consistency.
3. Place in the refrigerator overnight to rest (this will give you a better lift in the oven).
4. Preheat the oven to 180°C.
5. Heat oil in a Yorkshire pudding tray by placing a small amount in the bottom of each well, and place the tray in the oven for 5 minutes.
6. Carefully fill the wells on the tray to two-thirds full and return to the oven.
7. When the puddings have risen, and are golden brown, remove from the oven and keep warm.

For the beef

1. Preheat the oven to 195°C.
2. Place the dripping in a heavy roasting tray and heat on the stove top.
3. Place the beef in the tray and brown well on all sides.
4. Place in the oven on 195°C for 15 minutes then turn down to 75°C for 2 hours.
5. Remove and allow to rest before carving.

For the gravy

1. Remove the beef. Place the tray with the fat, sediment and the juice back on the stove.
2. Add the mirepoix and brown well.
3. Add the red wine and reduce by two-thirds.
4. Mix the flour and a little stock together to form a viscous batter-like mix.
5. Add the stock to the roasting tray and bring to the boil.
6. Pour in the flour mix and whisk into the liquid in the tray.
7. Bring to the boil, simmer and correct the seasoning.
8. Pass through a sieve and retain for service.

To complete

1. Slice the beef and warm the Yorkshire puddings, serve with the gravy, horseradish and mustard.

This dish would work well with most vegetables or potatoes. As an alternative, why not add slightly blanched root vegetables to the roasting tray at the start of the beef cooking, remove and reheat for service? They will get maximum flavour from the beef and juices.

29 Slow-cooked beef fillet with onion ravioli

energy	kcal	fat	sat fat	carb	sugar	protein	fibre
5119 KJ	1221 cal	52.5 g	25.3 g	116.4 g	9.1 g	77.2 g	6.9 g

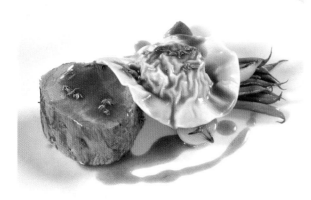

	4 portions	10 portions
Beef		
corn oil		
centre cut fillet	1 × 600 g	2 × 750 g
strands of thyme	3	7
garlic clove, thinly sliced	1	2
Ravioli pasta		
Flour	550 g	1400 g
egg yolks	5	12
eggs	4	10
Chicken mousse		
breast of chicken	300 g	1 kg
salt to taste		
cream	200 ml	500 ml
Ravioli mix		
chicken mousse (see above)	300 g	750 g
Lyonnaise onions	100 g	250 g
parsley	25 g	60 g
sherry vinegar	50 ml	125 ml
seasoning		
To finish		
haricot verts, cooked	200 g	500 g
button onions, cooked	12 (100 g)	30 (250 g)
sherry jus	200 ml	500 ml
picked lemon thyme	1 tsp	2 tsp

For the beef

1. Preheat the oven to 59°C.
2. Heat a pan with a little corn oil and carefully put the beef fillet in it, browning on all sides. Add thyme and garlic at the end (this operation should take no more than 2 minutes).
3. Remove from the pan and allow to cool.
4. Wrap the fillet in cling film and place in an oven already pre-set at between 55 and 60°C (the theory behind this cooking is that, for a medium rare 'doneness', the core temperature will be between 57 and 59°C; therefore, to achieve this preferred cooking degree throughout the fillet, the oven should be set at between 55 and 60°C).
5. It will take approximately 50–60 minutes for the temperature to penetrate to the core of the fillet. This will then last for an extra 1–1½ hours after this time (obviously the longer in the oven, the more it will dry out).
6. When ready to serve, remove from the oven and re-seal the fillet in a hot pan – this should take no more than 30 seconds. There is no need to rest the meat as the proteins will not have shrunk to a degree that requires it to be rested.

For the mousse

1. Blitz the chicken for 1 minute with the salt.
2. After standing for 30 seconds, add the cream.
3. Pass through a fine sieve and reserve.

For the ravioli pasta

1. Place the flour in a food processor.
2. Whisk the eggs together and pass through chinois to get rid of any membrane.
3. Slowly incorporate the egg mix into the flour.
4. When all the liquid is used, take out of the food processor.
5. Work together on the bench, as though working bread dough, for 5 minutes.
6. Rest for 1 hour before rolling out to your required thickness.

For the ravioli mix

1. Place the chicken mousse, lyonnaise onions and parsley in a bowl. Mix well.
2. Add the sherry vinegar and check the seasoning.
3. Weigh out into 25 g balls and reserve until you need to make the raviolis.

To make the raviolis

1. Roll the pasta very thinly and cut into discs approx. 12 cm in diameter.
2. Cover the 8 discs in cling film to prevent them drying out.
3. Lay a disc on the workbench and dab with a little water.
4. Place in the centre a ball of mousse and top with another disc ensuring that all the air is removed and an even shape is formed.
5. When all raviolis are complete, blanch in boiling water for 2 minutes then arrest the cooking with iced water.

6. Drain, store and cover in cling film to prevent drying.

To finish

1. Reheat the haricots verts, button onions and sauce, keeping them all warm. Meanwhile, reheat the raviolis in boiling water for 2 minutes. Remove and allow to drain. Carve the beef into equal slices (2 per portion).
2. Place the button onions and haricots verts in the centre of the plate, top with the beef, then the ravioli on top of the beef. Finish with the sauce and serve garnished with lemon thyme.

> A modern cooking method is adopted here. The risk involved in cooking at high heat for a short period of time and getting the degree of cooking correct has always been an issue, however with this method the beef can stay in the oven for up to 2 hours and still be able to be served due to the protein shrink temperature.

30 Slow-cooked sirloin with Lyonnaise onions and carrot purée

energy	kcal	fat	sat fat	carb	sugar	protein	fibre
1949 KJ	467 cal	25.3 g	6.9 g	16.0 g	14.0 g	44.8 g	4.3 g

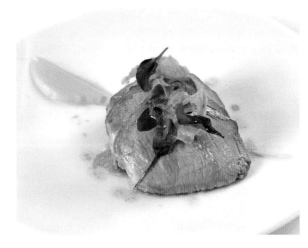

	4 portions	10 portions
Beef		
sirloin, denuded with fat tied back on	1.2 kg	3 kg
seasoning		
oil	50 ml	125 ml
garlic clove, sliced	1	2
sprigs thyme	1	2
bay leaves	1	2

Lyonnaise onions		
onions	200 g	500 g
seasoning		
Carrot purée		
medium-sized carrots	600 g	1½ kg
star anise	1	2
To serve		
jus de viande (meat juice)	150 ml	375 ml
sprigs of chervil		

For the beef

1. Preheat the oven to 180°C. Season the beef and heat the oil in the pan. Add the garlic, thyme, bay leaves and the beef.
2. Place the beef in the oven for 15 minutes. Remove, and turn the oven down to 69°C. When the oven has reached this new temperature, return the beef to it for a further 1 hour 10 minutes.
3. While the beef is cooking make the carrot purée and the Lyonnaise onions (see below) and keep warm.

For the onions

1. Finely slice the onions and put them into a large induction pan while cold.
2. Put on medium heat and season.
3. When the onions are starting to colour, turn down and cook slowly for approximately 2 hours.
4. Cool and refrigerate.

For the carrot purée

1. Peel the carrots and juice just over half of them into a small pan.
2. Cut the remaining carrots into equal slices of about 1 cm and place into the carrot juice.
3. Boil the carrots, ensuring that you scrape down the sides of the pan.
4. For the last 8 minutes of cooking, before all the liquid has completely evaporated, drop in the star anise. Pass, retaining the juice.

5. Remove the star anise pod(s) and blitz the purée for 7 minutes, adding the retained juice.

To finish

1. When the beef is cooked, remove from the oven and carve evenly. Place a portion of carrot purée and Lyonnaise onions on each plate. Top with the beef and pour over the jus de viande (meat juice), garnish with sprigs of chervil and serve.

i This recipe uses the same slow cooking method used in recipe 29 for beef fillet, but a slightly higher temperature is needed because there is a little more collagen in sirloin than in fillet.

---

31 Tournedos Rossini (classical)

energy	kcal	fat	sat fat	carb	sugar	protein	fibre
2591 KJ	619 cal	36.4 g	14.7 g	30.3 g	1.9 g	44.7 g	1.5 g

	4 portions	10 portions
Tournedos		
butter	50 g	125 g
olive oil	1 tsp	2 tsp
beef tournedos, 7–8 cm across and 4 cm deep (approx. 150 g each), at room temperature	4	10
seasoning	4	10
thick slices of foie gras	4	10
thick slices of good white bread, each slice cut into a circle the size of the steak	4	10
field mushrooms, slightly larger than the steaks	4 × 50 g	10 × 50 g
To serve		
chervil sprigs		
watercress sprigs		
red wine jus		

1. Heat the butter and olive oil in a large, heavy-based frying pan. Add the beef tournedos and fry, without moving them, for 3 minutes.
2. Turn the tournedos over and cook for a further 3 minutes, until the steaks are crusted on the outside but rare inside. Season with salt and freshly ground pepper, and set aside to rest.
3. Heat the frying pan the tournedos were cooked in. Add the foie gras and fry until just caramelised.
4. Remove the foie gras and keep warm.
5. Add the bread slices to the pan and fry until crisp.
6. Meanwhile, grill the field mushrooms until tender.
7. Place the fried bread slices in the centre of two plates; top each serving with the steak, then the foie gras, then the mushroom.
8. To finish, garnish with the chervil, and watercress, and pour over the jus.

32 Tournedos Rossini (modern)

energy	kcal	fat	sat fat	carb	sugar	protein	fibre
3532 KJ	848 cal	59.4 g	21.5 g	17.9 g	3.2 g	57.3 g	2.2 g *

	4 portions	10 portions
Tournedos		
oil	50 ml	125 ml
tournedos of beef (approx. 200 g each)	4	10
girolles, washed and prepared	500 g	1¼ kg
butter	50 g	125 g
slices white bread, without crusts and trimmed to the size of the beef	2	5
garlic cloves, thinly sliced	1½	3
slices foie gras (approx. 30 g each)	4	10
shallot sauce	200 ml	500 ml
truffle, sliced	1	2
Madeira jelly (see below) cut into 1 cm dice	100 g	250 g
thin slices Parma ham (baked in an oven until crisp)	4	10
chervil		
seasoning		
Jelly		
Madeira	125 ml	300 ml
port	100 ml	250 ml
brandy	50 ml	125 ml
agar-agar (powdered)	2.1 g	5.25 g

For the jelly

1. Mix all the ingredients together.
2. Place in a pan and bring to the boil, whisking for 1 minute.
3. Pour into a shallow container and allow to set at room temperature.
4. Store in the refrigerator until ready.

For the tournedos

1. In a small frying pan, add the oil and heat it, lightly season the tournedos and seal well in the pan. Cook until desired cuisson is achieved. Remove from the pan and rest on a wire rack somewhere warm.
2. In the same pan, add the girolles and butter and bring to a foam. Carefully remove the girolles from the butter using a slotted/perforated spoon. Keep warm.
3. In the same pan add the bread slices and cook until golden and crisp. Remove and put them on the draining tray next to the beef.
4. Remove the butter from the pan, leaving a small amount of residue in the bottom. Heat up and then place in the garlic slices. Cook gently for 1–2 minutes.
5. Add the foie gras slices and cook gently.
6. Meanwhile, reheat the sauce and slice the truffle.

To finish

1. Place the tournedos on top of the bread croute, then the crisp ham slice on top of the beef with the foie gras topping the Parma ham.
2. Finally, arrange the girolles and jelly around the plate with the beef stack in the centre. Drizzle the sauce over and around, and finish with freshly sliced truffle and chervil.

* Liver pâté was used instead of foie gras and mushrooms instead of truffles for this analysis.

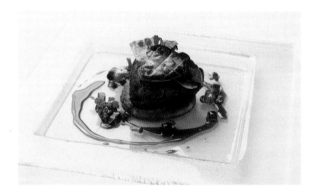

i The modernisation comes from the use of wild mushrooms instead of field, and Madeira jelly instead of Madeira jus.

Why not try a pork variation and use fillet, with a roast apple croute, and top with black pudding instead of foie gras: 'pork Rossini'?

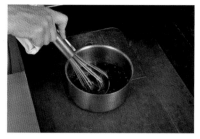
Whisk the jelly

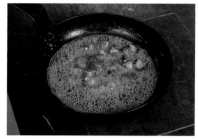
Fry the girolles in foaming butter

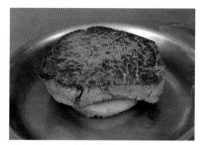
Place the meat on the bread

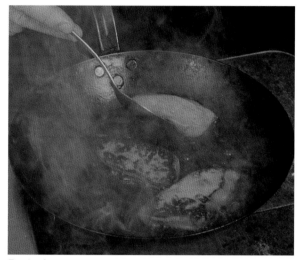
Fry the foie gras

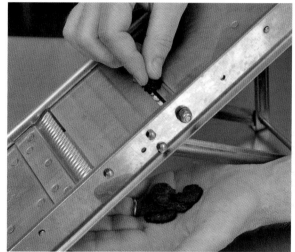
Carefully slice the truffle on a mandolin

33 Braised short rib with horseradish couscous

energy	kcal	fat	sat fat	carb	sugar	protein	fibre
3019 KJ	726 cal	44.91 g	11.2 g	46.2 g	6.6 g	36.3 g	2.1 g

	4 portions	10 portions
Rib meat		
rib meat off the bone	400 g	1 kg
vegetable oil	50 ml	125 ml
onion } mirepoix, medium cut	125 g	300 g
carrot }	125 g	300 g
garlic clove	1	2
sprigs of thyme	1	2
red wine	400 ml	1 litre
brown stock	300 ml	750 ml
sherry vinegar	25 ml	60 ml
Couscous		
water	300 ml	750 ml
olive oil	50 ml	125 ml
salt and cayenne pepper		
couscous	150 g	375 g
fresh horseradish, grated	20 g	50 g
lemon, juice of	½	1

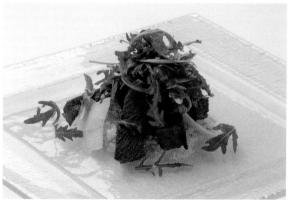

To finish		
salad rocket	260 g	625 g
shaved Parmesan	100 g	250 g
vinaigrette	50 ml	125 ml

For the rib meat

1. Preheat the oven to 130°C. Trim any excess fat from the meat.
2. Heat the oil in a heavy casserole and add the rib meat, mirepoix, garlic and thyme. Cook for 5–6 minutes until brown.
3. Add the wine, bring to the boil and simmer until reduced by half. Add the stock, then cover with foil and cook in the oven for 2 hours.
4. Remove from the oven and leave the meat to cool in the liquor. Remove the ribs and set aside. Strain the sauce into a clean pan and bring to the boil.
5. Simmer until it has reduced to a thick sauce, but be careful not to over-reduce.
6. Meanwhile, trim any elastin or connective tissue from the rib meat, being careful to leave it whole and keep warm.
7. The sauce may need to be adjusted with the vinegar to cut through the richness – be careful not to add too much as you want only an undertone of vinegar.

For the couscous

1. Bring the water, oil, salt and cayenne pepper to the boil.

2. Place the couscous in a bowl with the finely grated horseradish and pour on the liquid. Place cling film tightly over the top and leave for 5 minutes.
3. Remove the cling film and add a little more oil to help free the grains.
4. Allow to infuse.
5. Finish with lemon juice and check the seasoning.

To finish

1. Mix the rocket, Parmesan and vinaigrette together and check the seasoning.
2. Place a mould of couscous on the plate and divide the rib meat equally between the plates.
3. Pour over the sauce, top the ribs with the salad and serve.

i Ribs are full of flavour due to the amount of collagen in them – the animal breathes continuously, working the muscle group a great deal, hence the amount of flavour. This is a very versatile piece of meat.

34 Beef with mango and black pepper

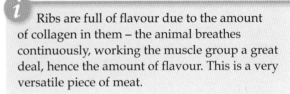

	4 portions	10 portions
beef, cut into strips	500 g	1½ kg
oyster sauce	3 tbsp	8 tbsp
hoisin sauce	3 tbsp	8 tbsp
sweet soy sauce	3 tbsp	8 tbsp
sesame oil	1 tbsp	2 tbsp
potato starch	1 tbsp	2½ tbsp
onion, sliced	1 medium	2 large
young ginger, cut into fine julienne	50 g	120 g
garlic, finely chopped	50 g	120 g
green mango, sliced	300 g	800 g
carrot, cut into julienne	100 g	240 g
red chilli, sliced	1	2
coriander, roughly sliced	20 g	50 g
spring onion, cut into 5 cm lengths	50 g	120 g
Chinese sao sing wine	3 tbsp	8 tbsp
salt and crushed black and white pepper		

1. Marinade the beef strips with the oyster sauce, hoisin sauce, sweet soy sauce, sesame oil and potato starch: set aside for an hour.
2. In a sauté pan, sauté the onion, ginger and garlic over heat.
3. Add in the marinated beef strips and stir-fry for 5–10 minutes or cook to medium.
4. Gently fold in the green mango, carrot, red chilli, coriander and spring onion. If the beef is dry, add water as needed.
5. Add the Chinese wine and season with salt and pepper to taste.

35 *Rendang* (beef curry)

	4 portions	10 portions
cooking oil	70 ml	150 ml
onion, finely chopped	100 g	250 g
garlic cloves, crushed	2	5
fresh ginger, finely chopped	12 g	30 g
hot Thai curry blend	2 tsp	5 tsp
ground lemon grass	1 tsp	2½ tsp
desiccated coconut	100 g	250 g
rump or sirloin cut into thin strips	400 g	1 kg
creamed coconut	100 g	250 g
hot water	¼ litre	¾ litre
salt, to taste		

1. Heat the oil in a suitable pan. Fry the onions, garlic and ginger until lightly coloured.

2. Add the curry blend and lemon grass. Continue to fry for a further 2 minutes.
3. Add the desiccated coconut and fry for a further 1 minute.
4. Quickly fry the beef in a separate pan. Drain off excess oil.
5. Place the beef in a clean saucepan. Season and add the coconut milk (creamed coconut and hot water blended together).
6. Add the other prepared ingredients to the beef.
7. Bring to the boil, then simmer until the beef is tender and the liquid has evaporated. Stir occasionally.
8. This curry should be served quite dry. Serve with prawn crackers.

36 *Daging masak merah* (beef in red spicy sauce)

	4 portions	10 portions
beef, sliced thinly	500 g	1.2 kg
red onions, large	2	4
cloves of garlic	8	20
young ginger	50 g	120 g
lemon grass stalks	3	8
galangal	30 g	75 g
fresh turmeric	30 g	75 g
tomato paste	3 tbsp	8 tbsp
red chillies	5	12
coriander	50 g	120 g
kaffir lime leaves	3	8
star anise	2	5
cinnamon stick	1	3
cardamom pods	3	7
kerisik (toasted dessicated coconut paste)	50 g	125 g
salt to taste		
sugar to taste		

1. Boil the beef in water until tender.
2. Blend all the other ingredients, except the star anise, cinnamon stick, cardamom pods and kerisik, with enough cooking oil until they form a smooth paste.
3. In a frying pan, sauté the paste over a moderate heat with the star anise, cinnamon stick and cardamom pods until it is fragrant and the oil starts to split from the paste.
4. Add the sliced beef and simmer for 15 minutes. Add some liquid to the beef if it is too dry.
5. Stir in the kerisik and continue to simmer until the sauce thickens.
6. Season with salt and sugar to taste.

37 Bok choy with beef in black bean sauce

	4 portions	10 portions
beef, thinly sliced	350 g	1 kg
black bean paste	2 tbsp	5 tbsp
oyster sauce	2 tbsp	5 tbsp
sesame oil	1 tsp	3 tsp
sweet dark soy sauce	1 tbsp	2 tbsp
Chinese sao sin wine	1 tbsp	2½ tbsp
potato starch	2 tbsp	5 tbsp
onion	50 g	140 g
young ginger	5 slices	12 slices
cloves of garlic, chopped	2	3
salt and pepper		
spring onion, sliced	30 g	75 g
coriander, chopped	50 g	120 g
red chilli, sliced	1	2
bok choy stalks	10	25

1. Marinade the beef with the black bean paste, oyster sauce, sesame oil, soy sauce, Chinese wine and some of the potato starch. Set aside for 1 hour.
2. Heat enough oil in a frying pan to sauté the onion, ginger and garlic until fragrant.
3. Stir in the beef and cook until medium well done.
4. Add some water to make the sauce, and thicken with some potato starch.
5. Season well with salt and pepper. Gently fold in the spring onion, coriander and red chilli.
6. In another pot, boil some water with cooking oil and salt.
7. Blanch the bok choy and place them in the centre of a plate.
8. Spoon the black bean beef on top of the bok choy.

38 Stuffed squash

	4 portions	10 portions
Hubbard squash	1	2 large
soft butter	20 g	50 g
salt	1 tsp	2 tsp
smoked bacon, diced	100 g	250 g
onion, diced	50 g	120 g
green pepper, chopped	75 g	180 g
tomato juice	50 g	120 ml
soft, stale breadcrumbs	200 g	500 g
egg	1	2
minced beef	340 g	1 kg
sausage meat	115 g	260 g
grain mustard	1 tbsp	2 tbsp
seasoning and sage to taste		

1. Peel the squash and cut it in half lengthways. Discard the seeds and any stringy pulp. Cut off a small slice of the underside so that the squash will rest flat.
2. Parboil for 8 minutes in boiling salted water. Drain, and dry with absorbent paper.
3. Brush the inside with soft butter and sprinkle with salt.
4. Sauté the bacon until crispy, add the onion and cook for 3 minutes. Remove from the heat.
5. Combine the bacon and onion with all the remaining ingredients.
6. Pile the mixture into the squash cavity. Place in a baking dish containing 2 cm of boiling water.
7. Bake at 180°C for 50 minutes or until the squash is tender when tested with a fork.
8. To serve, cut into wedges to make equal portions.

Piononos (deep-fried plantain rings with spiced minced-beef filling)

39

	4 portions	10 portions
large ripe plantains	2	5
butter or margarine	50 g	125 g
vegetable oil	2 tsp	5 tsp
vegetable oil mixed with 1 (2½) tsp annatto	2 tbsp	5 tbsp
lean minced topside of beef	400 g	1¼ kg
onion, finely chopped	50 g	125 g
green pepper, finely chopped	50 g	125 g
red chilli, finely chopped	1	2–3
garlic clove, crushed and chopped	1	2–3
plain flour	25 g	60 g
ham, chopped	100 g	250 g
tomato concassée	100 g	250 g
seasoning		
brown stock or water	125 ml	300 ml
olives, chopped	6	15
capers, chopped	25 g	60 g
malt vinegar	1 tbsp	2–3 tbsp
eggs, beaten	4	10

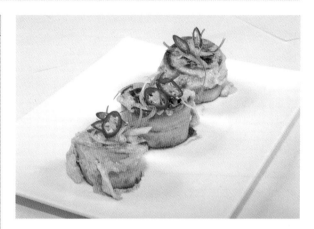

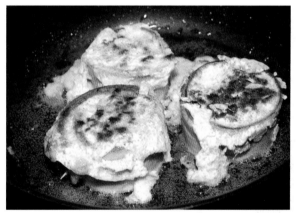

1. Peel the plantains and cut each one lengthways into thick strips, approximately 6 mm.
2. Place the butter in a suitable pan and fry the plantains both sides until golden brown, drain well.
3. Heat the vegetable oil and annatto in a suitable pan, quickly fry the minced beef.
4. Add the onions, peppers, chillies and garlic, and cook for 5 minutes stirring frequently.
5. Add the flour, stir well and cook for a further 5 minutes.
6. Stir in the ham, tomatoes and seasoning.
7. Moisten with a little water or brown stock.
8. Continue to cook until the mixture resembles a paste-like consistency.
9. Add the chopped olives and capers, the vinegar and the correct seasoning.
10. To make the piononos, shape each strip of plantain into a ring about 7.5 cm in diameter, overlap by 8 mm. Secure with a cocktail stick.
11. Fill each with the beef mixture. Do not overfill.
12. Dip each of the piononos into seasoned flour, brush off excess flour. Dip into beaten egg.
13. Carefully deep-fry in a suitable pan at 180°C for approximately 3 minutes.
14. Serve immediately with red beans and rice.

40 Bresaola (cured silverside)

energy	kcal	fat	sat fat	carb	sugar	protein	fibre
1395 KJ	332 cal	10.2 g	4.0 g	0.2 g	0.2 g	43.3 g	0.0 g

	4 portions	10 portions
beef silverside, trimmed of all fat	400 g	1 kg
red wine, inexpensive Burgundy	400 ml	1 litre
coarse salt	120 g	250 g
branches of rosemary (each about 15–23 cm)	1	2
sprig of thyme	1	1
bay leaves	1	2
carrots, quartered	½	1
onions, white	½	1
garlic cloves, crushed	1	1
black peppercorns	3	6
juniper berries, crushed	3	6
zest of orange	1	1

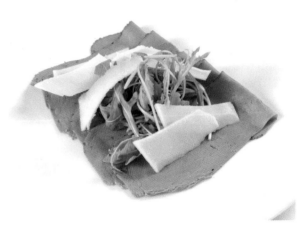

For the marinade

1. Put all the ingredients, except the meat, into a tub (plastic or otherwise) large enough to hold the marinade and the meat. Mix well for a minute or two.

For the bresaola

1. Place the meat in the marinade. All the meat should be covered. Cover the container and place at the back of the refrigerator.
2. Leave for a week, or until the meat feels quite firm. Turn the beef over once at the mid-cycle of the process. At the end of the marinating period, remove from the marinade, dry and wrap in two layers of muslin. Hang in a cool place to dry. Place paper on the floor as the meat drips a bit during the first few days of drying.
3. The meat should be hanged for at least 3 weeks. At the end of this time the meat should feel firm, with no give when you press it with your fingers. For a 5 kg piece of silverside, three weeks should be sufficient. The firmness test is the best method to judge readiness. Mould may form during the drying process.
4. When drying is complete, remove any white mould with a brush and scraper. Wash the bresaola with vinegar. Pat dry and rub the entire bresaola with olive oil. Wrap in greaseproof paper and keep in the refrigerator.
5. Serve sliced very thinly with rocket salad and shaved Parmesan.

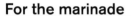

Bresaola della Valtellina takes its name from the famous geographical district in which it was first produced. Since ancient times, techniques for preserving meat by salting and drying have been known. The use of such techniques in the Valtellina district of Italy is noted in writings dating back as far as 1400.

Bresaola is made from raw beef that has been salted and naturally aged. The meat, which is eaten raw, has a delicate flavour and a capacity to melt in the mouth that is highly appreciated by consumers.

41 Traditional braised oxtail with garlic mash

energy	kcal	fat	sat fat	carb	sugar	protein	fibre
2457 KJ	587 cal	27.0 g	12.2 g	41.7 g	20.4 g	46.5 g	8.68 g

	4 portions	10 portions
Oxtail		
oxtails, trimmed of fat	4	10
seasoning		
beef dripping	100 g	250 g
carrots, chopped	225 g	550 g
onions, chopped	225 g	550 g
celery sticks, chopped	225 g	550 g
leeks, chopped	225 g	550 g
tomatoes, chopped	450 g	1 kg
sprig of thyme	1	2
bay leaf	1	2
garlic clove, crushed	1	3
red wine	570 ml	1½ litres
veal/brown stock	2¼ litres	6 litres
Garnish		
carrot, finely diced	100 g	250 g
onion, finely diced	100 g	250 g
celery sticks, finely diced	75 g	185 g
small leeks, finely diced	75 g	185 g
tomatoes, skinned, deseeded and diced	4	10
cooked mashed potato with garlic	500 g	1¼ kg
fresh parsley, chopped	1 heaped tbsp	3 tbsp

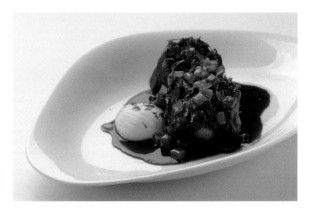

1. Preheat the oven to 200°C.
2. Separate the trimmed tails between the joints and season with salt and pepper.
3. In a large pan, fry the tails in the dripping until brown on all sides, then drain in a colander.
4. Fry the chopped carrots, onions, celery and leeks in the same pan, collecting all the residue from the tails.
5. Add the chopped tomatoes, thyme, bay leaf and garlic, and continue to cook for a few minutes.
6. Place the tails in a large braising pan with the vegetables.
7. Pour the red wine into the first pan and boil to reduce until almost dry.
8. Add some of the stock then pour onto the meat in the braising pan and cover with the remaining stock.
9. Bring the tails to a simmer and braise in the pre-heated oven for 1½–2 hours until the meat is tender.
10. Lift the pieces of meat from the sauce and keep to one side.
11. Push the sauce through a sieve into a pan, then boil to reduce it, skimming off all impurities, to a good sauce consistency.
12. While the sauce is reducing, quickly cook the diced garnish carrot, onion, celery and leek in 1 tbsp water and a little butter for 1–2 minutes.
13. When the sauce is ready, add the tails and vegetable garnish, and simmer until the tails are warmed through.
14. Add the diced tomato, and spoon into hot bowls allowing 3 or 4 oxtail pieces per portion.
15. Serve a large bowl of garlic mash in the centre of the table and a large sourdough loaf.
16. Sprinkle the oxtail with chopped parsley and serve.
17. Serve with the garlic mash.

Choose oxtails that clearly have plenty of flesh around the bone: one complete oxtail will serve two people.

Oxtail is particularly good with haricot or cannellini beans, which seem to absorb a great deal of the flavour.

42 Pickled ox tongue

energy	kcal	fat	sat fat	carb	sugar	protein	fibre
2128 KJ	513 cal	41.8 g	16.9 g	0.0 g	0.0 g	34.1 g	0.0 g *

	4 portions	10 portions
ox tongues	1 kg	2½ kg
pink salt	380 g	950 g
star anise	2	3
Mirepoix		
carrot	250 g	625 g
onions	250 g	625 g
leeks	250 g	625 g
celery	250 g	625 g
red wine vinegar	500 ml	1¼ ml
chicken stock	1 litre	2½ litres
red wine	500 ml	1¼ ml

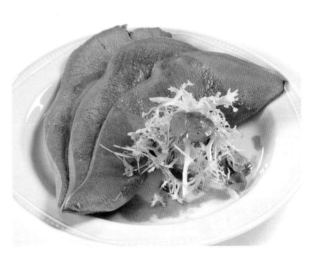

1. Wash the ox tongues and place in 2 litres of water with the pink salt and star anise for 3 hours.
2. Roast the mirepoix in a heavy-duty pan until golden brown.
3. Add the red wine vinegar and bring to the boil.
4. Add the chicken stock and red wine.
5. Pour onto the ox tongues and cook for 3 hours.
6. Remove the tongues from the liquid and pass the liquor.
7. Peel off the skin and store in retained liquor until cold. Remove from the liquid and wrap tightly in cling film.

Data on saturated fats was estimated based on other data about ox tongue.

Uses

Ox tongue can be sliced thinly when cold and served with pickled beetroot salad or, alternatively, diced and put through a meat sauce for either fish or meat preparations.

The texture of ox tongue is quite spongy, so when using warm in certain dishes something with a crisp, crunchy texture should be added to the dish to balance out the plate.

i Tongue has been cooked, pressed, pickled and canned since before the Second World War and remains an under-utilised product.

43 Veal chops with cream and mustard sauce

energy	kcal	fat	sat fat	carb	sugar	protein	fibre
1390 KJ	331 cal	12.74 g	7.3 g	29.2 g	4.5 g	26.7 g	2.6 g

	4 portions	10 portions
veal chops	4	10
butter or oil	50 g	125 g
dry white wine	125 ml	300 ml
veal stock	125 ml	300 ml
bouquet garni		
salt and pepper		
double cream	60 ml	150 ml
French mustard, to taste		
parsley, chopped		

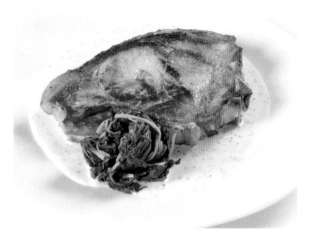

1. Shallow-fry the chops on both sides in hot butter or oil, pour off the fat.
2. Add white wine, stock, bouquet garni and season lightly; cover and simmer gently until cooked.
3. Remove chops and bouquet garni, reduce liquid by two-thirds, then add cream, the juice from the chops and bring to boil.
4. Strain the sauce, mix in the mustard and parsley, correct seasoning, pour over chops and serve.

44 Sautéed veal kidneys with shallot sauce

energy	kcal	fat	sat fat	carb	sugar	protein	fibre
2212 KJ	536 cal	53.1 g	31.5 g	2.2 g	2.0 g	12.1 g	0.2 g

	4 portions	10 portions
veal kidneys, free from fat and cut into individual nodules	250 g	625 g
shallots, sliced	50 g	125 g
butter	75 g	180 g
white wine vinegar	50 ml	125 ml
cream	250 g	625 g
tarragon, chopped	1 tsp	2 tsp
vegetable oil	1 tbsp	3 tbsp
brandy	75 ml	180 ml

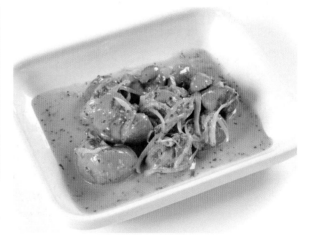

For the sauce

1. Place a hot pan in the middle of the stove for the kidneys.
2. Sweat the shallots in butter in a pan and add the white wine vinegar. Reduce by half.
3. Add cream and bring to the boil. Reserve to finish.

To sauté the kidneys

1. Place the vegetable oil and the kidneys in the hot pan.
2. Caramelise to a golden-brown colour.
3. Turn over and remove the pan from the stove.
4. Let the residual heat carry on cooking for 3–4 minutes.

To finish

1. Remove the kidneys from the pan, drain off the liquid, return the pan to the stove and deglaze with the brandy.
2. Reduce slightly and add the shallot sauce.
3. Bring to the boil, add the tarragon, return the kidneys to the pan and serve.

Uses

This dish would traditionally be served with sautéed potatoes and haricots verts, but due to the versatility of the kidneys, pretty much most things will suit (excluding salad).

Ox kidneys were used instead of veal for this analysis.

The offal in veal has a subtle flavour due to the age of the animal, and pairing it with the shallots here offers an undertone of sweetness to the slightly bitter note of the kidney.

45 Roast shoulder of pork with crackling and apple sauce

energy	kcal	fat	sat fat	carb	sugar	protein	fibre
1711 KJ	410 cal	28.6 g	9.6 g	29.1 g	11.7 g	10.9 g	0.8 g

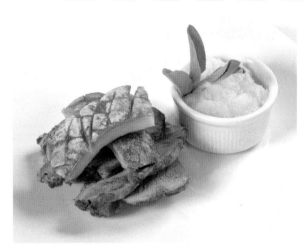

	4 portions	10 portions
Pork		
pork shoulder joint	450 g	1–1½ kg
olive oil to rub on joint		
fine sea salt and freshly ground black pepper		
Bramley apple sauce		
Bramley cooking apples	200 g	500 g
butter	10 g	25 g
caster sugar	1 tbsp	3 tbsp
Gravy		
plain flour	1 tsp	2 tsp
meat or vegetable stock	100 ml	450 ml

1. Preheat the oven to 180°C.
2. Rub the pork skin all over with kitchen paper. Leave for half an hour for the skin to dry (if the skin is moist it will not make crackling). Check the skin is evenly scored. If it is not, make further cuts in the flesh with a large, very sharp knife.
3. Brush the skin very lightly with oil. Sprinkle the skin with a thin, even layer of salt and a little pepper. Set the joint in a roasting tin and place in a preheated oven for 30 minutes, then reduce the temperature to 160°C for a further 1 hour 20 minutes.
4. Meanwhile, make the Bramley apple sauce. Cut the apples into quarters using a small, sharp knife. Peel, core and slice the quarters then place in a pan with 3 tbsp cold water and bring to the boil. Reduce the heat to medium, cover the pan with a lid and cook for 6–8 minutes, until the apples are soft and pulpy.
5. Remove the apples from the heat and beat with a wooden spoon until smooth, then beat in the butter and sugar. If the sauce is too thin, return it to the heat and cook gently, stirring until it thickens slightly. Transfer to a serving bowl.
6. When the pork is cooked, remove from the oven and rest. Cover loosely with foil and leave for 15 minutes while you make the gravy. Using a large spoon, remove as much surface fat from the pan juices as you can. Place the roasting tin on the hob and reheat the juices. Remove from the heat and stir in the flour. Return to the hob and cook gently for 2 minutes. Gradually add the stock, stirring all the time until the gravy is slightly thickened. Simmer for 5 minutes. Pass and check seasoning.
7. Using a sharp carving knife and a fork to steady the meat, remove the crackling from the joint and

place on a board. Cut the crackling into pieces (you can do this with kitchen scissors). Carve the pork into thick slices and serve each portion with some crackling, gravy and a generous spoonful of apple sauce.

* Separate figures were used for the pork crackling and the meat, based on estimated serving sizes.

As this is a traditional roast, most seasonal vegetables will go with it. This is a pure autumnal dish in every way – rich, flavoursome and a traditional Sunday lunch.

How to get the best crackling on roast pork is the subject of much debate in the kitchen. The secret of success is a good layer of fat beneath the rind. Also, the rind should be scored evenly all over. It helps if you choose a larger joint like this shoulder so there is more time in the oven to develop crisp crackling.

46 Herb pasta with Parma ham

	4 portions	10 portions
Chlorophyll (natural green colour)		
watercress, picked	40 g	90 g
parsley, picked	2 g	6 g
baby spinach	10 g	25 g
rocket	3 g	6 g
water	5 ml	12 ml
Pasta		
00 pasta flour	240 g	550 g
egg yolks	5	12
chlorophyll (see instructions below)	12 g	35 g
Parma ham, sliced	50 g	125 g

Chlorophyll

1. Pick the vegetables. Blanch for 3 minutes and refresh.

2. Blitz and pass through a chinois.
3. Add water to the required consistency.

To complete the dish

1. Place the pasta into the Robo Coupe and turn on.
2. Slowly pour the whisked egg yolks and chlorophyll into the flour until it forms a paste.
3. Turn out of the Robo Coupe and work and knead on a bench for 5 minutes to work the gluten and make the pasta more pliable for use.
4. Roll in a pasta machine and turn into linguini.
5. Cook for 2 minutes in boiling salted water, then toss in a little oil.
6. Finish with some sliced Parma ham.

47 Eggs on the dish with sliced onion, bacon and potato

energy	kcal	fat	sat fat	carb	sugar	protein	fibre
2053 KJ	496.5 cal	44.7 g	16.9 g	9.9 g	1.3 g	14.2 g	0.8 g

	4 portions	10 portions
onion, shredded	50 g	125 g
oil	60 ml	150 ml
small potatoes	2	5
lardons of bacon	100 g	250 g
butter	50 g	125 g
eggs	4	10
salt and pepper		
cream	4 tbsp	10 tbsp
chopped parsley		

1. Sauté the onions in oil until they are lightly coloured.

2. Peel and slice the potatoes then fry them separately in oil until cooked and golden brown; drain.
3. Add the onions to the potatoes.
4. Blanch the lardons; quickly fry in the butter, do not drain.
5. Divide the potatoes, onions and lardons into individual egg dishes.
6. Break in the eggs, season with salt and pepper and mask with cream. Cook in a moderate oven until the eggs are set.
7. Sprinkle with chopped parsley and serve immediately.

48 Eggs Benedict

energy	kcal	fat	sat fat	carb	sugar	protein	fibre
3501 KJ	840.5 cal	61.9 g	28.8 g	34.0 g	2.0 g	39.0 g	1.4 g

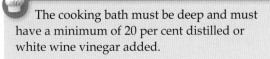

The cooking bath must be deep and must have a minimum of 20 per cent distilled or white wine vinegar added.

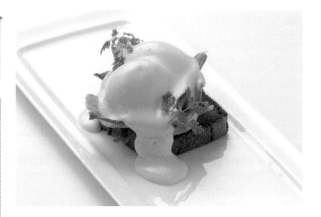

	4 portions	10 portions
cooking medium (see note)		
large eggs	8	20
unsalted butter	2 tbsp	5 tbsp
plain English muffins, split and toasted	4	10
slices smoked bacon or sweet cure bacon, cooked	12	30
Hollandaise sauce (see recipe 49)	200 g	500 g

1. Bring the cooking medium to a slight simmer.
2. Crack an egg into a cup and carefully slide it into the hot poaching liquid. Quickly repeat with all the eggs.
3. Poach the eggs for 3 minutes, turning them occasionally with a spoon, until the whites are firm.

4. Using a slotted spoon, remove the eggs and transfer to a kitchen towel. Lightly dab the eggs with the towel to remove any excess water.
5. While the eggs are poaching, butter the muffins and place 2 halves on each plate.
6. Reheat the bacon and place on top of the muffins, then top with the drained eggs.
7. To finish, lightly spoon over a generous helping of hollandaise sauce and serve immediately, or serve the hollandaise separately.

49 Hollandaise sauce

energy	kcal	fat	sat fat	carb	sugar	protein	fibre
972 KJ	236 cal	25.3 g	15.0 g	0.2 g	0.2 g	1.8 g	0.0 g

	Makes 500 g
peppercorns, crushed	12
white wine vinegar	3 tbsp
egg yolks	6
melted butter	325 g
salt and cayenne pepper	

1. Place the peppercorns and vinegar in a small pan and reduce to one-third.
2. Add 1 tablespoon of cold water and allow to cool. Add the egg yolks.
3. Put on a bain-marie and whisk continuously to a sabayon consistency.
4. Remove from the heat and gradually whisk in the melted butter.
5. Add seasoning. Pass through muslin or a fine chinois.
6. Store in an appropriate container at room temperature.

Egg-based sauces should not be kept warm for more than 2 hours. After this time, they should be thrown away. They are best made fresh to order.

Variations

- Mousseline sauce: hollandaise base with lightly whipped cream.
- Maltaise sauce: hollandaise base with lightly grated zest and juice of one blood orange.

50 Cumberland sauce

energy	kcal	fat	sat fat	carb	sugar	protein	fibre
336 KJ	1410 cal	0.3 g	0.0 g	78.8 g	78.6 g	1.1 g	1.2 g

	4 portions	10 portions
redcurrant jelly	100 ml	250 ml
chopped shallots	5 g	12 g
lemon juice	¼	½
port	2 tbsp	5 tbsp
juice and zest of orange	1	2
English mustard	¼ level tsp	½ tsp

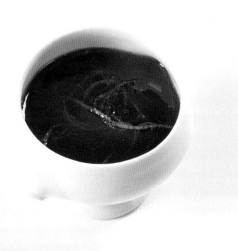

1. Warm and melt the jelly.
2. Blanch the shallots well and refresh.
3. Add the shallots to the jelly with the remainder of the ingredients, except the orange zest.
4. Cut a little fine julienne of orange zest, blanch, refresh and add to the sauce.

May be served with cold ham.

51 Smitaine sauce

	Makes ½ litre
butter or margarine	25 g
onion, finely chopped	50 g
white wine	60 ml
sour cream	½ litre
seasoning	
lemon, juice of	¼

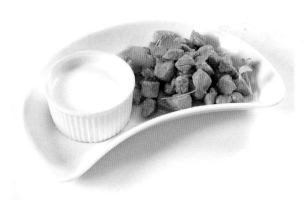

1. Melt butter or margarine in a sauteuse and cook onion without colour.
2. Add the white wine and reduce by half.
3. Add sour cream and season lightly; reduce by one-third.
4. Pass through a fine strainer and finish with lemon juice.

Use with a hached or diced beef steak as shown here or with sausages, etc.

52 Parma ham and cranberry stuffing

	4 portions	10 portions
fresh cranberries	150 g	340 g
sugar	2 tbsp	6 tbsp
water	75 ml	200 ml
butter		30 g
shallots, finely chopped	2	6
cloves of garlic, chopped	2	4
sage, finely chopped	1 tsp	
sprigs of thyme, leaves picked	2	6
salt and freshly ground black pepper		
pork sausage meat, high quality	200 g	500 g
streaky bacon rashers, finely chopped	150 g	400 g
fresh white breadcrumbs	75 g	200 g
walnuts, lightly crushed	1½ tbsp	4 tbsp
zest of lemon, finely grated	½	1
Parma ham, large slices	6	16
vegetable oil		

1. Put the cranberries and the sugar into a small saucepan. Add in the water and stir, then heat until simmering and stir again until the sugar has dissolved.

2. Turn off the heat and leave to go cold. The berries should have softened and deflated slightly.

3. Heat the butter in a frying pan. Add the shallots and garlic and fry gently until the shallots have softened but not coloured. Remove from the heat.

4. Mix in the sage and thyme, then season with salt and freshly ground pepper.

5. Mix in the sausage meat, chopped bacon, breadcrumbs, walnuts and lemon zest. Wear latex gloves and use your hands to ensure everything is well mixed together.

6. Drain away the syrup from the cranberries, then stir the berries into the stuffing mix.

7. Shape the stuffing into 8 balls, each the size of a large golf ball.

8. Wrap each one in two slices of Parma ham. Cover with cling film and put in the fridge to firm up, ideally overnight.

9. Place the balls into a shallow roasting tin, leaving lots of space between them.

10. Dab them all over with a little oil and roast for 30 minutes or so until crisped and cooked through.

53 Pork, sage and onion forcemeat

large onion, finely chopped (approx. 100 g)	1
dried sage	1 heaped tsp
white breadcrumbs	4 heaped tbsp
boiling water	2–3 tbsp
sausage meat	900 g
salt and freshly ground black pepper	

1. Mix the onion, sage and breadcrumbs in a large bowl, then add the boiling water and cool thoroughly.

2. Work the sausage meat into it and season.

Used with turkey. Makes enough for an 8 kg bird.

Poultry and game

This chapter covers Unit 306: Advanced Skills and Techniques in Producing Poultry and Game Dishes. In this chapter you will learn to:

1. Prepare cuts and joints of poultry and game

2. Prepare associated products

3. Produce poultry and game dishes, associated products and garnishes.

6.1 Poultry

Choosing and buying

Nowadays poultry is readily available both fresh and frozen, and suppliers sell birds either oven-ready or fresh (with the entrails still in). Generally a large bird gives better value because the meat-to-bone proportion is higher. As well as being available whole, poultry can be bought jointed and portioned, to save on labour and preparation time. Chicken and turkey are also frequently available smoked, as gourmet items.

Crowns are the breasts of the bird without the legs on the bone. For example, turkey crowns are easier and quicker to cook than whole birds and it is less likely that the breast meat will overcook, which often happens when the bird is roasted with the legs on.

Chicken is available as chicken legs, chicken wings, chicken breast, single and double, suprêmes are also sold as separate units, as are thighs, drumsticks and wings. Chicken meat is also available diced or minced. The small fillets from the underside of chicken breasts are now frequently sold separately for goujons or stir-fry.

Turkey can also be purchased as boneless breast meat, escalopes, minced, diced, strips for goujons, legs or boned legs (thigh and drumstick may be separate) and wings.

Duck steaks (breasts) are breasts of duck without bone and are very popular purchased as portion controlled items. Duck legs have become increasingly popular for such menu items as confit duck and other slow-cooked products.

Preservation

Poultry and game are most usually sold chilled but can also be purchased as frozen items and increasingly in vacuum packs and modified air packs. These methods are a flexible way of extending the shelf life of many kinds of fresh foods up to two to three times the normal levels. Modified air packs involve replacing the normal surrounding or dead space atmosphere within the food packages with specific mixtures of gases or a single gas. The objective is to inhibit the growth of pathogenic bacteria and moulds and to extend the shelf life of chilled and certain ambient food products.

Some poultry and game products (e.g. foie gras) are available in cans.

Cooking

Chicken

Chicken is a delicate meat and needs considerate cooking due to its high protein content (especially the breast). A high heat would render the fibres tough and dry; therefore consideration needs to be applied in order to deliver the desired result. Much depends on the age of the bird: tender, young poultry can be grilled, roasted or fried; older birds or poultry that has special high-worked muscle groups (for example, guinea fowl, poulet noir) would need slower cooking. For example, the French dish coq au vin would tend to be made from older birds – not necessarily cockerels, but birds of 3 kg-plus. Therefore, the age and type of the poultry determines the method and recipe.

Turkey

Turkeys can vary in weight from 3½–20 kg. They are cleaned and trussed in the same way as chicken. The wishbone should always be removed before trussing. The sinews should be drawn out of the legs. Allow 200 g per portion raw weight.

Note: When cooking a large turkey the legs may be removed, boned, rolled, tied and roasted separately from the remainder of the bird. This will reduce the cooking time and enable the legs and breast to cook more evenly.

Forcemeat

Forcemeat is minced or chopped meat, e.g. chicken, pork, veal, beef, often seasoned with a variety of herbs and spices sometimes bound with eggs and/or extended with breadcrumbs.

Forcemeat is used in poultry and game dishes to retain shape after boning etc, to enhance flavour, to assist in retaining moisture, to add a different texture or simply used as an accompaniment or garnish.

For food safety reasons* it is not recommended that the cavities of whole birds are stuffed with forcemeat (unless they are very small birds); stuff the smaller neck cavity only.

*stuffing the cavity prevents the centre of the birds getting hot enough to effectively destroy pathogenic bacteria.

See recipes 5, 6 and 8 for instructions on preparing forcemeat.

Storage

Fresh, uncooked poultry should be used within two to three days of purchase, provided it has been kept in a refrigerator. Poultry must be covered at all times and kept below all other food items, mainly on the bottom shelf, to ensure that no cross-contamination occurs. If the poultry has been purchased frozen, it should be removed from the freezer, placed directly into the fridge on a drip tray, covered and allowed to defrost thoroughly in the fridge. Cooked poultry too should be used within two to three days and kept separately from all other raw products.

6.2 Game

Origins

The word game is used, for culinary purposes, to describe animals or birds that are hunted for food, although many types of categorised game are now being bred domestically – squab (pigeon), ducks, venison and so on. Wild animals, because of their diet and general lifestyle, have select enzymes in their tissues, which are more abundant in game than in poultry. These tissues break down or metabolise meat proteins; they become active about 24 hours after the animal has been killed, softening the meat and making it gelatinous and more palatable, as well as giving the characteristic 'gamey' flavour. They also contain micro-organisms (anaerobes), which also help to break down the proteins.

Food value

As it is less fatty than poultry or meat, game is easily digested, with the exception of water fowl, owing to their oily flesh. Game is useful for building and repairing body tissues and for energy.

Choosing and buying

The most important factor when buying game is to know its life age and its hanging age since this will determine the method of cookery. Indications of age are by no means infallible, but there are some general guidelines when buying young birds – soft-textured feet, pliable breastbones – and young partridges have pointed flight feathers (the first large feather of the wing), while in older birds, the feathers are more rounded. There are many other distinctive guidelines you can use when selecting game, however the grading of game is a specialised subject and best left to the experts.

Although game birds are usually purchased whole or just gutted it is now possible to buy the specific cut or joint required e.g. crown of squab or pheasant. This allows the cut to meet the menu requirements and reduces time and resources needed in preparation.

Quality points for buying

Venison

Joints of venison should be well fleshed and a dark brownish-red colour.

Venison is the meat of the red deer, fallow deer and roebuck. Of these three, the meat of the roebuck is considered to have the best and most delicate eating quality. The prime cuts are the legs, loins and best ends. The shoulders of young animals can be boned, rolled and roasted, but if in any doubt as to their tenderness, they should be cut up and used for stewed or braised dishes.

After slaughter, carcasses should be hung well in a cool place for several days and when cut into joints are usually marinated before being cooked.

Hares and rabbits

The ears of hares and rabbits should tear easily. With old hares the lip is more pronounced than in young animals. The rabbit is distinguished from the hare by shorter ears, feet and body.

Young hares 2½ to 3 kg in weight should be used. To test a young hare it should be possible to take the ear between the fingers and tear it quite easily; also the hare lip, which is clearly marked in older animals, should be only faintly defined.

A hare should be hung for about a week before cleaning it out.

Wild boar

Buy from suppliers using as near as possible to completely pure breeding stock and allowing the boars to roam freely and forage for food.

Animals between 12 and 18 months old, weighing 60–75 kg on the hoof, are best slaughtered in late summer when the fat content is lower. The meat should be hung for 7–10 days before being used. Prime cuts (leg, loin, best end) can be marinated and braised.

Young boar, up to the age of 6 months, are sufficiently tender for cooking as noisettes and cutlets or roasting as joints.

Birds

You should check the following:
1. The beak should break easily.
2. The breast plumage ought to be soft.
3. The breast should be plump.
4. Quill feathers should be pointed, not rounded.
5. The legs should be smooth.

Hanging game

Game bought from a main dealer will probably have been hung correctly. If, however, you require your game (or any other meat that benefits from hanging) to be hung specifically for you, speak to your butcher or game dealer. The general rules are to hang in a cool, dry, airy place, protected from flies to prevent maggot infestation. However, there is no real need to hang certain types of game, due to the metabolic enzymes present, so if you object to the strong flavour hanging promotes, a short hanging period, or no hanging at all, may be preferable. As a general rule you should hang the carcass until you detect the first whiff of tainting. In Britain, birds are usually hung from their heads, feet down, and rabbits and other game hung with their heads down.

Storage of game

It would be wise to allow game to be hung at specific game dealers as current legislation does not allow a normal kitchen environment to hang or pluck game. Game should be wrapped well and careful consideration given to its age; strict labelling is essential because, when in prime condition, the meat may have a slightly tainted smell, which may be difficult to discern from the smell that denotes the meat is past its best.

Storage requirements:
1. Hanging is essential for some game. It drains the flesh of blood and begins the process of disintegration, which is vital to make the flesh soft and edible, and also to develop flavour.
2. The hanging time is determined by the type, condition and age of the game, and the storage temperature.
3. Old birds need to hang for a longer time than young birds.

Table 6.1 Seasons for game

	JAN	FEB	MAR	APR	MAY	JUN	JUL	AUG	SEP	OCT	NOV	DEC
Furred												
Hare	B	B	A				B	B	A	A	B	B
Rabbit	A	A	A	A	A	A	A	A	A	A	A	A
Venison	A	A	A	A	A	A	A	A	A	A	A	A
Feathered												
Goose (wild)	A									B	B	B
Goose (farmed)	A								A	B	B	B
Grouse								12th	B	B	B	A
Mallard	A								A	A	A	A
Moorhen	A								A	A	A	A
Partridge (English grey leg)	B								A	B	B	B
Partridge (French red leg)	A								A	A	B	B
Pheasant	B									A	B	B
Pigeon (farmed)	A	A	A	A	A	A	A	A	A	A	A	A
Pigeon (English wood)	A	A	A	A	B	B	B	B	B	B	B	B
Quail	A	A	A	B	B	B	B	A	A	A	A	A
Snipe	B							12th	A	B	B	B
Teal	B								A	A	A	B
Woodcock	B									B	B	A

Code:

Available

At best

4. Game birds are not plucked or drawn before hanging.
5. Venison and hare are hung with the skin on.
6. Game must be hung in a well-ventilated, dry, cold storeroom; this need not be refrigerated.
7. Game birds should be hung by the neck with the feet down.

Cooking game

Game meat responds best to roasting. Young game birds in particular should be roasted and it is traditional to leave them unstuffed. Due to the low fat content of game, especially wild non-domestic varieties, added fat in the form of sliced streaky bacon, lardons and the like can be wrapped around the bird to help baste while cooking, retaining moisture. Older, tougher game or high-worked muscle groups, such as a haunch of venison, should be casseroled or made into pies or terrines.

Marinating in oil, vinegar or wine with herbs and spices helps make tough meat more tender; it may also enhance the taste and it speeds up the action of the metabolic enzyme that breaks the game down.

Feathered game

Grouse, pheasant, partridge are the most popular game birds. Woodcock, snipe, wild duck and plover are used but much less so. All these birds are protected by game laws and can only be shot in season. Quail is a game bird, but large numbers of quail are reared and are available all year round.

The term includes all edible birds that live in freedom, but only the following are generally used in catering today:

- Pheasant
- Partridge
- Woodcock
- Snipe
- Wild duck
- Teal
- Grouse.

The flavour of most game birds is improved by their being hung for a few days in a moderate draught before being plucked. Hanging is to some degree essential for all game. It drains the flesh of blood and begins a process of disintegration, which is essential to make the flesh tender and develop flavour – this is due to the action of enzymes. Game birds should be hung with the feet down.

Care should be taken with the water birds – wild duck, teal, etc. – not to allow them to get too high, because the oiliness of their flesh will quickly turn them rancid.

Guinea fowl

Guinea fowl can be used in a similar manner to chicken. The flesh is of a dry nature and has little fat, therefore when roasted or pot roasted it is usual to bard the guinea fowl and not to overcook it.

Increasingly, just the crown or breast is purchased for specific menu requirements.

Pheasant

Young birds have a flexible beak, pliable breast bone, grey legs and underdeveloped spurs or none at all. The last large feather in the wing is pointed.

- They may be roasted or braised or pot roasted
- Season – 1 October to 1 February
- They should be hung well.

Partridge

Young birds indicated as for pheasant, the legs should also be smooth.

- May be roasted, braised, etc.

- Season – 1 September to 1 February
- Three to five days' hanging is ample time.

Woodcock

A good-quality bird should have soft supple feet, clean mouth and throat, fat and firm breast. It has a distinctive flavour that is accentuated by the entrails being left in during cooking. The vent must be checked carefully for cleanliness.

- Usually roasted
- Season – September to April
- Hang for three to four days.

Snipe

Snipe resemble woodcock but are smaller. Points of quality are the same as for woodcock. The flavour of the flesh can be accentuated in the same way as for the woodcock.

- May be roasted and are sometimes cooked in steak puddings or pies
- Season – October to November
- Hang for three to four days.

Snipe and woodcock are prepared with the head left on and the beak is used for trussing. The head is prepared by removing the skin and eyes.

Wild duck

The most common is the mallard, which is the ancestor of the domestic duck. The beak and webbed feet should be soft and pliable.

- They may be roasted, slightly underdone or braised
- Season – August to February.

It is particularly important that water birds be eaten only in season; out of season the flesh becomes coarse and acquires a fishy flavour.

Teal

This is a smaller species of wild duck. Select as for wild duck.

- May be roasted or braised
- Season – October to January.

Grouse

This is one of the most popular game birds.

Young birds have soft downy plumes on the breast and under the wings. They also have pointed wings and a rounded, soft spur knob; the spur becomes hard and scaly in older birds.

- Usually served roasted, left slightly underdone
- Grouse is equally popular hot or cold
- Season – 12 August to 10 December.

Stuffing

In the interests of food safety, stuffing should be used only in small birds (e.g. poussins or ballotines), where a savoury stuffing is required. For larger birds (e.g. turkeys, chickens, geese, ducks) it is safer to cook the stuffing separately and the term 'forcemeat' can be used in place of stuffing.

Leg removal and crowning
See photos.

Preparation of poultry and game birds
Drawing and washing

This is the process that is carried out when the bird is sold with all its entrails still inside. To remove, make a small lateral incision into the backside of the bird, then insert your forefinger and middle finger, and roll them around the inner cavity of the bird, thus loosening the membrane that holds the innards in. When loose, remove from the wider backside and discard. Ensure that all the innards are removed, wash and dry well.

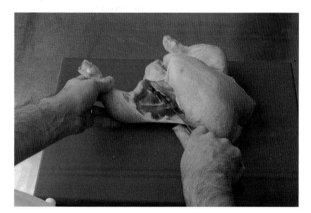

a) Starting to remove the leg

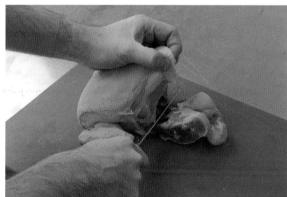

c) Preparing the crown

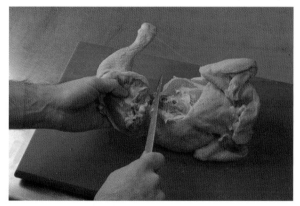

b) Cutting off the leg

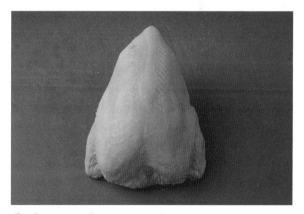

d) A prepared crown

White chicken stock

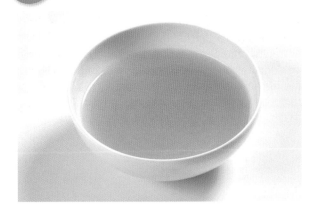

1. Remove any excess fat from the chicken carcasses and wash off under cold water.
2. Place all the bones into a pot that will hold all the ingredients, leaving 5 cm at the top to skim.
3. Add all the other ingredients and cold water, and bring to a simmer; immediately skim all the fat that rises to the surface.
4. Turn the heat off and allow the bones and vegetables to sink. Once this has happened turn the heat back on, skim and bring to just under a simmer, making as little movement as possible to create more of an infusion than a stock. Skim continuously.
5. Leave to simmer (infuse) for 10 hours then pass through a fine sieve into a clean pan; reduce down rapidly, until you have about 2 litres remaining.

	Makes 2 litres
chicken carcass/wings	20 kg
onions, peeled	6
carrots, peeled	8
bulb of garlic	1
leeks, washed and blemishes removed	4
celery sticks	8
bay leaves	2
sprigs of thyme	6
whole white peppercorns	30 g

Cutting for sauté, fricassée, pies, etc.

1. Remove the feet at the first joint.
2. Remove the legs from the carcass.
3. Cut each leg in two at the joint.
4. Remove the wishbone. Remove winglets and trim.
5. Remove the wings carefully, leaving two equal portions on the breast.
6. Remove the breast and cut in two.
7. Trim the carcass and cut into three pieces.

Preparation for suprêmes

1. Use chicken weighing 1¼–1½ kg.
2. Cut off both legs from the chicken.
3. Remove the skin from the breasts.
4. Remove the wishbone.
5. Scrape the wing bone bare adjoining the breasts.
6. Cut off the winglets near the joints leaving 1½–2 cm of bare bone attached to the breasts.
7. Cut the breasts close to the breast bone and follow the bone down to the wing joint.
8. Cut through the joint.
9. Lay the chicken on its side and pull the suprêmes off, assisting with the knife.
10. Lift the fillets from the suprêmes and remove the sinew from each.
11. Make an incision lengthways, along the thick side of the suprêmes, open and place the fillets inside.
12. Close, lightly flatten with a bat moistened with water and trim if necessary.

The suprême is the wing and half the breast of a chicken with the trimmed wing bone attached, i.e. the white meat of one chicken yields two suprêmes.

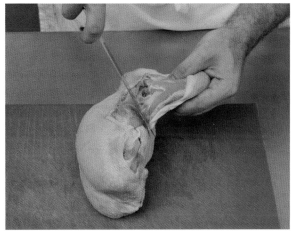

Cut off each leg

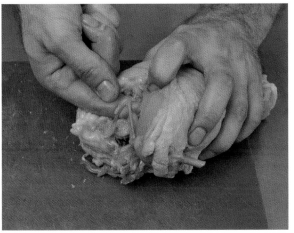

Remove the wishbone

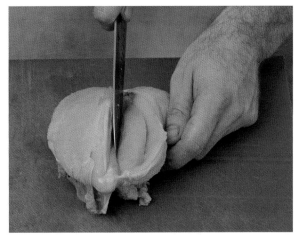

Cut the breast

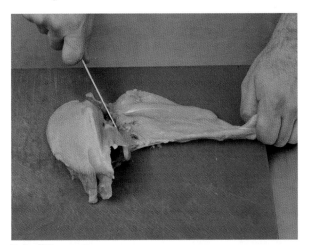

Pull off the suprême

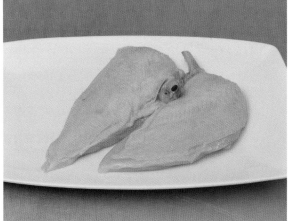

Chicken suprêmes ready for cooking

4 Chicken escalopes

Escalopes can be prepared in a number of ways.

- 75–100 g slices of chicken breast thinly beaten out using a little water, then left plain, or flour, egg and crumbed.
- Boned and skinned chicken thighs treated as above.
- Minced raw breast and/or leg of chicken bound with a little egg white, shaped, flattened and either left plain, or egg and crumbed.

Chicken escalopes can then be cooked and served in a wide variety of ways using different garnishes and sauces.

Any recipe using a cut of chicken can be adapted to use chicken escalopes, but often the simpler recipes are most effective, e.g. egg and crumbed chicken escalope with asparagus tips.

5 Chicken forcemeat or farce

energy	kcal	fat	sat fat	carb	sugar	protein	fibre
2407 KJ	581.6 cal	52.4 g	31.9 g	1.6 g	1.6 g	26.0 g	0.0 g

	4 portions	10 portions
prepared chicken (without skin or bone)	400 g	1 kg
salt and pepper		
whites of egg	3	8
double cream, very cold	225–350 ml	500–600 ml
nutmeg		

1. Remove all the sinew from the flesh of the chicken.
2. Lightly season and process to a purée.
3. Gradually add the egg whites, mixing thoroughly.
4. Place mixture in a bowl on ice until very cold.
5. While on ice, gradually combine with the cream and nutmeg, mixing thoroughly. Test a little of the mixture by gently cooking in simmering water. If the mixture is too light add a little more white of egg; if too stiff, add a little more cream. Check seasoning.

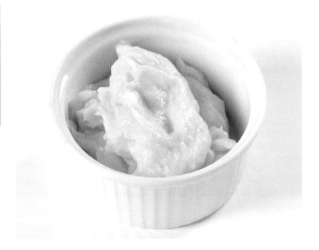

6 Chestnut and apple forcemeat

eating apples, peeled and cored	450 g
tinned whole unsweetened chestnuts, roughly mashed	900 g
salted or fresh belly of pork, cut into small dice	175 g
shallots, finely chopped (approx. 50 g)	2
garlic cloves, crushed	2
parsley, finely chopped	3 tbsp
egg	1

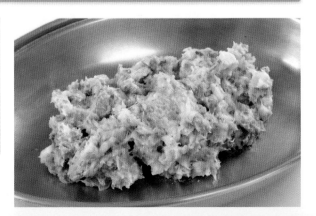

1. Gently stew the apples, covered, in 1 tbsp water until reduced to a pulp.
2. Add to the roughly mashed chestnuts, pork, shallots, garlic and parsley, and bind with the egg.

Used with turkey. Makes enough for an 8 kg bird.

 ## Prune and foie gras stuffing

prunes, stoned and soft	49–50
white wine *or*	300 ml
dry white vermouth	150 ml
beef stock	425 ml
goose liver, finely chopped (approx. 200 g)	1
shallots, finely chopped	2 tbsp
butter	10 g
port	150 ml
foie gras, chopped	110 g
breadcrumbs	2–3 tbsp
allspice	pinch
thyme	pinch
salt and pepper, to taste	

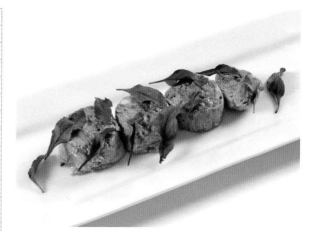

1. Simmer the prunes with the wine and stock in a covered pan for about 10 minutes, until tender. Drain them, reserving the cooking liquid.
2. Sauté the goose liver and shallots in butter in a small sauté pan for 2 minutes. Scrape into a mixing bowl.
3. Boil the port in the sauté pan until reduced to 2 tbsp. Add to the mixing bowl.
4. Add the foie gras to the bowl and mix well until everything is incorporated. If the mixture is too wet for easy stuffing, beat in the breadcrumbs.

5. Season to taste with the allspice, thyme, salt and pepper. Fill each prune with 1 tsp stuffing, then stuff them into the cavity, and skewer or tie closed.

Used with goose. Makes enough for a 6 kg bird.

 ## Game farce

	4 portions	10 portions
butter or margarine	50 g	125 g
game livers	100 g	250 g
onion, chopped	25 g	60 g
sprig of thyme		
bay leaf	1	2–3
salt, pepper		

1. Heat half the butter in a frying pan.
2. Quickly toss the seasoned livers, onion and herbs, browning well but keeping underdone. Pass through a sieve or mincer.
3. Mix in the remaining butter. Correct the seasoning.

9 Serving of cold roast chicken and duck

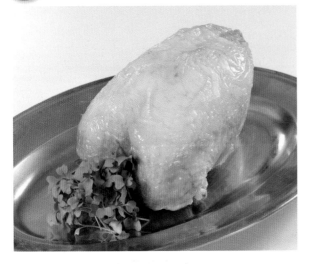

If the chicken is to be displayed whole at a buffet it may be brushed with aspic or oil. It is then dressed on a suitably sized oval dish with watercress and a little diced aspic jelly.

When serving individual portions it is usual to serve either a whole wing of chicken neatly trimmed, or a half chicken. If a half is served, the leg is removed, the wing trimmed, and the surplus bone removed from the leg, which is then placed in the wing (1½ kg chickens).

Larger chickens may be cut into four portions, the wings in two lengthwise and the legs in two joints.

Sometimes the chicken may be requested sliced; it is usual to slice the breast only and then reform it on the dish in its original shape.

To keep roast chicken or duck moist and succulent, roast 2–3 hours before it is required and do not refrigerate.

The serving of cold duck

Use the same methods as for chicken. Serve with sage and onion dressing and apple sauce.

10 Ballotines

Ballotines are boned-out stuffed legs of poultry, usually chicken, duck or turkey, which can be prepared, stuffed with a variety of forcemeat stuffings, cooked, cooled and prepared for service cold with a salad.

Ballotines may also be served hot, with a suitable sauce such as chasseur (red wine, tomato and mushroom).

 When preparing ballotines, keep the skin long as this will help to form a good shape; the shape can be long, round or like a small ham.

11 Chicken, bacon and water chestnut salad

	4 portions	10 portions
chicken suprêmes	4	10
back bacon, cut into lardons	100 g	250 g
water chestnuts, canned, drained	200 g	500 g
celery sticks, finely diced	1	3
white grapes, cut in half, deseeded	50 g	125 g
parsley, chopped	1 tsp	2½ tsp
onion, finely chopped	50g	125 g
lemon juice	1 tsp	2½ tsp
ground ginger	½ tsp	1¼ tsp
Worcestershire sauce	¼ tsp	1 tsp
mayonnaise	125 ml	300 ml

1. Poach the suprêmes of chicken. Allow to cool. Cut into fine strips.
2. Gently fry the lardons of bacon in a little oil. Drain and allow to cool.
3. Mix the chicken, bacon, water chestnuts cut in half, celery and grapes in a suitable bowl.
4. In another bowl, mix together the remaining ingredients.
5. Bind the chicken, bacon, etc. with this mixture. Chill well.
6. Serve in suitable individual dishes or in a salad bowl with the mixed salad leaves.

The salad may also be garnished with tomato, radish and slices of fresh avocado.

Grilled chicken escalopes with asparagus and balsamic vinegar

12

energy	kcal	fat	sat fat	carb	sugar	protein	fibre
1329 KJ	318 cal	17.0 g	2.4 g	3.5 g	2.9 g	37.8 g	1.2 g

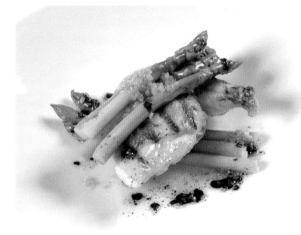

1. Cook the prepared asparagus in boiling salted water for approx. 4 minutes, refresh in ice water.
2. Sweat the shallots without colour until soft, drain and mix with the vinaigrette and lemon juice to form a dressing.
3. Place the escalopes on an oiled tray and season with salt and pepper.
4. Place the escalopes on a preheated grill and grill gently for 3–4 minutes either side, ensuring an even bar mark on the sides.
5. Warm the asparagus through in boiling water, drain and place in the shallot dressing.
6. Take the cooked chicken escalopes and place on a plate or serving dish, lay the asparagus on top, finish with the dressing and balsamic vinegar.
7. Serve immediately.

	4 portions	10 portions
asparagus pieces	20	50
banana shallots, finely diced	2	5
vinaigrette	20 ml	50 ml
lemon, juice of	1	3
chicken breast escalopes (see recipe 4)	4 × 150 g	10 × 150 g
vegetable oil	50 ml	125 ml
salt and pepper		
aged balsamic vinegar	20 ml	50 ml

If a grill is unavailable it is possible to obtain the same marking effect with the use of a bar-marking iron – this process is known as quadrillage.

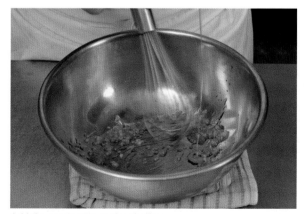

Add the vinaigrette to the shallots

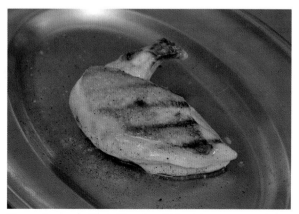

Bar marks created by grilling the chicken

13 Chicken sauté

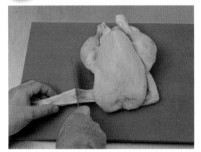
Remove the winglets

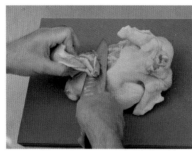
Remove each leg around the oyster

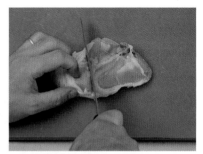
Separate the drumstick from the thigh

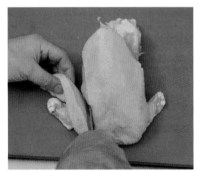
Remove the wings

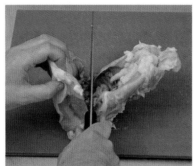
Cut into the cavity

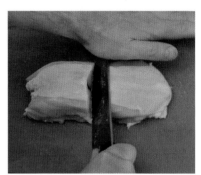
Split the breast

Chickens 1¼–1½ kg in weight are suitable to cut into 8 pieces for 4 portions.

Chicken is prepared in this manner for fricassée, blanquette and chicken pies; the winglets, giblets and carcass are used for chicken stock.

There are many garnishes for chicken sauté. Further variety can be introduced by using herbs (e.g. tarragon, basil, rosemary etc.), wines (e.g. dry white, dry sherry, vermouth) and different garnishes (e.g. wild mushrooms and ceps).

The pieces can be prepared on the bone or skinned and boned out. Boning out slightly increases shrinkage, the portions look smaller and preparation time is increased, but they are easier to eat.

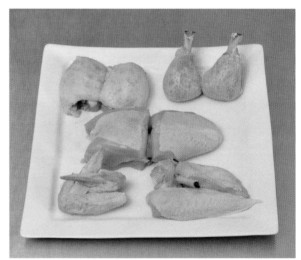
Chicken pieces ready to sauté

14 Chicken with peppers and black bean sauce

	4 portions	10 portions
boneless chicken, cubed	500 g	1 ½ kg
oyster sauce	5 tbsp	275 ml
dark sweet soy sauce	5 tbsp	275 ml
potato starch	1 tbsp	3 tbsp
sesame oil	1 tsp	3 tbsp
leeks, sliced	100 g	250 g
onion, sliced	1	2 large
garlic, chopped	10 g	25 g
young ginger, chopped	20 g	50 g
black bean paste	3 tbsp	200 ml
brown bean paste	1 tbsp	3 tbsp
red pepper, diced	50 g	120 g
green pepper, diced	50 g	120 g
yellow pepper, diced	50 g	120 g
spring onion, sliced	50 g	120 g
coriander, chopped	30 g	75 g
Chinese sao sing wine	3 tbsp	7 tbsp
salt and pepper		

1. Marinate the chicken cubes with the oyster sauce, sweet soy sauce, potato starch and sesame oil for 1 hour.
2. In a frying pan, sauté the leeks, onion, garlic and ginger until fragrant.
3. Add the black and brown bean paste and stir-fry for 2–5 minutes over a moderate heat. Be careful not to burn the paste.
4. Add the marinated chicken and simmer with enough water until it is cooked.
5. Stir in the diced peppers, spring onion, coriander and Chinese wine.
6. Mix the potato starch with enough water and add to the pan to thicken the sauce.
7. Season with salt and pepper accordingly.

15 Lemon and ginger chicken

	4 portions	10 portions
egg, beaten	1	3
sugar	1 tsp	3 tsp
potato starch	3 tbsp	170 g
lemon, zest of	1	1
oyster sauce	5 tbsp	275 ml
cloves of garlic, finely chopped	2	5
young ginger, finely chopped	20 g	45 g
sesame oil	2 tsp	5 tsp
salt and pepper		
boneless chicken legs	4 (180–200 g each)	10
potato starch for coating		
oil for frying		
Lemon and ginger sauce		
young ginger, cut into fine julienne	50 g	120 g
sesame oil	1 tsp	3 tbsp
water	500 ml	1.2 litres
plum sauce (ready-made)	200 ml	500 ml
lemon juice to taste		

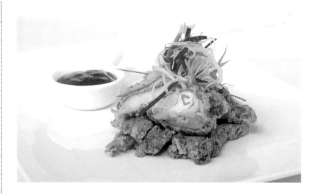

sugar to taste		
salt to taste		
egg yellow colouring		
potato starch	1 tbsp	3 tbsp

1. Mix together the beaten egg, sugar, 3 tablespoons of potato starch, lemon zest, oyster sauce, garlic, ginger, sesame oil, salt and pepper.
2. Marinate the chicken with the mixture and set aside for 3 hours.

3. Dredge the chicken pieces in more potato starch, shaking off excess.
4. Heat the cooking oil in a frying pan and deep fry the chicken over high heat for the first 5 minutes, and then on a moderate heat until it is cooked.
5. Rest the chicken on kitchen paper to remove excess cooking oil.
6. To make the sauce, lightly sauté the young ginger with the sesame oil in a non-stick pan.
7. Add the rest of the ingredients, except the potato starch, and bring to the boil.
8. Mix some water with the potato starch to make a slurry. Thicken the lemon and ginger sauce, and adjust the sweetness and sourness to taste with lemon juice, salt and sugar.
9. Slice the chicken and pour over lemon and ginger sauce to serve.

16 *Ayam kicap asam* (Malaysian spiced fried chicken with plum sauce)

	4 portions	10 portions
boneless chicken, cubed	500 g	1½ kg
salt		
turmeric powder	1 tbsp	2½ tbsp
sesame oil	1 tsp	2 tsp
chilli powder	1 tsp	2½ tsp
oyster sauce	3 tbsp	150 ml
Chinese sao sin wine	1 tbsp	3 tbsp
flour for dusting		
cloves of garlic, chopped	5	12
yellow onion, sliced	1	2
leeks, sliced	50 g	120 g
dried chillies	10 g	22 g
young ginger pieces, thinly sliced	10	22
sweet dark soy sauce	2 tbsp	5 tbsp
plum sauce	3 tbsp	7–8 tbsp
spring onion, cut into 5 cm lengths	50 g	120 g
coriander, chopped	10 g	25 g
salt and black pepper to taste		
sesame seeds, toasted	1 tsp	3 tsp

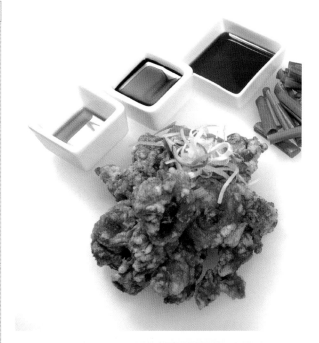

1. Marinate the chicken with the salt, turmeric powder, sesame oil, chilli powder, oyster sauce and Chinese wine for 2–3 hours.
2. Dust with some flour and deep fry the chicken until it is crispy and cooked.
3. Heat a small quantity of oil and add the garlic, onion, leek, dried chillies and ginger.
4. Add the soy sauce and plum sauce. If it is too thick, dilute with some water.
5. Once it is ready, stir in the spring onion and coriander and season to taste.
6. Sprinkle toasted sesame seeds over the chicken and serve.

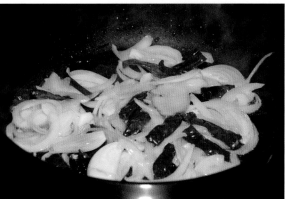

Fry the garlic, leeks, chillies, ginger and onion

17 Chicken stir-fry with bok choy and garlic

	4 portions	10 portions
chicken suprêmes	4	10
bok choy	3	8
Marinade		
Chinese rice wine or sherry	1 tbsp	2½ tbsp
onion, chopped	50 g	125 g
cornflour	2 tsp	5 tsp
Sauce		
chicken stock	125 ml	300 ml
water	2 tbsp plus 4 tsp	5 tbsp plus 10 tsp
white rice vinegar	1 tsp	2½ tsp
black rice vinegar	½ tsp	1¼ tsp
garlic clove, crushed, chopped	1	3
seasoning		
cornflour	1 tsp	2½ tsp
water	4 tsp	10 tsp
vegetable oil	5 tbsp	12 tbsp

Method

1. Cut the chicken into thin strips. Marinate in the rice wine and chopped onion, and sprinkle with the cornflour.
2. Shred the washed bok choy coarsely.
3. For the sauce, mix the stock, vinegars and garlic together with 2 tablespoons of water (5 tablespoons for 10 portions). Disperse the cornflour in the remaining 4 or 10 teaspoons of water.
4. Heat half the oil in a wok and stir-fry the chicken until cooked. Drain and keep warm.
5. Add the remaining oil to the wok. Heat and stir-fry the bok choy. Drain the bok choy and put to one side.
6. Add the sauce ingredients to the wok and bring to the boil. Then add the cornflour and water and stir well to thicken.
7. Add the chicken and the bok choy to the sauce. Stir well.

18 Chicken and coriander satay

chicken breast	3 kg (4 breasts)
cream	130 g
egg whites	300 g
chillies, cut into fine brunoise	30 g
ginger, grated on a micro plane	55 g
lemon grass, soft centre only, cut into brunoise	50 g
garlic, crushed	11 g
coriander leaves, cut into fine julienne	3 g
soy sauce	25 g
peanut butter, crunchy	350 g

1. Chill the Robo Coupe in a freezer.
2. Remove all the fat and sinew from the chicken breasts.
3. Place the chicken in the Robo Coupe and blitz with the cream and then with the egg whites added, until smooth (do not overheat as the mixture will start to cook).
4. Place the chicken mixture in a large mixing bowl and add the rest of the ingredients one by one, mixing well together.
5. Form one piece as a tester and deep fry. Taste for seasoning and flavour, and adjust the seasoning in the remaining mixture accordingly.
6. Form into pieces and deep fry.

Serve as an appetiser or canapé.

19   Ballotine of chicken leg with lentils and tarragon

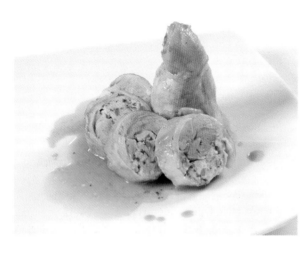

	4 portions	10 portions
chicken legs, large	4	10
chicken mousse (recipe 23)	300 g	750 g
cooked lentils, dry	75 g	185 g
chives, chopped	1tsp	3 tsp
tarragon, chopped	2tsp	5 tsp
chicken stock	125 ml	500 ml

1. Bone out the chicken legs for ballotines.
2. Combine all the other ingredients well, taking care not to overwork the mousse so that it does not split.
3. Fill the chicken leg cavity with the mousse and carefully wrap in foil, making sure the mousse is well encased in the chicken leg.
4. Place the leg in the preheated oven for 25 minutes. Remove and allow to rest for 5 minutes.
5. Remove from the foil and place in a hot pan with oil. Cook until golden brown, then rest for 3 minutes.
6. While resting, deglaze the pan with the chicken stock, scraping the base of the pan for residual cooking matter. Reduce by two-thirds.
7. Carve each ballotine into 3 pieces. Serve with a seasonal garnish and pour over the roasting juices.

Variations

- Ballotine of chicken leg with black pudding: substitute 200 g chopped black pudding for the lentils.
- Ballotine of chicken leg with morels: substitute 150 g chopped, cooked morels for the lentils, and use parsley instead of tarragon.
- Ballotine of chicken leg with smoked bacon: substitute 150 g cooked, chopped pancetta for the lentils, and use parsley instead of tarragon.

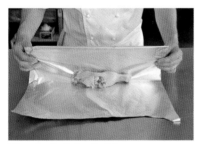
Wrap the ballotine in foil

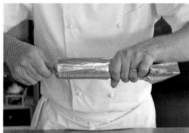
Seal the foil package

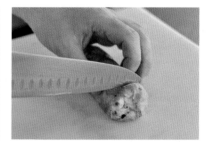
Carve the cooked ballotine into slices to serve

20 Confit chicken leg with leeks and artichokes

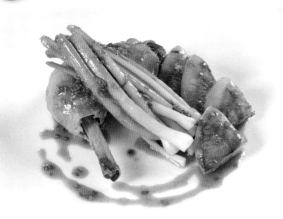

> *i* Confit oil is 50/50 olive oil and vegetable oil infused with herbs, garlic, whole spice or any specific flavour you wish to impart into the oil; then, through slow cooking in the oil, the foodstuff picks up the flavour.

	4 portions	10 portions
confit oil	1 litre	2½ litres
garlic cloves	4	10
bay leaf	1	3
sprig of thyme		
chicken legs	4 × 200 g	10 × 200 g
vegetable oil	50 ml	125 ml
globe artichokes, prepared, cooked and cut into quarters	4	10
whole leeks, blanched	2	5
brown chicken stock	250 ml	625 ml
butter	50 g	125 g
chives, chopped	1 tbsp	3 tbsp
seasoning		

1. Gently heat the confit oil, add the garlic, bay and thyme.
2. Put the chicken legs in the oil and place on a medium to low heat, ensuring the legs are covered.
3. Cook gently for 3–3½ hours.
4. To test if the legs are cooked, squeeze the flesh on the thigh bone and it should just fall away.
5. When cooked, remove the legs carefully and place on a draining tray.
6. Heat the vegetable oil in a medium sauté pan, add the artichokes and leeks, colour slightly and then add the brown chicken stock.
7. Reduce the heat to a simmer and cook for 4–5 minutes; meanwhile, place the confit leg on a baking tray and place in a preheated oven at 210°C; remove when the skin is golden brown (approx. 5 minutes), taking care as the meat is delicate.
8. Place the chicken in a serving dish or on a plate, check the leeks and artichokes are cooked through, and bring the stock to a rapid boil, working in the butter to form an emulsion.
9. Add the chopped chives to the sauce and nap over the chicken leg.

> This dish utilises the by-product of the chicken crown; it is not only very cost-effective but has great depth of flavour due to the work the muscle group has done.

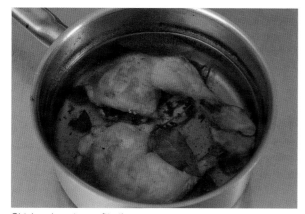

Chicken legs in confit oil

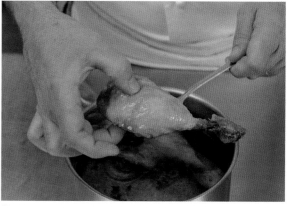

Check whether the chicken is done using the squeeze test

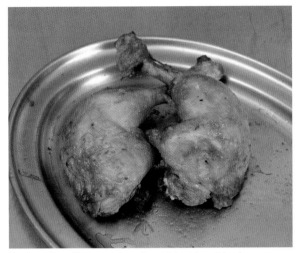

Remove from the oven once the chicken is golden brown

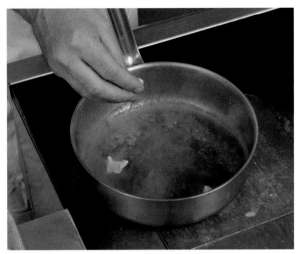

Add the butter to the stock to form an emulsion

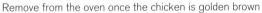

21 Five spice chicken spring roll filling

	For 20–25 small rolls
Chinese dried mushrooms	4
chicken, minced	325 g
baby sweetcorn, finely chopped	100 g
soy sauce	1 tbsp
sesame oil	¼ tsp
shallots, finely chopped	2
five spice powder	½ tsp
fresh ginger, finely grated	1 tsp

1. Place the mushrooms in a bowl and cover with boiling water. Leave to stand for 20 minutes, drain and chop finely.
2. Mix with all the remaining ingredients.

22 Poached eggs with chicken and tomato and cream sauces

energy	kcal	fat	sat fat	carb	sugar	protein	fibre
1624 KJ	390.8 cal	30.4 g	13.9 g	15.8 g	1.9 g	14.5 g	1.0 g

	4 portions	10 portions
eggs	4	10
short pastry	100 g	250 g
cooked chicken, diced	50 g	125 g
tomatoes, peeled, deseeded and diced	50 g	125 g
butter or margarine	50 g	125 g
chicken velouté	125 ml	300 ml
double cream	1 tbsp	2–3 tbsp
tomato sauce	125 ml	300 ml
meat glaze		

1. Poach the eggs and retain in cold water.
2. Line tartlet moulds with short pastry, bake blind.
3. Reheat the diced chicken and tomatoes in the butter or margarine.
4. Place the chicken and tomato in the bottom of the tartlet cases.
5. Reheat the eggs in simmering salted water; drain well. Arrange the eggs on top of the chicken and tomato.
6. Boil the chicken velouté, add the cream and strain.
7. Mask each egg with the two sauces: tomato sauce on one half and suprême sauce on the other.
8. Separate the two sauces with a thin line of warm meat glaze and serve.

23 Chicken mousse

chicken breast	350 g
whipping cream	250 ml
salt and pepper to season	

1. Roughly dice the chicken and place in the freezer for 10 minutes to chill.
2. When the chicken is cold, place in a food processor and blend slightly, then season with a little salt.
3. Pour in the cold cream gradually until all of it has emulsified with the chicken.
4. Form the mousse into quenelles using 2 tablespoons. Dip the spoons into water after each quenelle. Place on a tray lined with cling film and chill.
5. Poach in a little simmering water, adjust the seasoning, drain and store well cling filmed in the refrigerator. Serve with a suitable sauce or as an accompaniment to another dish.

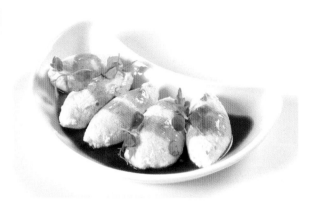

24 Chicken soufflé

energy	kcal	fat	sat fat	carb	sugar	protein	fibre
397 KJ	94.6 cal	5.1 g	3.2 g	0.4 g	0.4 g	11.7 g	0.0 g

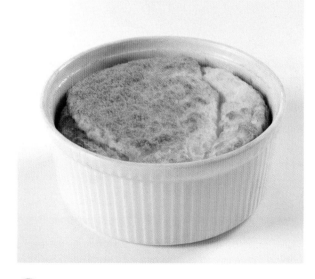

	4 portions	10 portions
raw chicken, without skin or sinew	250 g	600 g
butter	50 g	125 g
thick velouté	250 ml	600 ml
salt and pepper		
egg, separated	3	8

1. Finely dice the chicken and cook in the butter.
2. Add to the velouté and purée in a food processor. Check seasoning.
3. Beat the yolks into the warm mixture.
4. Fold in the stiffly beaten whites carefully.
5. Place into individual buttered moulds or one mould.
6. Bake at 170°C for approximately 15 minutes and serve.
7. Serve a suitable sauce separately, for example mushroom or suprême sauce.

For a lighter soufflé use 3 egg yolks and 4 egg whites.

Add a little egg white powder to the fresh egg whites to strengthen them, which will develop a better foam and improve the rise.

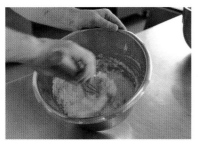
Mix the chicken and the velouté

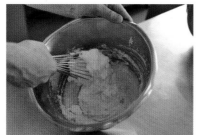
Fold in the egg whites

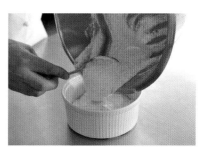
Place the mixture into greased moulds

25 Stuffed leg of turkey

Ensure that the sinews are withdrawn from the turkey leg, remove the leg from the turkey and bone out.

Season and stuff, then tie with string.

Roast, braise or pot roast, remove the string and allow to stand before carving in thick slices.

Suitable stuffings include chestnut, walnut, peanuts or mixed nuts in pork sausage meat or those stuffings suggested for chicken or duck ballotines.

Stuffings may be rolled in foil, steamed or baked and thickly sliced. If a firmer stuffing is required, mix in one or two raw eggs before cooking.

Sauces such as jus-lié, containing cranberries, black-currants or redcurrants, may be served.

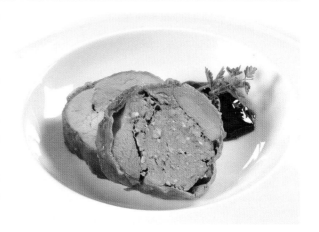

26 Turkey escalopes

100 g slices cut from the boned-out turkey breast can be beaten out using a little water, then flour, egg and crumbed. They may then be shallow-fried on both sides and served with a variety of sauces and garnishes.

The escalopes can also be left in a thicker cut, stuffed and then egg and crumbed.

For simpler dishes they can be lightly coated in sea-soned flour and cooked gently in butter, margarine or oil on both sides with the minimum of colour.

27 Roast goose

Goose, average weight 5–6 kg
Gosling, average weight 2½–3½ kg

The preparation for cleaning and trussing is the same as for chicken.

Roast goose is traditionally served with sage and onion dressing and apple sauce. Other dressings

include peeled apple quarters and stoned prunes, and peeled apple quarters and peeled chestnuts.

For roasting goose proceed as for roast duck using a moderate oven 200–230°C, allowing 15–20 minutes per ½ kg.

28 Serving of cold turkey or goose

For display, cold turkey or goose may be brushed with jelly or oil, but otherwise it is normally served sliced, with the dark meat under the white, chopped jelly and watercress.

Serve turkey with a dressing and cranberry sauce. Serve goose as for duck (see recipe 9).

29 Serving of cold game

Larger birds, such as pheasant, may be sliced or served in halves or quarters; small birds, whole or in halves.

The birds are served with watercress and game chips. Most of the smaller birds are served on a fried bread croûte spread with a little of the corresponding pâté, farce au gratin or pâté maison.

30 Game pies

These can be made from hare, rabbit or any of the game birds.

	4 portions	10 portions
Forcemeat		
game flesh	200 g	500 g
fat bacon	200 g	500 g
beaten egg	1	2–3
salt	10 g	25 g
spices		
Filling		
game fillets	300 g	750 g
larding bacon	200 g	500 g
brandy or Madeira	60 ml	150 ml
salt	15 g	35 g
spices		

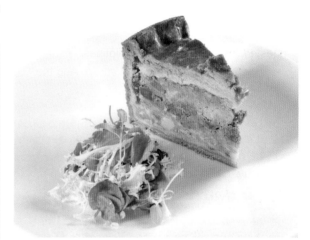

1. Marinate the game fillets in the liquor, salt and spices for 1–2 hours.
2. Prepare, cook and finish as for pâté en croûte (see page 154).

31 Guinea fowl *en papillote* with aromatic vegetables and herbs

energy	kcal	fat	sat fat	carb	sugar	protein	fibre
1540 KJ	370 cal	23.82 g	9.15 g	1.81 g	1.43 g	37.2 g	0.46 g *

	4 portions	10 portions
guinea fowl breasts	4 × 150 g	10 × 150 g
butter	50 g	125 g
shallots, chopped	25 g	65 g
onions, sliced	25 g	65 g
carrots, cut into julienne	25 g	65 g
leeks, cut into julienne	25 g	65 g
sticks of lemon grass	1	2½
sprigs of lemon thyme	3	7
oil	25 g	65 g
dry white wine	100 ml	250 ml
seasoning		
coriander, chopped	15 g	35 g

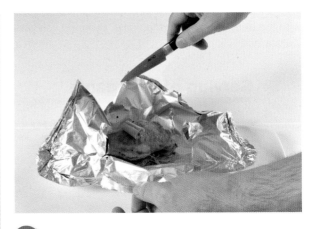

1. In a pre-heated pan seal off the guinea fowl breasts in butter.
2. Sweat the shallots, onions, carrots, leeks and herbs in half the butter without colour. Add the wine and allow to reduce.
3. Season and add the coriander.
4. Cut greaseproof paper or aluminium foil into large heart shapes, big enough to hold one breast each. Oil the paper or foil liberally.
5. Place a small pile of the vegetable and herb mix to one side of the centre of the paper or foil. Place a breast on top and a piece of lemon grass on the breast, and cover with a little of the wine mix. Fold or pleat the paper or foil tightly. Place on

This method of cookery is very healthy as little oil or fat is used, therefore it can be adopted for most poultry preparations.

The choice of aromats or herbs used will obviously reflect the end product. One thing to bear in mind, though, is that hard herbs and big pieces of aromats will not release their flavour quickly enough to penetrate the protein.

an oiled tray in a hot oven (240°C) until the bag expands. Cook for approximately 8 minutes. Serve immediately.

* Partridge was used instead of guinea fowl for this analysis.

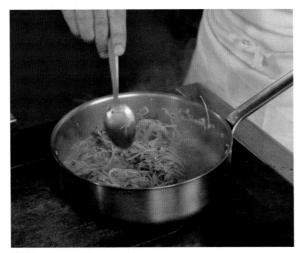

Reduce the cooking liquid

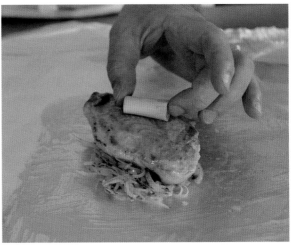

Place the ingredients on the foil, topping with lemon grass

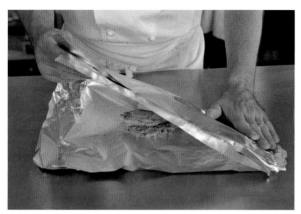

Fold over the foil

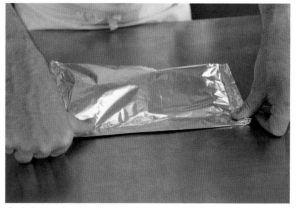

Seal the package

32 Poached guinea fowl with muscat grapes and salsify

	4 portions	10 portions
chicken stock	2 litres	5 litres
guinea fowl crowns	2 (300 g)	5 (750 g)
vegetable oil	50 ml	125 ml
button onions	12	30
reduced chicken stock	250 g	625 g
natural yoghurt	100 g	250 g
juice of lemon	1	3
cooked salsify batons	200 g	500 g
salt and pepper		
peeled muscat grapes	250 g	625 g

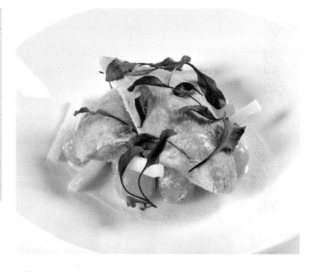

1. Bring the stock up to a simmer; place the crowns in the stock and simmer for 11 minutes.
2. Meanwhile, place the oil in a medium pan and heat to a moderate heat. Place the onions in the pan and colour slightly. Add the reduced chicken stock and cook the onions gently.
3. When the onions are cooked put to one side and retain. Remove the guinea fowl crowns and rest for 2–3 minutes, breast-side down.
4. Remove the breasts from the crown (see page 195) and check if cooked; if not quite cooked place back in the cooking liquor for 1–2 minutes. Then place the breasts on a plate or in a serving dish and keep warm.
5. Add the yoghurt, lemon juice and salsify to the onions with the reduced stock. Warm slightly – do not boil – adjust the seasoning, add the peeled grapes and pour over the guinea fowl.

This recipe may also be used with roast poultry. If using with a roast bird, why not emulsify some of the fat from the roasting pan to increase the flavour of the sauce?

If muscat grapes are unavailable, normal green table grapes will suffice.

33 Confit duck leg rillette

1. Place the duck confit meat in the oven to warm through, which will allow the food processor to break down the meat more easily.
2. Combine all the ingredients, except the fat, in the bowl of an electric mixer fitted with a dough hook. Beat at low speed for about 1 minute, or until everything is well mixed. Or use a food processor, taking care not to purée the mixture or let it turn into a paste. The texture should be like finely shredded meat.
3. Place in ramekins and press down lightly, ensuring an even top. Pour over the reserved confit fat ensuring that it covers the meat to form a seal when set.
4. Use immediately (if doing so, serve without topping off with the oil), or cling film well and store in the refrigerator for up to 1 week.
5. Serve with a chutney or a relish as an hors d'oeuvre (starter).

This preparation can be made with either guinea fowl, pheasant or chicken, and offers a use for surplus legs.

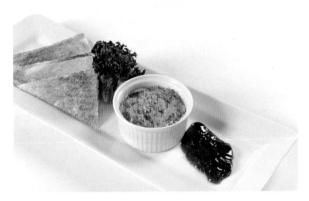

	4 portions	10 portions
duck confit legs, skin and bone removed	4 × 200 g	10 × 200 g
shallots, cooked and chopped	200 g	500 g
parsley, chopped	15 g	40 g
cognac	15 ml	35 ml
orange zest (optional)	1	3
freshly ground black pepper		
sea salt flakes		
fat reserved from the confit	30 g	75 g

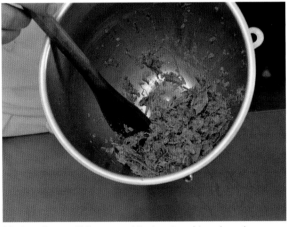

Mix together until the correct texture is achieved as shown here

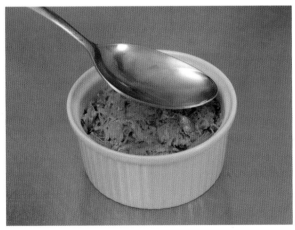

Spoon fat over the meat

34 Garbure of duck

	4 portions	10 portions
duck legs confit, with skin and bone removed	4 × 150 g	10 × 150 g
small green cabbage	½	3
small onion	½	3
Napoli salami in thin batons	40 g	100 g
chicken stock	200 ml	500 ml
haricots blanc, half-cooked	25 g	65 g
flageolet, half-cooked	25 g	65 g
butter	75 g	185 g
leek, in rounds	1	3
bouquet garni	small	large
potatoes, cut into 1 cm dice	250 g	625 g
chopped parsley	2 tsp	6 tsp

1. Place all ingredients in a pan (except the potatoes and parsley) and cook slowly for 1 hour, stirring frequently.
2. After 1 hour add the potatoes and cook for a further 25 minutes.
3. Remove the bouquet garni, add the parsley and work in the butter on a high heat.
4. Serve in a bowl with traditional country French bread, toasted.

This recipe can be used as a secondary protein element on most duck dishes. This is a cost-saving addition as you will be able to reduce the amount of prime breast meat that is needed.

35 Duck and raisin raviolis

	4 portions	10 portions
confit duck, flaked	350 g	1 kg
smoked duck, diced	150 g	350 g
golden raisins soaked in jasmine tea	275 g	650 g
shallots, very finely diced	50 g	120 g
thyme, very finely chopped	10 g	25 g
foie gras, cooked	100 g	225 g
nutmeg, grated, to taste		
salt, pepper		
won ton paste		

1. Mix all the ingredients together except the foie gras.
2. When the mixture is soft, fold in the foie gras and season with nutmeg, salt and pepper.
3. When the mixture is ready, place a small bit of the mix into the centre of a won ton wrapper.
4. Place another sheet on top and then form into a ravioli.
5. Deep fry for 3 minutes at 170°C.
6. Take out of the fryer and place on a plate with paper to take off the excess oil. Add a little more seasoning. Rest for 2 minutes.

36 Peking duck

Peking duck, whole	1
water	4 litres
wolf berries	20 g
dan gui	30 g
dan shen	10 g
yu zhu	10 g
young ginger	100 g
lemon grass	100 g
honey	200 g
cloves of garlic	10
dark soy sauce	100 ml
salt	100 g
five spice powder	20 g
white pepper powder	50 g
sesame oil	2 tbsp
Sauce	
cloves of garlic, minced	3
shallots, chopped	20 g
young ginger, chopped	20 g
sesame oil	1 tsp
hoisin sauce	200 ml
oyster sauce	200 ml
brown bean paste	100 g
Chinese sao sin wine	50 ml
water	1 litre
sweet dark soy sauce	1 tbsp
potato starch	2 tbsp
salt and pepper	

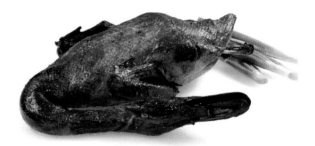

1. Clean the duck, removing and discarding any excess fat from the cavity. Tie a piece of string around its neck.
2. Bring the water to the boil and add the wolf berries, dan gui, dan shen, yu zhu, ginger, lemon grass, honey, garlic and soy sauce. Simmer for 20 minutes.
3. Place the duck into the water and turn it backwards and forwards for about 15 minutes. Remove.
4. In a frying pan, sauté the salt, white pepper and five spice powder in the sesame oil for 10–15 minutes over a moderate heat.
5. Rub the duck with the spiced salt mixture. Hang the duck in a cool, draughty place for about 5 hours.
6. Preheat the oven to 200°C.
7. Place a roasting pan in the oven with a wire rack in it, making sure that there is a space of about 5 cm between the rack and the pan base.
8. Place the duck on the rack, breast-side up, and roast for 40–55 minutes, depending on the size of the duck. Always watch carefully to make sure the skin of the duck does not burn.
9. To make the sauce, sauté the garlic, shallots and young ginger in the sesame oil until fragrant.
10. Stir in the rest of the sauce ingredients (except the potato starch) and bring to the boil. Simmer for 5 minutes.
11. Mix the potato starch with cold water to make a slurry. Use this to thicken the sauce as needed. Season with salt and pepper.

i   Dan gui, dan shen and yu zhu are available from Chinese grocery stores and specialist suppliers. Wolf berries are also known as goji berries; they are sold in health food shops and Chinese supermarkets.

37 Roast pigeon with red chard, celeriac and treacle

energy	kcal	fat	sat fat	carb	sugar	protein	fibre
2735 KJ	655 cal	40.56 g	18.35 g	6.24 g	3.25 g	66.9 g	2.08 g *

i As pigeons do not have gall bladders it is not necessary to remove the livers when they are drawn and cleaned.

	4 portions	10 portions
celeriac, peeled and cut into 2½ cm dice	1	2
milk and water, to cook the celeriac		
squab pigeon crowns (350–400 g each)	4	10
butter, to place in the squab cavity	50 g	125 g
parsnip batons	12	30
butter, to cook the parsnips	75 g	185 g
vegetable stock	200 ml	500 ml
reduced brown stock	100 ml	250 ml
red chard, picked and washed	200 g	500 g
black treacle	5 g	15 g

1. In a saucepan, cook the chopped celeriac until soft in a mixture of half milk and half water.
2. Drain off all the liquid, then purée the celeriac in a food processor.
3. When smooth, place in a clean pan and return to the stove. Cook until thick, letting as much moisture evaporate as possible.
4. Preheat the oven to 180°C. Adjust the seasoning to taste.
5. Roast the squab on the bone for 3 minutes on its back and 3 minutes on its breast.
6. Remove and rest with the butter evenly placed in the cavity to add extra moisture to the bird.
7. Cook the parsnips in butter and vegetable stock, place to one side and keep warm.
8. Wilt the chard, season and drain.
9. Warm the celeriac purée and place on the plate with the chard and the parsnip batons.
10. Carefully remove the two breasts from the bone, place on the chard and liberally drizzle the sauce over the breasts and the plate.
11. If red chard is unavailable you can substitute with spinach or pak choi.
12. Reduce brown stock by half again, add treacle sauce and plate.

* Chicken was used for the saturated fat analysis.

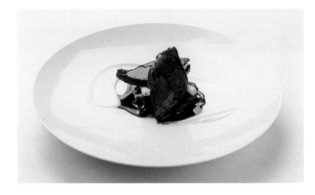

All elements of this dish can be used elsewhere – for example, the celeriac purée is a suitable component for most poultry dishes.

38 *Pot au feu* of pigeon

energy	kcal	fat	sat fat	carb	sugar	protein	fibre
1545 KJ	367 cal	11.29 g	3.44 g	11.12 g	9.98 g	56.2 g	4.79 g *

	4 portions	10 portions
squabs, legs removed	6 (approx. 2 kg)	10 (approx. 3½ kg)
carrot, peeled and cut into 4 laterally	1	3
celery stick, cut into 4	1	3
baby turnips	8	20
medium turnips, peeled and blanched	2	4
leek, washed, cut in rounds	1	3
small shallots, peeled and left whole	8	20
smoked streaky bacon, rind removed	100 g	250 g
chicken/game stock	400 ml	1 litre
bouquet garni with 4 black peppercorns and 1 clove garlic	1	3
salt		

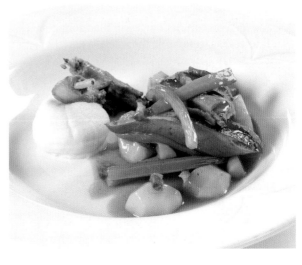

1. Place the squab legs in a large casserole and arrange the vegetables tightly in one layer with the legs, add the bacon, then cover with the stock to about 4 cm above the ingredients (you may need to top this up with water).
2. Add the muslin-wrapped bouquet garni. Season with salt and bring to a gentle boil.
3. Skim off any impurities, cover with a lid (leaving a small gap), and simmer gently for 50 minutes.
4. Skim off any fat or impurities, then add the squab breasts and cook for a further 12 minutes.
5. Taste the broth, correct the seasoning and serve with rich mashed potato or minted new potatoes, depending on the season.

* *Chicken was used for the saturated fat analysis.*

> This is a family or social dish, designed to be placed in the middle of the table and served with warm, crusty bread, mashed potato or buttered new potatoes.

39 Poached pheasant crown with chestnuts and cabbage

energy	kcal	fat	sat fat	carb	sugar	protein	fibre
2417 KJ	581 cal	37.35 g	17.48 g	22.70 g	9.40 g	39.7 g	5.74 g

	4 portions	10 portions
chicken stock	2 litres	5 litres
pheasant crowns	2	5
butter	50 g	125 g
savoy cabbages, cored, shredded and blanched	2	5
cooked bacon lardons	75 g	187 g
reduced chicken stock	250 ml	625 ml
cooked chestnuts	175 g	437 g
double cream	50 ml	125 ml
parsley, chopped	5 g	12.5 g
salt and pepper		
lemons, juice of	1	2½

1. Bring the stock up to a simmer and place the crowns in it; simmer for 11 minutes.
2. Meanwhile, place the butter in a medium pan on a moderate heat and melt. Add the cabbage and bacon lardons and 100 ml of reduced chicken stock.
3. When the cabbage and bacon have formed an emulsion with the butter and stock, put to one side and retain.
4. Remove the pheasant crowns and rest for 2–3 minutes breast-side down.
5. Remove the breasts from the crown (see page 195) and check if cooked; if not quite cooked place back in the cooking liquor for

1–2 minutes. Then place the cooked breasts in a serving dish and keep warm.

6. Add the cooked chestnuts to the remaining reduced chicken stock and bring to the boil, adding the cream. At this point add the chopped parsley and check the seasoning – if the sauce appears to be rich this can be modified with a little lemon juice. You should not be able to taste the lemon but using it allows the deep flavours of the sauce to come through.

7. Place the cabbage mix in the centre of the plate and top this with the pheasant; finish with the sauce over and around, ensuring an even distribution of chestnuts.

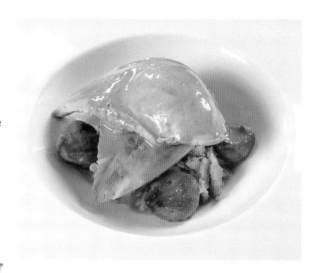

With the legs from the crowns, why not make a pheasant leg garbure (see recipe 34) and serve as a secondary part of the preparation, taking the dish from four portions to eight?

40 Traditional roast grouse

energy	kcal	fat	sat fat	carb	sugar	protein	fibre
3874 KJ	916 cal	23.87 g	8.60 g	104.16 g	7.49 g	77.9 g	3.48 g

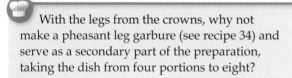

	4 portions	10 portions
Grouse		
young grouse (approx. 750 g each), wings removed	4	10
hearts and livers from the grouse		
sage leaves	4	10
butter	20 g	50 g
salt and pepper		
Stock		
oil	30 ml	80 ml
grouse wings		
giblets		
large onion	1	2
celery stick	1	3
carrot	1	3
red wine	250 ml	625 ml
water		
sprig of thyme		
bay leaf	1	3
brandy		
Toast		
small slices of bread	16	40
duck fat		

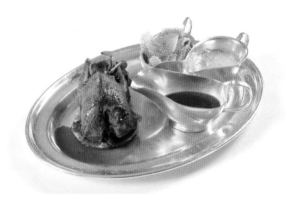

To serve		
bread sauce		
bunches watercress	1	2
game chips		

1. Trim the wings from the young grouse, draw and reserve the livers, hearts and giblets. Season birds liberally inside and out, and put the livers and hearts back in with a sage leaf and a knob of butter. Preheat the oven to its maximum (240°C).

2. Brown the wings and the remaining giblets with the diced onion, celery and carrot. Deglaze pan with red wine, cover with water and simmer for 30 minutes with the thyme and bay leaf. Strain and reserve.
3. Meanwhile, fry the bread in duck fat. Make bread sauce and pick through watercress.
4. To cook, place birds at top of oven and leave for 6 minutes, by which time the legs should be starting to brown.
5. Put bird back in oven for another 7 minutes until, when inserted into the deepest point above the wing, a temperature probe reads 57–60°C.
6. Remove from the pan and leave the birds to rest for 10 minutes in a warm place, on top of the toast, so that the blood drips into it.

7. Put the roasting tray over a flame, add a splash of brandy and the stock, and allow to bubble down to a thin gravy.
8. To serve, scoop out the liver and heart, mash these up and serve on the toast. Stick a bunch of the watercress into the grouse's cavity and put the bird and toast onto a plate with some bread sauce and game chips. Pour a little of the gravy over each bird and serve remaining gravy separately.

Partridge was used for the saturated fat analysis.

Good-quality grouse is essential for this dish – birds that have not been over-hung.

41 Braised partridge with cabbage

energy	kcal	fat	sat fat	carb	sugar	protein	fibre
750 KJ	3137 cal	57.6 g	14 g	11.5 g	6.2 g	47.8 g	1.15 g

*

Older or red-legged partridges are suitable for this dish.

	4 portions	10 portions
old partridges	2	5
lard, butter, margarine or oil	100 g	250 g
Savoy cabbage	400 g	1¼ kg
belly of pork or bacon (in the piece)	100 g	250 g
carrot, peeled and grooved	1	2–3
studded onion	1	2–3
bouquet garni		
white stock	1 litre	2½ litres
frankfurter sausages or pork chipolatas	8	20

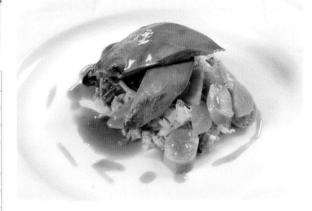

1. Season the partridges, rub with the fat, brown quickly in a hot oven and remove.
2. Trim the cabbage, remove the core, separate the leaves and wash thoroughly.
3. Blanch the cabbage leaves and the belly of pork for 5 minutes. Refresh and drain well to remove all water. Remove the rind from the pork.
4. Place half the cabbage in a deep ovenproof dish; add the pork rind, the partridges, carrot, onion, bouquet garni, the remaining fat, and stock, and season lightly.

5. Add the remaining cabbage and bring to the boil, cover with greased greaseproof paper or foil and a lid, and braise slowly until tender, approximately 1½–2 hours.
6. Add the sausages halfway through the cooking time by placing them under the cabbage.
7. Remove the bouquet garni and onion, and serve everything else, the pork and carrot being sliced.

Based on 100 g cooked meat and oil.

42 Pot-roasted quail with roast carrots and mashed potato

energy	kcal	fat	sat fat	carb	sugar	protein	fibre
2839 KJ	680 cal	41.89 g	16.61 g	9.99 g	2.47 g	66.1 g	1.15 g *

	4 portions	10 portions
quails (approx. 75 g each)	12	30
pancetta, thinly sliced	12 (approx. 250 g)	30 (approx. 625 g)
fresh sage leaves	12	30
vegetable oil	15 ml	50 ml
salt and freshly ground pepper		
carrots, peeled and cut into quarters	3 (100 g)	8 (250 g)
dry white wine	125 ml	310 ml
red wine	125 ml	310 ml
brown stock	250 ml	625 ml
unsalted butter	50 g	125 g
portions of mashed potato	4 (200 g)	10 (500 g)
chives, chopped	1 tsp	2 tsp

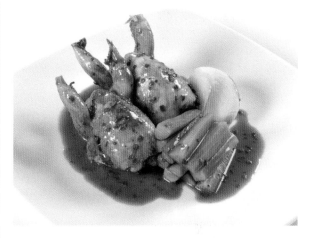

1. Wash the quails thoroughly inside and out, then place them in a large colander to drain for at least 20 minutes; pat the quail dry.
2. Stuff the cavity of each bird with 1 slice of pancetta and 1 sage leaf.
3. Put the oil in a large thick-bottomed roasting pan on high heat. When the fat is hot, add all the quails in a single layer and cook until browned on one side, gradually turning them, and continue cooking until they are evenly browned all over.
4. Lightly sprinkle the quails with salt and pepper, then add the carrots and cook for a couple of minutes until a slight colour appears.
5. Add the wine and brown stock then turn the birds once, let the wine bubble for about 1 minute, then lower the heat to moderate and partially cover the pan. Cook the quails until the meat feels very tender when poked with a fork and comes away from the bone (approx. 35 minutes).
6. Check from time to time that there are sufficient juices in the pan to keep the birds from sticking; if this does occur, add 1 to 2 tbsp of water at a time. When the quails are done, transfer them to a warmed tray and reserve.
7. Turn up the heat and reduce the cooking juices to a glaze – enough to coat all the birds, scraping the bottom of the pan with a wooden spoon to loosen any cooking residues.
8. Add the butter and whisk in to form an emulsion; at this point if the sauce splits or is too thick add a little water and re-boil.
9. Remove the carrots from the pan and place neatly on the plate with the potato purée.
10. Pour the juices over the quail, sprinkle with chopped chives and serve immediately.

Partridge was used for the saturated fat analysis and streaky bacon used instead of pancetta.

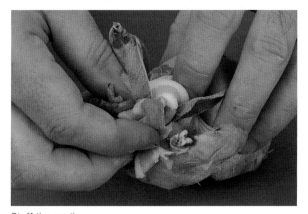

Stuff the quail

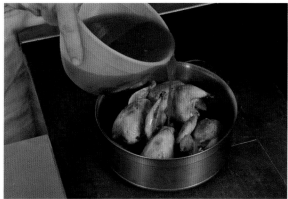

Add stock

43 Stuffed roast quail

Only plump birds with firm white fat should be selected. When prepared the entrails are drawn but the heart and liver are retained inside the birds.

Bone out from the back, stuff with a forcemeat, made as follows, then cook by roasting, spit-roasting, in casserole or by poaching in a rich stock.

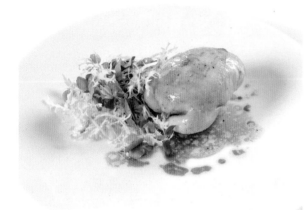

	4 portions	10 portions
Forcemeat		
finely minced pork (half lean, half fat)	200 g	500 g
quail and chicken livers	400 g	900 g
shallot or onion, chopped	50 g	125 g
mushroom, chopped	25 g	60 g
pinch of thyme, half bay leaf		
salt, pepper, mixed spice		

1. Gently fry the pork to extract the fat.
2. Increase the heat, add the livers and the remainder of the ingredients.
3. Fry quickly to brown the livers but keep them pink.
4. Allow to cool and pass through a sieve or mince finely.

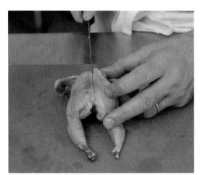

Cut down the back of the bird

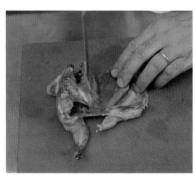

Bone it out from the back

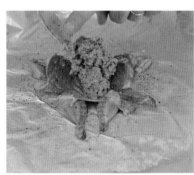

Stuff the quail with farce

44 Quail with pomegranate and blood orange

energy	kcal	fat	sat fat	carb	sugar	protein	fibre
1118 KJ	267 cal	13.30 g	2.59 g	8.24 g	8.01 g	29.2 g	2.49 g *

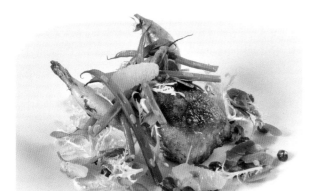

1. Preheat the oven to 180°C.
2. Heat a medium saucepan and add the oil and butter.
3. Season the quails and place in the pan, backs down, colour evenly all over, place in a roasting tray and cook for 6 minutes.
4. Meanwhile, segment the oranges and set aside.
5. Remove the seeds from the pomegranate and also set aside.
6. When cooked, remove the quails from the oven and rest for 2–3 minutes.
7. Remove the quail breasts from the bone and slice into 4 pieces.
8. On the centre of the plate combine the dressed leaves, beans and oranges with a dessertspoon of vinaigrette.
9. Place the quail around the leaves, finish with the pomegranate seeds and serve immediately.

Partridge was used for the saturated fat analysis.

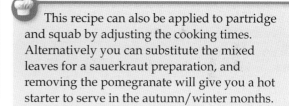

This recipe can also be applied to partridge and squab by adjusting the cooking times. Alternatively you can substitute the mixed leaves for a sauerkraut preparation, and removing the pomegranate will give you a hot starter to serve in the autumn/winter months.

	4 portions	10 portions
oil	10 ml	25 ml
butter	50 g	125 g
salt and pepper		
oven-ready quails (approx. 75 g each)	8	20
blood oranges	2	5
pomegranate	1	2
mixed leaves	200 g	650 g
split cooked green beans	100 g	250 g
vinaigrette		

45 Rabbits

 Rabbits are available wild or farm reared.

Preparation

1. Carefully remove the fur.
2. Cut an incision along the belly.
3. Remove the intestines.
4. Clean out the forequarter removing all traces of blood.

Depending on the required use and size of rabbit, it can be cut as follows.

1. Legs, forelegs, forequarter (well trimmed) into two pieces each, saddle into two or three pieces.
2. Saddles can be removed and left whole for roasting, braising or pot roasting.
3. The two nuts of meat can be removed from the saddle, half cut through lengthwise and carefully beaten out using a little cold water to form escalopes.

Rabbit can be used in a wide variety of dishes, e.g. pâtés, terrines, pies, salads, roast, braised, pot roasted, white and brown stews, curries.

46 Braised baron of rabbit with olives and tomatoes

energy	kcal	fat	sat fat	carb	sugar	protein	fibre
2365 KJ	568 cal	40.98 g	8.42 g	5.47 g	4.75 g	44.6 g	0.87 g

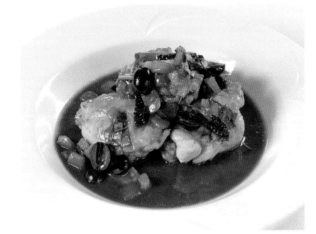

	4 portions	10 portions
farm-raised rabbit barons (approx. 750–800 g each), including bones and trim for gravy	2	5
carrot	1	3
onion	1	3
celery stick	1	3
olive oil	90 ml	225 ml
balsamic vinegar	15 ml	40 ml
caster sugar	10 g	25 g
bottle (750 ml) dry white wine	1	2½
butter, to brown the meat		
basil leaves	12	30
black olives	32	80
pieces home-dried tomato	8	20
salt and pepper		

'Mediterranean influence'

i A baron is the rear end of the rabbit – the rack and the two hind legs.

1. Well ahead of time, prepare the sauce; cut the rabbits across at the point where the ribs end and chop the forequarters into small pieces.
2. Cut the vegetables into a mirepoix.
3. In a large saucepan, brown the forequarter bones and mirepoix in 2 tbsp/5 tbsp of the olive oil.
4. Add the vinegar and sugar, and toss to coat. Cook until light brown.
5. Pour over almost all the white wine, reserving about 1 glass/2½ glasses (150 ml/375 ml) for deglazing the roasting pan later. Boil to reduce until the liquid has a syrupy consistency.
6. Just cover with cold water, return to the boil and skim.
7. Simmer for 1½ hours.
8. Pass the resulting stock into a bowl, wash out the saucepan and return the stock to it.
9. Bring back to the boil, skim again and, once more, return to a slow simmer until reduced by half. Reserve.
10. Cut the rabbit legs into two (thigh and drumstick), and the rack into two.
11. In a large saucepan, brown the meat cuts in foaming butter; when golden brown add the finished stock and cook for a further 1½ hours (approx.).
12. When cooked, pass the sauce through a fine strainer, bring to the boil and reduce by half.
13. While reducing, put the rabbit into a serving dish, shred the basil and remove the stones from the olives.
14. When the sauce is reduced by half, add the tomatoes, olives and basil. Correct the seasoning, pour over the rabbit and serve.

Variation

The 'Mediterranean influence' can be omitted, substituted with a British theme – woodland mushrooms, parsnips – and served with braised cabbage.

Rabbit saddle stuffed with its own livers

energy	kcal	fat	sat fat	carb	sugar	protein	fibre
1393 KJ	333 cal	18.21 g	2.66 g	6.64 g	2.47 g	36.0 g	2.66 g

	4 portions	10 portions
Saddle		
long saddles rabbit (approx. 400 g each), livers retained	3	5
spinach leaves	100 g	250 g
thin slices Parma ham	9	23
Lentil sauce		
brown chicken stock	300 ml	750 ml
cold butter, diced	40 g	100 g
plum tomatoes, cut into concassée	3	8
cooked umbri or puy lentils	30 g	75 g
chives, chopped	1 tsp	4 tsp
sherry vinegar, to taste		
To serve		
spinach, picked, washed and wilted	300 g	750 g

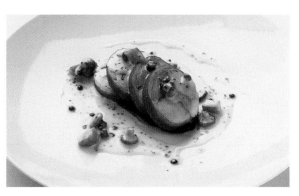

For the rabbit

1. Split the two natural halves of the rabbit liver with a sharp knife.
2. Keeping them as whole as possible, remove any sinew. Wrap the livers in the spinach leaves.
3. Trim off any excess fat from the belly flaps of the rabbit.
4. Lay the spinach-wrapped livers in the cavity of the rabbit.
5. Lay 2 pieces of the Parma ham on a 30 cm-square sheet of kitchen foil and place the rabbit saddle with the livers facing upwards on the ham.
6. Roll into a sausage shape, twisting the ends of the foil to ensure a tight parcel.
7. Repeat with the remaining rabbits and place in the fridge overnight to rest.

For the lentil sauce

1. Place the chicken stock in a saucepan, bring to the boil and simmer until the volume has reduced to 150 ml.
2. Add the butter to the reduced stock and whisk to an emulsion, add the tomatoes, lentils and chives, and adjust the seasoning to taste. Finish with the sherry vinegar so you can just taste the acid in the background.

To complete

1. Preheat the oven to 180°C. Place the rabbit saddles on a baking tray and roast for 17 minutes, turning after 10 minutes.
2. Remove the rabbit from the oven and rest for 3–4 minutes in the foil.
3. Remove the foil from the rabbit and slice each saddle into 4 equal pieces.
4. Lay the sliced rabbit on wilted spinach and garnish the dish with the lentil sauce. Serve immediately.

If thinking ahead, the best approach for this dish is to prepare the rabbit saddle the day before or at least 8 hours before cooking, to allow the meat to rest and form an even cylinder – otherwise, when sliced, it will tend to spring open.

48   Rabbit, truffle and tarragon boudin

	4 portions	10 portions
white bread, no crusts (soaked in the milk)	65 g	160 g
milk	100 ml	230 ml
chicken breasts, diced	2	5
egg white	1	3
cream	150 ml	350 ml
foie gras, diced	100 g	230 g
confit rabbit, diced	125 g	280 g
chopped tarragon, chopped	5 g	15 g
chopped truffle, chopped	5 g	15 g
seasoning		

1. Soak the bread in the milk.
2. Blitz the chicken in the food processor and then add salt.
3. When tight, add the bread and egg white, and mix until smooth.
4. Add the cream and then pass.
5. Fold in all the other ingredients.
6. Poach a little piece and check for seasoning.
7. Roll into ballotines and cook at 68°C for 60 minutes.

49   Venison cutlets, chops and steaks

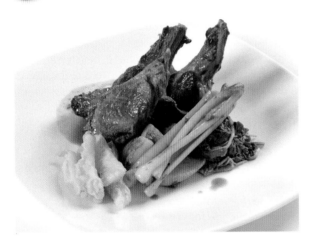

1. Venison cutlets, cut from the best end, and chops, cut from the loin, are usually well trimmed, and cooked by shallow-frying, provided that the meat is tender. If in doubt they should be braised.
2. After they are cooked they should be removed from the pan, the fat poured off and the pan deglazed with stock, red wine, brandy, Madeira or sherry, which is then added to the accompanying sauce.
3. A spicy, peppery sauce is usually offered, which can be varied by the addition of any one or more extra ingredients, e.g. cream, yoghurt, redcurrant jelly, choice of cooked beetroot, sliced button or wild mushrooms, cooked pieces of chestnut, etc.
4. Accompaniments can include, for example, a purée of green, brown or yellow lentils, a purée of any other dried bean, purée of braised chestnuts, braised red cabbage, or purée of a root vegetable, e.g. celeriac, turnip, swede, carrot, parsnip or any combination of these.
5. Venison steaks or escalopes are cut from the boned-out nuts of meat from the loins, well trimmed and slightly thinned with a meat bat.
6. The escalopes can be quickly shallow-fried and finished as for cutlets and chops, with a variety of accompanying sauces and garnishes.

50 # Medallions of venison with red wine, walnuts and chocolate

energy	kcal	fat	sat fat	carb	sugar	protein	fibre
1834 KJ	439 cal	26.96 g	5.62 g	8.38 g	8.18 g	43.7 g	0.66 g

	4 portions	10 portions
vegetable oil	50 ml	125 ml
trimmed venison loin	750 g	1.8 kg
salt and pepper		
Merlot sauce (see recipe 54)	200 ml	500 ml
broken walnut pieces	40 g	100 g
70 per cent bitter chocolate in small broken pieces	50 g	125 g

1. Preheat the oven to 190°C. Heat the oil in a heavy frying pan and seal the venison loin, add salt and pepper, place on a baking tray and then in the oven, and cook for 6–8 minutes medium rare or according to taste.
2. Meanwhile, warm the sauce and add the broken walnuts.

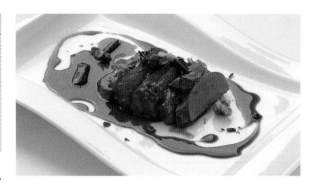

3. Slice the venison loin equally, nap over the sauce and sprinkle liberally with chocolate pieces.

This method of sprinkling the chocolate on afterwards allows you to taste the sauce and the chocolate separately.

51 # Medallions of venison with carrot purée and truffle mash

	4 portions	10 portions
medallions of venison	4	10
Carrot purée		
carrots, peeled	400 g	1 kg
butter	40 g	100 g
Truffle mash		
truffle oil	1 drop	4 drops
truffles, chopped	8 g	20 g
truffle trim, chopped	20 g	50 g
Maris piper potatoes	2 kg	5 kg
double cream	400 ml	1 litre
butter	80 g	200 g

Carrot purée

1. Slice half of the carrots very finely on a mandolin. Juice the remaining carrots.
2. Place the sliced carrots in a pan and then add the juice to cover. If there is not enough liquid, add a little water.
3. Bring to the boil and keep boiling until the carrots are cooked and nearly all the liquid is gone.
4. Add the butter to the cooked carrots and then blitz.
5. Season and store until needed.

Truffle mash

Diced, cooked wild mushrooms may be used instead of truffles.

1. Peel the potatoes, cut into 2 inch pieces and put into cold water.
2. Bring to the boil. Cook for 20–30 minutes, until soft.
3. Remove and wash in running cold water for 2 minutes.
4. Cover with cold water again. Bring up to approximately 80°C and cook for 1 hour 50 minutes.
5. Remove and allow to dry lightly on the pass for 10–15 minutes.
6. Put through a sieve. Mix in the cream and butter (no more than 35 per cent of the mixture should be cream and butter).

To complete the dish

1. Prepare the medallions of venison as for recipe 50.
2. Serve on a bed of truffle mash with a garnish of carrot purée.

52 Medallions of venison with buttered cabbage and haricots blancs

	4 portions	10 portions
medallions of venison	4	10
Haricots blancs		
beans, soaked	200 g	500 g
chicken stock	100 ml	250 ml
clove of garlic	½	1
bay leaf	½	1
thyme	1 g	2 g
Buttered cabbage		
shallots, finely sliced	200 g	500 g
garlic cloves, crushed and chopped	1	2
bay leaves	1	2
thyme	1 g	2 g
cabbage, stalk removed	600 g	1½ kg
salt	8 g	20 g
butter	240 g	600 g
chicken stock	240 ml	600 ml

Haricots blancs

1. Cook all the ingredients together in a vacuum pack bag in the steamer for 25–30 minutes (approx.).
2. Allow to chill on a bench for 1 hour, then place in the fridge until required for the buttered cabbage.

Buttered cabbage

1. Sweat the shallots, garlic and aromats in a little oil.
2. Add the cabbage and sweat for a further 5 minutes.
3. Add the butter and stock, and reduce until emulsified and cooked.
4. To finish, add the cooked haricots blancs.

To complete the dish

1. Prepare the medallions of venison as for recipe 50.
2. Serve on a bed of the buttered cabbage.

53 Medallions of venison with celeriac purée and braised red cabbage

	4 portions	10 portions
medallions of venison	4	10
Celeriac purée		
celeriac, in 2 cm dice	550 g	1.4 kg
milk	300 ml	750 ml
butter	50 g	125 g
cream	200 ml	500 ml
salt (approx.)	2 g	5 g
vinegar		
Braised red cabbage		
red cabbage	150 g	375 g
salt, pepper		
butter	50 g	125 g
cooking apples, finely chopped	100 g	250 g
caster sugar	10 g	25 g
vinegar or red wine	50 ml	125 ml
olive oil	25 ml	62 ml

2. Place the contents of the bag into the thermomix and add the cream.
3. Blitz for 8 minutes and then pass.
4. Season with salt and vinegar.
5. Chill and keep for service.

Braised red cabbage

1. Salt the cabbage for 10 minutes and then wash in water.
2. Dry in a cloth and then add the rest of the ingredients.
3. Place in a suitable pan, lightly oiled. Braise in the oven at 150–200°C for 1½ hours.

To complete the dish

1. Prepare the medallions as for recipe 50.
2. Serve with the celeriac and cabbage.

Celeriac purée

1. Cook the celeriac with the milk and butter in a vacuum pack bag for 40 minutes in the steamer.

Pot roast rack of venison with buttered greens and Merlot sauce

54

energy	kcal	fat	sat fat	carb	sugar	protein	fibre
2984 KJ	717 cal	49.99 g	23.21 g	10.39 g	9.17 g	60.2 g	5.44 g

	4 portions	10 portions
Venison		
venison rack, bones cleaned and trimmed	2 kg	5 kg
vegetable oil	50 ml	125 ml
small mirepoix	250 g	625 g
clarified butter	100 g	250 g
garlic cloves	2	5
sprig of thyme	1	3
salt and pepper		
Merlot sauce		
oil	100 g	200 g
venison trimmings and bones	450 g	1 kg
cracked pepper	½ tsp	1½ tsp
bay leaf	1	3
sprig of thyme	1	2
carrot, peeled and roughly chopped	1	3
onion, peeled and roughly chopped	½	2
garlic cloves, split	2	5
Merlot wine	330 ml	800 ml
chicken stock	1½ litres	2½ litres
Greens		
butter	50 g	125 g
spinach leaves	250 g	500 g
spring cabbage, cut into 1½ cm strips (blanched for 2 minutes and refreshed in an ice bath)	1	2
escarole, stalks removed	1	3

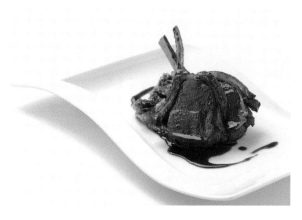

4. Boil rapidly until the volume of liquid has reduced by half. Add the chicken stock, return to the boil, then lower the heat right down and cook the sauce for about 1 hour.

5. Stir every 10 minutes to prevent sticking and skim off any sediment that rises to the surface.

6. When the sauce has reduced to approx. 400 ml (for 10 portions, 1 l), pour it through a fine strainer into a clean pan.

7. Bring to the boil and simmer until the volume of liquid has reduced to 200 ml/500 ml, giving a rich plum-coloured sauce.

For the venison

1. Preheat the oven to 180°C. Trim the venison so that the bones rise 5 cm above the meat. Tie the venison with kitchen string at intervals along the joint, tying 3 pieces of string between each bone.

2. Place a large pan with a tight-fitting lid over a high heat, add the oil and seal the venison, turning until it is a light golden colour all over.

3. Transfer the meat to a tray and cook the mirepoix in the same way.

4. Add the venison back to the pan, placing it on top of the mirepoix, and cover in the clarified butter. Add the garlic, thyme and seasoning. Place in the oven for 20–25 minutes until medium rare (the residual heat will cook it further).

5. Remove from the oven and set aside to rest for 10 minutes.

For the Merlot sauce

1. In a large saucepan, heat the oil over a medium heat. Working in batches to prevent steaming and give a good colour, cook the venison trimmings until brown, add the cracked pepper, bay leaf and thyme. Remove from the pan and set aside in a bowl.

2. Reduce the heat and, in the same pan, cook the carrots, onion and garlic for about 10 minutes or until brown. Return the meat to the pan and stir well.

3. Raise the heat and, when the pan is quite hot, add the wine. Bring to the boil.

To complete

1. Add the butter to a pan, place in the greens and heat through, warm the sauce and then slice the venison.
2. Lay the buttered greens in the centre of the plate with the venison on top and finish with the Merlot sauce.

The rich Merlot sauce can be used for other rich meat dishes; it can be made two or three days ahead and stored in an airtight container in the refrigerator.

55 Ragôut of wild boar with wild rice

	4 portions	10 portions
wild boar, diced	400 g	1¼ kg
butter	50 g	125 g
walnut oil	20 ml	62 ml
matignon	400 g	1¼ kg
flour (for roux)	100 g	250 g
wild boar brown stock	1 litre	2½ litre
smoked bacon strips	100 g	250 g
button onions	100 g	250 g
wild mushrooms	300 g	1 kg
brandy	1 measure	2½ measures
seasoning		
heart-shaped fried bread	4	10
croûtons		
Marinade		
red wine	½ litre	1¼ litre
red wine vinegar	3 tbsp	7½ tbsp
bay leaf	1	2½
onion, sliced	½	1¼
gin	1 measure	2½ measures
juniper berries, crushed	1 tbsp	2½ tbsp

1. Combine the marinade ingredients.
2. Place the diced wild boar in marinade for 24 hours. (Allow ½ litre for 4 portions, 1¼ litres for 10 portions.)

3. Remove the wild boar from the marinade and drain. Retain the marinade.
4. Seal the meat in butter and walnut oil and sweat off. Remove the meat from the pan.
5. Add the matignon to the pan with a little butter and cook the roux out.
6. Add the stock and the sieved marinade and cook for 1 hour.
7. Return the meat to the pan and cook for a further 1 hour.
8. Add the bacon, button onions and mushrooms and simmer for 15–20 minutes.
9. Add a measure of brandy and remove from the heat.
10. Correct the seasoning.
11. Serve with wild rice, chopped chives and heart-shaped fried bread croûtons.

Matignon is a vegetable mixture cooked slowly in butter, with suet, sugar, thyme and a bay leaf, until very soft. (Fortified wine may then be added.) Carrot, celery and onion would be a suitable mixture.

This recipe was contributed by Marc Sanders.

56 **Wild boar medallions with morels and lentils**

	4 portions	10 portions
medallions of wild boar	8 × 50–75 g	20 × 50–75 g
marinade (see recipe 55)	2 tbsp	5 tbsp
lentils	100 g	250 g
ham stock	½ litre	1¼ litre
onion	1	2–3
rashers of smoked bacon	3	7–8
walnut oil	50 ml	125 ml
butter	10 g	25 g
shallots, chopped	2	5
morels, washed	100 g	250 g
brandy	30 ml	75 ml
brown wild boar stock	¼ litre	600 ml
chopped chives	½ tsp	1 tsp
seasoning		

1. Place the wild boar medallions in the marinade and leave overnight. Soak the lentils overnight.
2. When thoroughly soaked, drain the lentils and add to the ham stock with the chopped onion and bacon. Bake in the oven for approximately 45 minutes.
3. Remove the medallions of wild boar from the marinade and retain the marinade. Sauté the boar in the walnut oil and butter, remove from the pan and place on top of the cooked lentils. Keep hot.
4. Add a little butter to the sauté pan and add the chopped shallots, morels, brandy, stock and marinade. Reduce to a sauce consistency, pour over the medallions and finish with chopped chives.

This recipe was contributed by Marc Sanders.

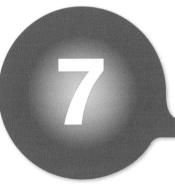

7 Fish and shellfish

This chapter covers Unit 307: Advanced Skills and Techniques in Producing Fish and Shellfish Dishes.

In this chapter you will learn to:

1. prepare fish and shellfish dishes

2. prepare associated products and garnishes.

Fish

Fish are vertebrates (animals with a back bone) and are split into two primary groups: flat and round. From this they can be split again, into sub- or secondary groups such as pelagic (oil-rich fish that swim mid-water, for example mackerel and herring) and demersal (white fish that live at or near the bottom of the sea, such as cod, haddock, whiting and plaice).

Flat fish

Examples of flat fish include:

- Halibut is a long and narrow brown fish, with some darker mottling on the upper side, up to 3 metres in length and weighing 20–50 kg. Much valued for its flavour, halibut is poached, boiled, grilled, shallow-fried or smoked.
- Sole is considered to be the best of the flat fish. It is cooked by poaching, grilling or frying, and served whole or filleted.
- Dover sole is well known to be excellent.
- Lemon sole is related to Dover sole, but broader in shape. Its upper skin is warm, yellowy-brown and mottled with darker brown. It can weigh up to 600 g.
- Turbot has no scales and is roughly diamond in

shape; it has knobs (tubercles) on its dark skin. The average weight is 3.5–4 kg. Turbot may be cooked whole, filleted or cut into portions on the bone. It is boiled, poached, grilled or shallow-fried.

Round fish

Examples of round fish include:

- Bass have silvery grey backs and white bellies; small ones may have black spots. They are usually about 30 cm long but may grow to 60 cm. They have an excellent flavour, and white, lean, quite soft flesh. Bass must be very fresh; it may be steamed, poached, stuffed and baked, or grilled in steaks. It is usually farmed, but sea bass (also called wild or natural bass) is available.
- Grey mullet has a scaly, streamlined body, which is silver-grey or blue-green. Deep-sea or offshore mullet has a fine flavour and firm, moist flesh. Some people believe that the flavour is improved if the fish is kept in a refrigerator for 2 or 3 days, without being cleaned. Grey mullet may be stuffed and baked or grilled in steaks. Its length is usually about 30 cm and the weight 50 g.
- Grouper has a light pink flesh that cooks to a grey-white colour, with a pleasant mild flavour.

Types of grouper include brown, brown spotted, golden strawberry and red speckled.

- Haddock looks similar to cod but with a 'thumb mark' on the side and is a lighter colour. The average weight is 0.5–2 kg. Every method of cooking is suitable for haddock.

Oily fish

Examples of oily fish include:

- Common eels live in fresh water; some are farmed. They grow up to 1 m in length. They are found in many British rivers and are also imported from Holland. Eels must be kept alive until the last minute before cooking, and are generally used in fish stews.
- Salmon is a river fish, caught in British rivers like the Dee, Tay, Severn and Spey, and also extensively farmed in Scotland and Norway. Salmon is also imported to Britain from Canada, Germany and Japan. It is used fresh in a variety of dishes, or tinned or smoked.
- Sardines are small fish of the pilchard family. They are usually tinned and used for hors d'oeuvre or sandwiches. Fresh sardines are also available and may be grilled or fried.
- Tuna has a dark red-brown flesh that, when cooked, turns a lighter colour. It has a thin texture and a mild flavour. If overcooked, it dries out, so it is best cooked medium rare. It is used fresh or tinned in oil.

Checklist for choosing and buying fish

Whole fish

Check for:

- Clear, bright eyes, not sunken
- Bright red gills
- Scales should not be missing and they should be firmly attached to the skin
- Moist skin (fresh fish feels slightly slippery)
- Shiny skin with bright natural colouring
- Tail should be stiff and the flesh should feel firm
- A fresh sea smell and no trace of ammonia.

Fillets

Check for:

- Neat, trim fillets with firm flesh
- Fillets should be firm and closely packed together, not ragged or gaping
- White fish should have a white translucent colour with no discoloration.

Smoked fish

Check for:

- Glossy appearance
- Flesh should feel firm and not sticky
- Pleasant, smoky smell.

Frozen fish

Check for:

- Fish that is frozen hard with no signs of thawing
- The packaging should not be damaged
- No evidence of freezer burn (i.e. dull, white, dry patches).

Storage of fish

Spoilage is mainly caused by the actions of enzymes and bacteria. Enzymes are present in the gut of the living fish and help to convert its food to tissue and energy. When the fish dies, these enzymes carry on working and help the bacteria in the digestive system to penetrate the belly wall and start breaking down the flesh itself. Bacteria exist on the skin and in the fish intestine. While the fish is alive, the normal defence mechanisms of the body prevent the bacteria from invading the flesh. Once the fish dies, however, the bacteria invade the flesh and start to break it down – the higher the temperature the faster the deterioration. Note that although these bacteria are harmless to humans, eating quality is reduced and the smell will deteriorate dramatically.

Fish, once caught, have a shelf life of 6–8 days if kept properly in a refrigerator at a temperature of between 0–5°C. If the fish is delivered whole with the innards still in, then gut and wash the cavity well before storage.

Fresh fish

Fresh fish should be used as soon as possible, but it can be stored overnight. Rinse, pat dry, cover with cling film and store towards the bottom of the refrigerator.

Ready-to-eat cooked fish

Ready-to-eat cooked fish, such as 'hot' smoked mackerel, prawns and crab, should be stored on shelves above other raw food items to avoid cross-contamination.

Frozen fish

Frozen fish should be stored at −18°C to −20°C and thawed out overnight in a refrigerator. It should *not* be

Table 7.1 Seasons for fish

	JAN	FEB	MAR	APR	MAY	JUN	JUL	AUG	SEP	OCT	NOV	DEC
Bream					*	*	*					
Brill			*	*	*							
Cod			*	*								
Eel												
Mullet (grey)			*	*								
Gurnard												
Haddock												
Hake			*	*	*							
Halibut				*	*							
Herring												
John Dory												
Mackerel												
Monkfish												
Plaice			*	*								
Red mullet												
Salmon (farmed)												
Salmon (wild)												
Sardines												
Sea bass				*	*							
Sea trout								*	*	*	*	
Skate												
Squid												
Sole (Dover)	*											
Sole (lemon)												
Trout												
Tuna												
Turbot			*	*	*							
Whiting												

Code:

Available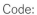

At best

* Spawning and roeing – this can deprive the flesh of nutrients and will decrease the yield.

thawed out in water, as this spoils the taste and texture of the fish, and valuable water-soluble nutrients are lost. Fish should not be refrozen as this will impair its taste and texture.

Smoked fish

Smoked fish should be well wrapped up and kept separate from other fish to prevent the smell and dye penetrating other foods.

Smoking

Fish can be either cold smoked or hot smoked. In either case if the fish are not to be consumed immediately they are salted before smoking. This can be done either by soaking them in a brine solution (strong enough to keep a potato afloat) or rubbing in dry salt. This is to improve flavour and help the keeping quality.

Cold smoking
This takes place at a temperature of approximately 24°C, which smokes but does not cook the fish. Smoke boxes can be bought or improvised. Sawdust is used and different woods can impart different flavours. Herbs, e.g. thyme and rosemary, can also be incorporated. Fish can be left either whole or filleted. Smoked salmon is prepared by cold smoking usually over a fire of oak chips and peat. Kippers, haddock and young halibut are also cold smoked, as are bloaters – these are lightly salted herring smoked without the gut being removed, which is what gives them their more pronounced gamey flavour.

Hot smoking
This takes place at approximately 82°C. Eel, trout, buckling, bloater (ungutted herring), sprats and mackerel are smoked and lightly cooked at one and the same time.

Cooking fish

Fish is very economical to prepare as it cooks quickly and thus can actually represent a fuel saving. When cooked, fish loses its translucent appearance and in most cases takes on an opaque white colour. It will also flake easily and has to be considered as a delicate product after preparation.

Fish easily becomes dry and loses its flavour if overcooked; for this reason, carefully considered methods of cookery need to be applied as certain fish will dry out too quickly before benefiting from the chosen cooking approach. It is important to avoid overcooking fish as this will reduce its eating quality.

Any fish or shellfish cooked by poaching can alternatively be cooked by steaming. Combination steam/convection ovens are commonly used in many kitchens; fish cooked in a controlled moist atmosphere at temperatures below 90°C benefits as shrinkage is kept to the minimum, overcooking is easier to control and the texture of the fish is moist and succulent.

An alternative cooking method for fish is the preparation of a ceviche (also known as *cebiche* or *seviche*). This is citrus-marinated seafood. Its true birthplace is unknown; some believe the dish was developed by the Spanish and then introduced into Latin America along with citrus fruits. Many countries in Latin America have adopted the ceviche, with variations. Both fish, such as sea bass or tuna, and shellfish, such as scallops, can be used in the preparation of ceviche.

Sauces for fish

The contemporary trend is for hot fish sauces to be lightly thickened, preferably without the use of a roux-based sauce. However, in large-scale cookery, when considerable quantities of fish sauces may be required, the use of fish velouté may be necessary.

Preparing fish

The following photos show how various cuts of fish are prepared.

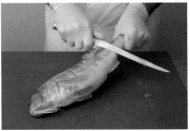

Scaling a red mullet

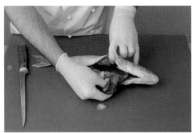

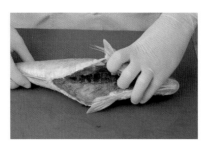

Gutting a red mullet

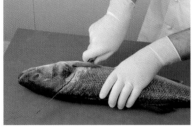
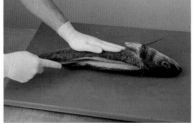
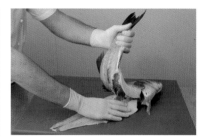

Filleting a sea bass

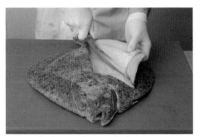
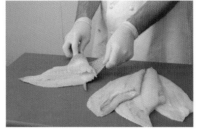
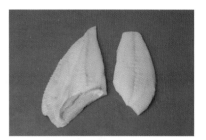

Filleting a turbot

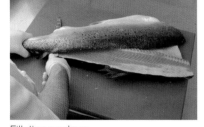
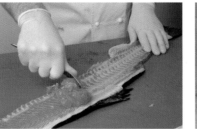
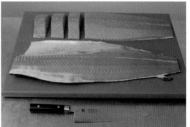

Filleting a salmon

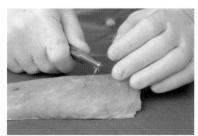
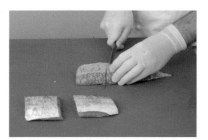

Pin boning a red mullet   Trimming a portion of red mullet

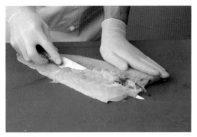 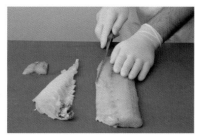

Trimming a sea bass

7.2 Shellfish

Shellfish, such as lobsters and crabs, are all invertebrates (i.e. they do not possess an internal skeleton) and are split into two main groups:

- Molluscs have either an external hinged double shell (e.g. scallops, mussels) or a single spiral shell (e.g. winkles, whelks), or have soft bodies with an internal shell (e.g. squid, octopus)
- Crustaceans have tough outer shells that act like armour, and also have flexible joints to allow quick movement (e.g. crab, lobster).

Choosing and buying shellfish

Shellfish are prized for their tender, fine-textured flesh. They can be prepared in a variety of ways, but are prone to rapid spoilage; the reason for this is that they contain quantities of certain proteins, amino acids, which encourage bacterial growth.

To ensure freshness and best flavour it is preferable to choose live specimens and cook them yourself. This is now often possible as a result of the expansion of globalisation, air freight and such like, which has created a healthy trade in live shellfish.

Bear in mind the following points when choosing shellfish:

- Shells should not be cracked or broken
- Shells of mussels and oysters should be tightly shut; open shells that do not close when tapped sharply should be discarded
- Lobsters, crabs and prawns should have a good colour and be heavy for their size
- Lobsters and crabs should have all their limbs.

Cooking shellfish

The flesh of fish and shellfish is different to meat and, as a consequence, their muscle make-up is very different too, making their connective tissue very fragile,

the muscle fibres shorter and the fat content relatively low. Generally, care should be taken when cooking and shellfish should be cooked as little as possible, to the point that the protein in the muscle groups just coagulate. Beyond this point the flesh tends to dry out, leading to toughening and a dry texture. Shellfish are known for their dramatic colour changing: from blue/grey to a vibrant orange colour. This is because they contain red and yellow pigments called carotenoids, bound to molecules of protein. The protein bonds obscure the yellow/red pigment and, once heat is applied, the bonds are broken and the vibrant pigmentation revealed.

Storage

All shellfish will start to spoil as soon as they have been removed from their natural environment; therefore, the longer shellfish are stored the more they will deteriorate due to the bacteria present (see the guidelines on choosing and buying, above). Best practice would be to cook immediately and store as for cooked fish. Shellfish can be blanched quickly to remove the shell and membrane (especially in lobsters), but they will still need to be stored as for a raw product, as they will require further cooking.

Types or varieties of shellfish
Cockles

These are enclosed in pretty cream-coloured shells of 2–3 cm. Cockles are soaked in salt water to purge and then steamed. They may be used in soups, salads and fish dishes, or served as a dish by themselves.

Cockles live in sand; therefore, it is essential to wash them well under running cold water and then leave them in cold salted water, ensuring that it is changed frequently until no traces of sand remain.

Table 7.2 Seasons for shellfish

	JAN	FEB	MAR	APR	MAY	JUN	JUL	AUG	SEP	OCT	NOV	DEC
Crab (brown cock)	At best	At best	At best	At best	Available	Available	Available	Available	Available	Available	Available	Available
Crab (spider)	Available	Available	Available	Available	Available	At best	At best	At best	At best	At best	Available	Available
Crab (brown hen)	At best	At best	Available	Available	Available	Available	At best	At best	At best	At best	At best	At best
Clams	At best	At best	At best	At best	Available	Available	Available	Available	Available	Available		
Cockles	At best	At best	At best	At best	Available	Available	Available	Available	Available	Available	Available	Available
Crayfish (signal)				Available	At best	At best	At best	At best	At best	At best		
Lobster	Available	Available	Available	Available	Available	Available	At best	At best	At best	At best	Available	Available
Langoustines			At best	At best	At best	At best	At best	Available				At best
Mussels	Available	Available	Available	Available	Available	Available	Available	Available	At best	At best	At best	At best
Oysters (rock)	Available	Available	Available	Available	Available	Available	Available	Available	At best	At best	At best	At best
Oysters (native)	At best	At best	At best	At best					At best	At best	At best	At best
Prawns	Available	Available	Available	Available	Available	At best	At best	At best	At best	At best	At best	At best
Scallops	Available	Available	Available	Available	Available	Available	At best	At best	At best	At best	Available	Available

Code:

Available

At best

Cockles are cooked:

- In unsalted water until the shells open
- On a preheated griddle
- As for any of the mussel recipes.

They can be used for soup, sauces, salads and as garnishes for fish dishes.

Shrimps

Shrimps are used for garnishes, decorating fish dishes, cocktails, sauces, salads, hors d'oeuvres, potted shrimps, omelettes and savouries.

Prawns

Prawns are larger than shrimps; they may be used for garnishing and decorating fish dishes, for cocktails, canapés, salad, hors d'oeuvres, and for hot dishes such as curried prawns.

Scampi, Dublin Bay prawns

Scampi are found in the Mediterranean. The Dublin Bay prawn, which is of the same family, is caught around the Scottish coast. These shellfish resemble small lobsters, about 20 cm long, and only the tail flesh is used.

Crayfish

Crayfish is a freshwater variant of the lobster, used for garnishing cold buffet dishes and for recipes using lobster. They are dark brown or grey, turning pink when cooked. Average size is 8 cm.

Lobster

Lobsters are served cold in cocktails, hors d'oeuvres, salads, sandwiches and on buffets.

When hot they are used for soup, and grilled and served in numerous dishes with various sauces. They are also used as a garnish to fish dishes.

Crawfish (rock lobster)

Crawfish are like large lobsters without claws, but with long antennae. They are brick red in colour when raw and cooked. Owing to their size and appearance they are used mostly on cold buffets but they can be served hot. The best size is 1½–2 kg in weight.

Both the body and the flesh of the crawfish are similar to the lobster, the main difference being that the crawfish does not have main claws. All the flesh is contained in the tail.

Crawfish are boiled in the same way as lobsters and the meat can be used for any of the lobster recipes. Because of its spectacular image the crawfish cooked, dressed and presented whole is a popular addition to cold buffets.

Crab

Crabs are used for hors d'oeuvres, cocktails, salads, dressed crab, sandwiches and bouchées. Soft-shelled crabs are eaten in their entirety. They are considered to have an excellent flavour and may be deep- or shallow-fried, or grilled.

Oysters

Whitstable and Colchester are the chief English centres for oysters; they occur here naturally and are also farmed. Since the majority of oysters are eaten raw it is essential that they are thoroughly cleansed before hotels and restaurants receive them.

The popular way of eating oysters is in the raw state. They may also be served in soups, hot cocktail savouries, fish garnishes, as a fish dish, and in meat puddings and savouries.

Quality and purchasing:

1. Oysters must be alive; this is indicated by the firmly closed shells.
2. They are graded in terms of size, and the price varies accordingly.
3. Oysters should smell fresh.
4. They should be purchased daily.
5. English oysters are in season from September to April (when there is an 'R' in the month).
6. During the summer months oysters are imported from France, Holland and Portugal.

Storage

Oysters are stored in barrels or boxes, covered with damp sacks and kept in a cold room to keep them moist and alive. The shells should be tightly closed; if they are open, tap them sharply – if they do not shut at once, discard them.

Scallops

Great scallops are up to 15 cm in size, bay scallops up to 8 cm and queen scallops ('queenies') the size of small cockles. Scallops may be steamed, poached, fried or grilled.

Note: when selecting scallops, always make hand-dived scallops your first choice as dredged ones are sometimes unethical. You pay a bit more for the hand-dived but the difference in quality is certainly worth it.

Preparing shellfish

The following photos show how mussels and scallops are prepared. For information about preparing a lobster, refer to recipe 51, and for oysters refer to recipe 66.

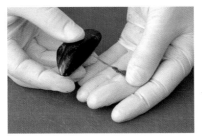

The beard, shown here, is removed from a mussel before use

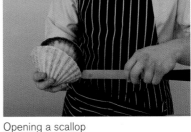

Opening a scallop

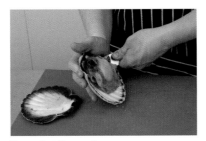

Removing the scallop

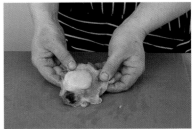

The scallop must be cleaned and trimmed before use

1 Fish stock

	Makes 2 litres
fish bones, no heads, gills or roe (turbot, sole and brill bones are best)	5 kg
olive oil	100 ml
onions, finely chopped	3
leeks, finely chopped	3
celery sticks, finely chopped	3
fennel bulb, finely chopped	1
dry white wine	350 ml
parsley stalks	10
sprigs of thyme	3
white peppercorns	15
lemons, finely sliced	2

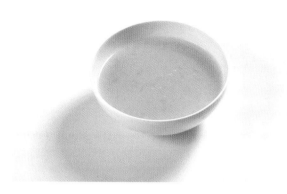

1. Wash off the bones in cold water for 1 hour. Heat the olive oil in a pan that will hold all the ingredients, leaving a 1 cm gap at the top for skimming.
2. Add all the vegetables and sweat off without colour for 3 minutes.
3. Add the fish bones and sweat for a further 3 minutes.
4. Next add the white wine and water to cover. Bring to a simmer, skim off the impurities, and add the herbs, peppercorns and lemon. Turn off the heat.
5. Infuse for 25 minutes, then pass into another pan and reduce by half. The stock is now ready for use.

2 Shellfish nage

	Makes 2 litres
olive oil	50 ml
unshelled prawns	500 g
cock crab body, no claws, gills removed (roughly smashed)	1 kg
carrots, chopped	2
onion, chopped	1
celery stick, chopped	1
fennel, chopped	½ bulb
garlic cloves	2
tomato purée	3 tbsp
dry white wine	200 ml
cold water	2 litres
fish stock	500 ml
star anise	2
bay leaf	1
sprigs of parsley	5
sprigs of thyme	5

1. Take a pan big enough to hold all the ingredients and put on a medium heat.
2. Heat the oil, then add the prawns and crab body.
3. Sweat off for 8 minutes. Add the vegetables and tomato purée, and continue to sweat for a further 8 minutes then add the wine, water, stock and herbs.
4. Bring to a simmer and skim off any impurities. Continue to cook for 30 minutes, skimming when a scum develops on the top of the nage.
5. When ready, pass the nage into a container through a fine sieve; do not force. Refrigerate and use as required.

i Shellfish nage can be used in soups, sauces and risottos, and can be reduced to a glaze. With a small amount of milk added, it can be 'cappuccinoed' using a hand blender.

Light and fragrant, with a hint of aromatic spices and herbs. It gives an excellent flavour to all types of fish dishes and sauces.

Store for up to 3 days in an airtight container in the refrigerator, or freeze for up to 1 month.

Butter thickened (*monter au beurre*)

Many sauces can be given a final finish to enrich flavour and given a sheen by thoroughly mixing in small pieces of butter at the last moment before serving.

The traditional way of making à la carte classic fish sauces:

1. Strain off the liquid in which the fish has been poached.
2. Reduce it to a glaze.
3. Away from the heat, gradually and thoroughly mix in small pieces of butter.
4. If the sauce is to be glazed then some lightly whipped double cream may be added.

Sabayon with olive oil (an alternative to hollandaise sauce)

	4–6 portions	8–12 portions
crushed peppercorns	6	15
vinegar	1 tbsp	2½ tbsp
egg yolks	3	8
olive oil	250 ml	625 ml
salt, cayenne pepper		

1. Place the peppercorns and vinegar in a small sauteuse or stainless-steel pan and reduce to one-third.
2. Add 1 tablespoon of cold water and allow to cool.
3. Add the egg yolks and whisk over a gentle heat in a sabayon.
4. Remove from heat. Cool.
5. Gradually whisk in the tepid olive oil.
6. Correct the seasoning.
7. Pass through a muslin or fine strainer.
8. Serve warm.

If the sauce curdles, place a teaspoon of boiling water in a clean sauteuse and gradually whisk in the curdled sauce.

If this fails to reconstitute the sauce then place an egg yolk in a clean sauteuse with a dessertspoon of water. Whisk lightly over gentle heat until slightly thickened. Remove from heat and gradually add the curdled sauce, whisking continuously.

To stabilise the sauce during service, 60 ml thick béchamel may be added before straining.

i This sauce is healthier than hollandaise because it does not contain the cholesterol of a hollandaise made with butter.

Lobster sauce

	Makes 1 litre
live hen lobster	¾–1 kg
butter or oil	75 g
onion	100 g
carrot } roughly cut (mirepoix)	100 g
celery	50 g
brandy	60 ml
flour	75 g
tomato purée	100 g
fish stock	1¼ litres
dry white wine	120 ml
bouquet garni	
crushed clove garlic	½
salt	

1. Wash the lobster well.
2. Cut in half lengthwise, tail first, then the carapace.
3. Discard the dark green sac from the carapace, clean the trail from the tail, remove any spawn into a basin.
4. Wash the lobster pieces.
5. Crack the claws and the four claw joints.
6. Melt the butter or oil in a thick-bottomed pan.
7. Add the lobster pieces and the onion, carrot and celery.
8. Allow to cook steadily without colouring the butter for a few minutes, stirring continuously with a wooden spoon.
9. Add the brandy and allow it to ignite.

10. Remove from the heat, mix in the flour and tomato purée.
11. Return to a gentle heat and cook out the roux.
12. Cool slightly, gradually add the fish stock and white wine.
13. Stir to the boil.
14. Add the bouquet garni and garlic, and season lightly with salt.
15. Simmer for 15–20 minutes.
16. Remove the lobster pieces.
17. Remove the lobster meat from the pieces.

18. Crush the lobster shells, return them to the sauce and continue simmering for ¼–¾ hour.
19. Crush the lobster spawn, stir into the sauce, reboil and pass through a coarse strainer.

> This sauce may be made in a less expensive way by substituting cooked lobster shell (not shell from the claws), which should be well crushed, in place of the live lobster.

6 Crispy seared salmon with horseradish foam and caviar

energy	kcal	fat	sat fat	carb	sugar	protein	fibre
2209 KJ	533.4 cal	41.7 g	18.3 g	4.8 g	4.1 g	34.7 g	3.5 g

	4 portions	10 portions
salmon fillet steaks, skin on, scaled	4 × 140 g	10 × 140 g
vegetable oil		
baby spinach, washed	400 g	1 kg
butter		
spears of asparagus, blanched	12	30
garlic cloves, chopped	1	3
caviar (optional)	50 g	125 g
chervil		
Foam		
shallots, sliced	2	5
sprig of thyme	1	3
butter	80 g	200 g
white wine	60 ml	150 ml
double cream	60 ml	150 ml
horseradish, grated	20 g	50 g
lemons, juice of	1	3

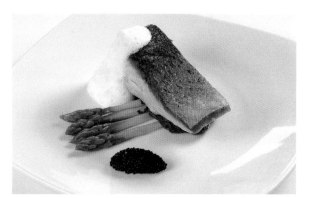

5. Wilt the spinach in a little butter, add the asparagus to re-heat and arrange neatly in the centre of each serving dish.
6. Place the seared salmon skin-side up on the asparagus and spinach, and finish with a quenelle of caviar. Garnish with chervil. Add the foam to the plate at the last minute.

1. Place salmon skin-side down in a hot pan with a little vegetable oil and cook on a medium heat until two-thirds of the salmon is cooked.
2. For the foam, sweat the shallots and thyme in half the butter, adding white wine after 2 minutes and reduce by half.
3. Add the cream and horseradish, bring to the boil and infuse for 15 minutes off the heat.
4. Pass through a fine chinois and work in the other half of the butter and the lemon juice while the mix is hot (this will stop it from splitting). Place into a pressurised container used to produce foams.

> This dish can be adapted in many ways. Substitute the caviar with avruga caviar to save the expense.
>
> Alternatively, if cost is not an issue, use smoked salmon (a smaller portion to replace the caviar) and sear that in the same way. The horseradish will be a great foil for this.

> i Foams are aerated sauces produced using either a siphon or a blender.

7 Salmon fish cakes

leek, in small, fine dice	½
fennel, in small, fine dice	½
onion, in small, fine dice	½
small stick of celery, in fine dice	1
Noilly Prat	120 ml
dry, warm potato purée	250 g
crème fraiche	75 g
egg	½
salmon, diced in small cubes	140 g
melted butter at room temperature	75 g
chives, chopped	10 g
dill, chopped	10 g
squeeze of lemon	
salt and pepper	
flour	
egg, beaten	
breadcrumbs	

1. Sweat the vegetables lightly in a little oil. Add the Noilly Prat and reduce until it just covers the vegetables. Season lightly and cool.
2. To the warm, dry potato purée, add the crème fraiche, egg, salmon, vegetables, melted butter, herbs, lemon juice and seasoning. Mix together and check seasoning.
3. Form the mixture into mini fish cakes and chill for 4 hours.
4. Prepare a pané of flour, egg and breadcrumbs, each with a little seasoning.
5. Add the fish cakes one at a time into the flour, then the egg and then the breadcrumbs. Go through this process twice with each fish cake.
6. Deep fry at 180°C when required.

8 Salmon marinated in dill (gravlax)

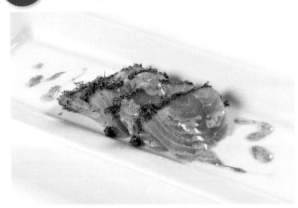

	4 portions	10 portions
middle-cut, fresh, descaled raw salmon	¾ kg	1¾ kg
bunch dill, washed and chopped	1	2
caster sugar	25 g	60 g
salt	25 g	60 g
peppercorns, crushed	1 tbsp	2 tbsp

1. Cut the salmon lengthwise and remove all the bones.
2. Place one half, skin-side down, in a deep dish.
3. Add the dill, sugar, salt and peppercorns.
4. Cover with the other piece of salmon, skin-side up.
5. Cover with foil, lay a tray or dish on top, and evenly distribute weights on the foil.
6. Refrigerate for 48 hours, turning the fish every 12 hours and basting with the liquid produced by the ingredients. Separate the halves of salmon and baste between them.
7. Replace the foil, tray and weights between basting.
8. Lift the fish from the marinade, remove the dill and seasoning, wash, dry and top with chopped dill.
9. Place the halves of salmon on a board, skin-side down.
10. Slice thinly, detaching the slice from the skin.
11. Garnish gravlax with lemon and serve with mustard and dill sauce.

 Gravlax can be sliced very thinly and served in appetisers, canapés, buffets, starters and open sandwiches.

Chervil gravlax

whole salmon fillets with scaled skin, pin boned	2 (about 2½ kg)
coarse salt	100 g
sugar	100 g
large bunch of chervil	

1. Mix the salt and sugar together in a small bowl and set aside. Coarsely chop the chervil and set aside.
2. Stretch out a length of foil about 15 cm longer than the fillets. Distribute one quarter of the salt and sugar curing mixture on the foil in an area just the size of the fillet. Place one fillet skin-side down on the mixture. Sprinkle two-thirds of the remaining curing mixture evenly on top of the fillet, along with the chopped herbs.
3. Place the second fillet flesh-side down on top of the herbs and curing mixture. Sprinkle the remaining curing mixture on the skin side of the second fillet.
4. Seal the fillets tightly in the foil and place on a large deep tray. Set another tray on top of the fillets and add something heavy to weigh them down.
5. Refrigerate for 2–3 days, turning the fish twice a day. The salmon will release juices as it cures. These can be drained off but it is not essential to do so.

 ## Beetroot gravlax

coarse salt	100 g
fresh, coarse ground black pepper	4 tsp
large beetroots, raw, grated	2
sugar	100 g
whole salmon fillets with scaled skin, pin boned	2 (about 2½ kg)
large bunch of fresh dill, chopped	

1. Mix the salt, pepper, grated beetroot and sugar together in a small bowl and set aside. Coarsely chop the dill and set aside.
2. Stretch out a length of foil about 15 cm longer than the fillets. Distribute one quarter of the beetroot curing mixture on the foil in an area just the size of the fillet. Place one fillet skin-side down on the mixture. Sprinkle two-thirds of the remaining curing mixture evenly on top of the fillet, along with the chopped herbs.
3. Place the second fillet flesh-side down on top of the herbs and curing mixture. Sprinkle the remaining curing mixture on the skin side of the second fillet.
4. Seal the fillets tightly in the foil and place on a large deep tray. Set another tray on top of the fillets and add something heavy to weigh them down.
5. Refrigerate for 2–3 days, turning the fish twice a day. The salmon will release juices as it cures. These can be drained off but it is not essential to do so.

 ## Gin and tarragon gravlax

coarse salt	100 g
cracked black pepper	1 tsp
sugar	100 g
whole salmon fillets with scaled skin, pin boned	2 (about 2½ kg)
London gin	120 g
bunch of dill, chopped	½
bunch of tarragon, chopped	1

1. Mix the salt, pepper and sugar together in a small bowl and set aside. Coarsely chop the herbs and set aside.
2. Stretch out a length of foil about 15 cm longer than the fillets. Distribute one quarter of the salt and sugar curing mixture on the foil in an area just the size of the fillet. Place one fillet skin-side down on the mixture. Drizzle half the gin over the salmon. Sprinkle two-thirds of the remaining

curing mixture evenly on top of the fillet, along with the chopped herbs. Drizzle the remaining gin over the cure.

3. Place the second fillet flesh-side down on top of the herbs and curing mixture. Sprinkle the remaining curing mixture on the skin side of the second fillet.

4. Seal the fillets tightly in the foil and place on a large deep tray. Set another tray on top of the fillets and add something heavy to weigh them down.

5. Refrigerate for 2–3 days, turning the fish twice a day. The salmon will release juices as it cures. These can be drained off but it is not essential to do so.

12   Braised tuna Italian style

energy	kcal	fat	sat fat	carb	sugar	protein	fibre
1557.25 KJ	373.11 cal	22.3 g	4.02 g	6.36 g	4.97 g	37.2 g	1.86 g

	4 portions	10 portions
piece of tuna	1 × 600 g	3 × 600 g
shallots, chopped	100 g	250 g
mushrooms, chopped	200 g	500 g
white wine	125 ml	300 ml
fish stock	125 ml	300 ml
Marinade		
lemon, juice of	1	2–3
olive oil	60 ml	150 ml
onion, sliced	100 g	250 g
carrot, sliced	100 g	250 g
bay leaf	½	1
thyme, salt and pepper		

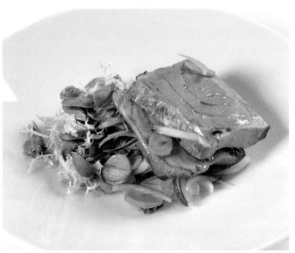

1. Mix together the ingredients for the marinade and marinate the pieces of fish for 1 hour.
2. Remove, dry well and colour in hot oil.
3. Place in braising pan, add shallots and mushrooms.
4. Cover with a lid, cook gently in oven for 15–20 minutes.
5. Add white wine and fish stock, cover, return to oven.
6. Braise gently for approximately 45 minutes until cooked.

7. Carefully remove the fish, correct the seasoning of the liquid (which may be lightly thickened with beurre manié, if required) and serve.

Variations

- Other ingredients that may be used when braising tuna include tomatoes, garlic, basil and vinegar.
- Slices of tuna can also be shallow-fried or cooked meunière with or without the meunière variations.

13   Baked stuffed sardines

1. Slit the stomach openings of the sardines and gut.
2. From the same opening carefully cut along each side of the back bones and remove by cutting through the end with fish scissors.
3. Scale, wash, dry and season the fish.

4. Stuff the fish. A variety of stuffings can be used – for example:
   (a) cooked chopped spinach with cooked chopped onion, garlic, nutmeg, salt, pepper
   (b) fish forcemeat
   (c) thick duxelle.

5. Place the stuffed sardines in a greased ovenproof dish.
6. Sprinkle with breadcrumbs and oil.
7. Bake in hot oven, 200°C, for approximately 10 minutes and serve.

Herring, mackerel, sea bass and trout can also be prepared and cooked in this way, and there is considerable scope for flair and imagination in the different stuffings and methods of cooking the fish.

14 Whole sole grilled with traditional accompaniments

energy	kcal	fat	sat fat	carb	sugar	protein	fibre
3320 KJ	798 cal	57.4 g	33.4 g	0.6 g	0.6 g	70.0 g	0.0 g

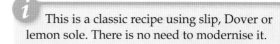

	4 portions	10 portions
whole sole, white and black skin removed	4	10
butter for grilling	200 g	500 g
seasoning		
parsley butter	100 g	250 g
lemons, peeled and cut into rondels	1	3

1. Ensure the fish is clean of roe, scales and skin.
2. Place on a buttered grilling tray and rub soft butter in to the flesh.
3. Season and place under the grill.
4. When the butter starts to brown slightly, remove from the grill and turn the fish over carefully using a roasting fork or a long palette knife.
5. With a spoon, baste the flesh of the uncooked side and continue cooking. Extra care should be taken as the tail end will cook faster than the head end, therefore the gradual reduction in heat towards the front of the grill is where the tail should be cooked.
6. To check whether the fish is done, place your thumb just behind the gill area and you should feel the flesh ease away from the bone.
7. Finish with parsley butter and a wedge of lemon.

i This is a classic recipe using slip, Dover or lemon sole. There is no need to modernise it.

15 Dover sole stuffed and baked with bacon, mushrooms and onion

button mushrooms	200 g
shallots	100 g
butter for frying	
lemon, juice	½
Dover sole	1
slices of pancetta	8

1. Slice the button mushrooms and shallots.
2. Melt some butter in a pan and start to sweat the shallots.
3. After 10 minutes, add the button mushrooms and lemon juice to the pan.
4. Cook for another 8 minutes. Remove from the heat and chill.
5. While the filling mixture chills, prepare the sole. Cut a pocket for the filling to go into.
6. Stuff the fish, wrap it in the bacon and place on a well-oiled tray.
7. Place in an oven at 160°C for 20 minutes.

16 Fillet of halibut madura (*kukus ikan sebalah madura*)

	4 portions	10 portions
pieces of halibut fillet	4 × 100 g	10 × 100 g
julienne of chillies	25 g	60 g
sweet basil leaves (kemangi)	25 g	60 g
seasoning		
fish stock	140 ml	300 ml
shallots	50 g	125 g
potatoes, small cubes or balls	50 g	125 g
carrots, small cubes or balls	50 g	125 g
green beans, small pieces	50 g	125 g
peanut oil	15 ml (3 tsp)	60 ml (7½ tsp)
garlic, peeled and chopped	6 g	15 g
banyuwangi sauce	140 ml	300 ml
sour turmeric sauce	70 ml	150 ml
whole green beans, blanched	4	10

1. Sprinkle the halibut with the chillies and chopped basil leaves and season.
2. Place in a suitable pan with enough fish stock to come halfway up the fish. Cover with greased paper, and poach in a moderate oven for approximately 5–8 minutes.
3. Keep warm.
4. Blanch the finely chopped shallots, potatoes and carrots for 1 minute.
5. Blanch and refresh the green beans.
6. Heat the peanut oil in a suitable pan. Sauté the blanched vegetables and garlic for approximately 2–5 minutes until tender.
7. Remove the vegetables. Keep warm.
8. On plates, place the banyuwangi sauce with a little sour turmeric sauce on top.
9. Carefully place the halibut on top.
10. Garnish with sautéed vegetables and the blanched whole green beans.

17 Poached hake with cockles and prawns

energy	kcal	fat	sat fat	carb	sugar	protein	fibre
974.6 KJ	232.71 cal	9.5 g	1.76 g	2.14 g	1.54 g	34.7 g	0.39 g

	4 portions	10 portions
onion, finely chopped	100 g	250 g
oil	1 tbsp	2½ tbsp
fish stock	250 ml	600 ml
parsley, chopped	1 tbsp	2½ tbsp
hake steaks or fillets	4 × 150 g	10 × 150 g
shelled cockles	8–12	20–30
shelled prawns	8–12	20–30
salt and pepper		
hard-boiled eggs, coarsely chopped	2	5
chopped parsley (for garnish)	½ tsp	1 tsp

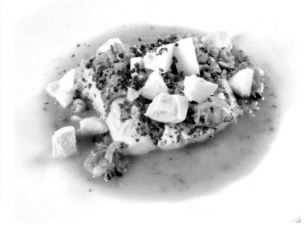

1. Lightly colour the onion in the oil, add the fish stock and parsley and simmer for 10–15 minutes.
2. Place the fish in a shallow ovenproof dish, and add cockles and prawns.
3. Pour on the fish stock and onion; season lightly.
4. Poach gently, and remove any bones and skin from the fish.
5. If there is an excess of liquid, strain and reduce.
6. Serve coated with the unthickened cooking liquor, sprinkled with the egg and parsley.

Red mullet on fine noodles with lobster sauce

	4 portions	10 portions
red mullet fillets (125 g each)	4	10
flour	25 g	60 g
salt, black pepper		
fine noodles	400 g	1 kg
olive oil	3 tbsp	7 tbsp
butter	25 g	60 g
garlic cloves, finely chopped	2	5
red chillies, deseeded, finely chopped	1	2
lobster sauce (see page 242)	250 ml	625 ml
parsley, chopped	½ tsp	1 tsp
lemon juice		
extra virgin olive oil, to serve		

1. Lightly flour the fillets and season with a little salt and black pepper.
2. Cook the fine noodles in boiling salted water, refresh under cold water and drain well.
3. Shallow fry the fillets in the olive oil, skin side up. When golden brown, turn over and cook the other side. Remove from the pan and drain on kitchen paper.
4. Heat the butter in a suitable pan and reheat the noodles in it. Add the garlic and the chillies, and bind with the hot lobster sauce.
5. Add the chopped parsley.
6. Place the noodles with the sauce on a suitable plate. Place the fillets on top and sprinkle with a little lemon juice. Finish with a drizzle of extra virgin olive oil.

 Grey mullet with green chutney (*policha meen*)

	4 portions	10 portions
grey mullets weighing about 500 g each, scaled and gutted (sea bass may be used as a substitute)	2	5
turmeric powder	½ tsp	½ tsp
salt	½ tsp	½ tsp
lemon, juice of	1	3
Chutney		
fresh green peppercorns, stripped from the stem	4 tbsp	10 tbsp
fresh coriander	½ bunch	1 bunch
green chillies, deseeded	2	5
cloves garlic, peeled	5	12
cumin powder	½ tsp	1½ tsp
lemon, juice of	½	1½
salt, to taste		
banana leaf to wrap the fish in (kitchen paper or foil may be used instead)	1	3
sprigs of fresh green pepper and fresh red chillies cut into fine julienne to garnish		

1. Cut 3 gashes on either side of the fish; rub in the turmeric powder, salt and lemon juice to coat the fish. Set aside for at least 1 hour.
2. Grind or process all the chutney ingredients (not too finely), incorporating the lemon juice and a pinch of salt.
3. Smear the fish with the chutney, making sure it goes into the gashes and the inside cavity.
4. Parcel the fish in two pieces of banana leaf cut to the appropriate size and moistened with vegetable oil. You can secure the parcels with string or with toothpicks (alternatively parcel the fish in oiled kitchen paper or foil).
5. Bake for 15 minutes in an oven heated to 180°C.
6. Serve hot in the banana leaf with tomato rougail as an accompaniment, and garnish with the green pepper and julienned red chillies.

This recipe was contributed by Mehernosh Mody.

20 Stuffed red snapper (*ikan bahan dengan kunyit celi padi*)

	4 portions	10 portions
red snapper	4	10
red chillies	12	30
red onions	300 g	750 g
turmeric powder	12g	25 g
salt	1 tsp	2 tsp
vegetable oil	4 tbsp	10 tbsp
red chillies to garnish	4	10
spring onions to garnish	8	20
fresh coriander sprigs to garnish	4	10

1. Prepare the red snapper by removing the scales, eyes and gills.
2. Gut the fish by making a cut from the stomach to the head, remove all the innards. Clean under running cold water to remove debris.
3. Across the back make three incisions (ciseler).
4. Remove the stalk and seeds from the first lot of chillies and chop them.
5. Finely chop the onions.
6. In a pestle place the chillies, onions, turmeric powder and salt, blend to a paste. (Alternatively use a food processor.)
7. Rub the fish with the paste inside and out.
8. Heat some oil in a suitable wok or pan, and gently fry the fish for 4–5 minutes on each side.
9. Serve on a suitable plate garnished with chilli, spring onion and coriander. Serve with plain boiled rice.

Note: Other fish that may be used include mackerel, trout and red mullet.

21 Whole sea bass baked with Swiss chard, spinach and scallops

sea bass 1.6 kg (after preparation, about 880 g)	
lemon butter	30 g
Swiss chard or spinach	65 g
scallops	280 g

1. Remove all the fins with scissors and scale thoroughly.
2. Wash the fish quickly and dry it thoroughly.
3. Remove the head with two neat cuts at 45° behind the gills.
4. Cut down the back bone about 2 cm from the tail on both sides.
5. Cut down to the rib cage.
6. After you reach the rib cage, go behind it and down to the flesh towards the tail.
7. Cut along the rib bones without breaking the flesh and trim right down to the tail. Trim by the belly.
8. Take the guts out and wash and dry the fish thoroughly.
9. Take out the pin bones.
10. Remove any pieces of silver skin from inside the belly.
11. Trim about 1 cm of flesh from the body where you made the first incision, so that when you tie it, it comes together.
12. Brush the inside of the fish with softened lemon butter and line it with spinach.
13. Lay the scallops in the centre and fold the spinach over so they are completely covered.
14. Bring the two sides of the bass together. Tie in the middle first, then either side of the middle.
15. At the head end, double-loop the string, hook it under the gills that you left on and tie it very tightly so as to close up the hole.
16. Tie the rest of the bass up, leaving about 3–4 mm between each tie.
17. Place in an oven at 170°C and cook for 40 minutes. Allow to rest for 10 minutes before serving.

After stuffing and tying the bass, leave it in a refrigerator for 24 hours to firm up, before use.

22 Barramundi with Moroccan spices

	4 portions	10 portions
barramundi	4 × 350 g	10 × 350 g
Spice dressing		
ground cumin	1 tsp	2½ tsp
paprika	½ tsp	1 tsp
chilli powder	½ tsp	1¼ tsp
garlic cloves, crushed and chopped	4	10
juice of lemons	2	5
olive oil	10 tbsp	15 tbsp
coriander, chopped	5 tbsp	7 tbsp
salt	pinch	pinch

1. Place all the spice dressing ingredients in a food processor. Blitz the ingredients.
2. Marinate the fish for 30 minutes in half of the dressing.
3. Place the cleaned fish in a suitable roasting tray. Cook in the oven for approximately 20 minutes at 200°C.
4. When the fish is cooked, brush it with the remainder of the dressing. Serve with steamed couscous or braised rice.

23 Steamed grouper with soy sauce and ginger

	4 portions	10 portions
grouper, whole	600 g	1½ kg
ginger, fresh, finely sliced	50 g	125 g
spring onions, finely shredded	4	10
vegetable oil	3 tbsp	7½ tbsp
Sauce		
soy sauce	2 tbsp	5 tbsp
water	180 ml	450 ml
Thai fish sauce	1 tsp	2½ tsp
sugar	1 tsp	2½ tsp

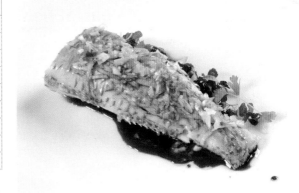

1. To make the sauce, bring the water to the boil and add the soy sauce, fish sauce and sugar. Stir well, then remove from the heat.
2. Steam the fish, spring onions and ginger in a suitable container such as an oriental steamer. Steam for approximately 8–10 minutes until cooked.
3. Serve the fish with the spring onions and ginger. Garnish with fresh coriander.
4. Heat the oil until slightly smoking, and drizzle it over the fish. Pour the sauce over the fish.

Bengali-style tilapia

	4 portions	10 portions
tilapia fillets	4 × 100–150 g	10 × 100–150 g
turmeric	½ tsp	1¼ tsp
ground coriander	½ tsp	1¼ tsp
cumin	¼ tsp	1 tsp
curry powder	1 tsp	2½ tsp
water	2 tbsp	5 tbsp
onion, finely shredded	50 g	125 g
vegetable oil	50 ml	125 ml
Kachumbar		
onion, finely shredded	1	2½
plum tomatoes, chopped	2	5
green chilli, finely chopped	1	2½
fresh coriander, chopped	1 tbsp	2½ tbsp

1. Place the tilapia fillets in a suitable dish.
2. Mix the turmeric, coriander, cumin, curry powder and water in a bowl and pour over the fillets of fish. Leave to marinate.
3. Heat the oil in a frying pan and sweat the shredded onion until slightly coloured.
4. Add the fish fillets to the pan. Cook until golden brown on both sides.
5. Prepare the kachumbar by combining all the ingredients in a bowl. Season.
6. Serve the fish on a plate with the kachumbar on the side. Garnish with fresh limes if desired.

Caribbean-style parrot fish

	4 portions	10 portions
parrot fish	4 × 225 g	10 × 225 g
seasoned flour		
butter	60 g	150 g
vegetable oil	1 tbsp	1½ tbsp
turmeric	½ tsp	
red pepper, cut into fine strips	½	1
yellow pepper, cut into fine strips	½	1
green pepper, cut into fine strips	½	1
dry white wine	300 ml	750 ml
double cream	1 tsp	2½ tsp
lemon juice	½ tsp	1¼ tsp
sugar	½ tsp	1¼ tsp
salt, pepper		
Caribbean dressing		
onion, finely chopped	1	1½
cloves of garlic, crushed and chopped	2	5
sprigs of thyme	3	7
mild fresh chilli powder	½ tsp	1¼ tsp
vinegar	½ tsp	1¼ tsp

1. Pass the cleaned fish through seasoned flour.
2. Carefully shallow fry the fish in the butter and oil. Fry on both sides until cooked.
3. When cooked, remove the fish and keep warm.
4. To the pan add the turmeric, the Caribbean dressing and the peppers. Cook for 2 minutes.
5. Deglaze the pan with the white wine. Add the cream, bring to the boil and reduce to a light consistency.
6. Finish with lemon juice and sugar.
7. Place the fish on a suitable dish and mask with the sauce.

26 ## Ackee and salted codfish

	4 portions	10 portions
vegetable oil or bacon fat	65 ml	150 ml
onion, chopped	1	2
bunch of spring onions, chopped (both green and white parts)		2
large tomato, chopped	1	3
Scotch bonnet pepper, minced	¼ tsp	½ tsp
salted codfish, desalted and cooked	240 g	600 g
sprig of thyme		
black pepper	½ tsp	1 tsp
can of ackee, well drained	1 (about 570 g)	2

1. Debone the cooked codfish and flake with a fork. Set aside.
2. Place a skillet over medium heat and add the vegetable oil. When the oil is hot, add the chopped onion and spring onions. Sauté until they are translucent, but not browned.
3. Add the chopped tomato, Scotch bonnet pepper, thyme and black pepper, and stir gently to combine with the onions. Continue to sauté for just a few minutes, or until the tomatoes are warmed through.
4. Add the salted codfish flakes to the vegetable mixture and stir gently. Reduce the heat to low and cook for 5–10 minutes, or until the water from the codfish has evaporated.
5. Add the ackee to the skillet and gently fold it into the codfish and vegetable mixture. Simmer for 5–10 minutes, or until the water from the ackee has evaporated.
6. Gently remove the ackee and salted codfish from the skillet with a slotted spoon, allowing any excess oil to drain off. Serve with cooked white rice or breadfruit.

i Ackee is a Caribbean fruit which may be purchased fresh or in cans.

To desalt and prepare the codfish, soak it in cold water overnight. Drain it, replace the water and simmer for 5–10 minutes.

27 ## Omelette with creamed smoked haddock and cheese (Arnold Bennett)

energy	kcal	fat	sat fat	carb	sugar	protein	fibre
1944 KJ	468.1 cal	37.2 g	16.2 g	3.3 g	1.4 g	30.4 g	0.1 g

	4 portions	10 portions
butter or margarine	12 g	30 g
cooked, flaked, smoked haddock	50 g	125 g
mornay sauce	90 ml	225 ml
egg flat omelette	4 × 3	10 × 3
Parmesan cheese	10 g	25 g

1. Melt the butter or margarine in a suitable pan, reheat the smoked haddock. Bind with a little of the mornay sauce.
2. Prepare a flat omelette and place on to a plate.
3. Arrange the fish on top of the omelette, coat with the remainder of the sauce, sprinkle with Parmesan cheese and glaze under the salamander. Serve immediately.

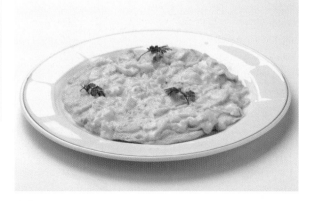

i An Arnold Bennett is always made with smoked haddock. However, the recipe could be adapted to use salmon, smoked salmon, shellfish, etc.

28 Smoked haddock pâté

	4 portions	10 portions
smoked haddock	570 g	1.4 kg
fresh bay leaves	2	2
milk	1 litre	2.2 litres
double cream	140 ml	350 ml
juice and zest of lemon	1	2
butter, melted (plus a little extra)	75 g	150 g
horseradish sauce	1 tbsp	2 tbsp
Worcestershire sauce	½ tbsp	1 tbsp
ground white pepper	½ tsp	1 tsp
cayenne pepper	½ tsp	1 tsp
salt		

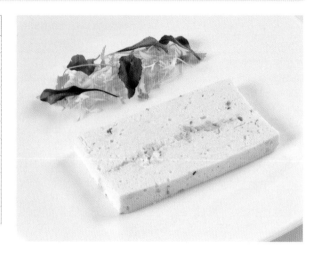

1. Place the haddock and bay leaves in a saucepan, and cover with milk.
2. Bring to the boil, then simmer over a low heat for 8–10 minutes.
3. Drain in a colander, then place the haddock in a bowl.
4. Remove the skin and any bones. Allow to cool.
5. Transfer to a food processor with the remaining ingredients, season with salt, and blend to a coarse paste.
6. Transfer to a ramekin or terrine lined with cling film. Pour over enough melted butter to cover.
7. Refrigerate overnight, then serve in the ramekins or turn out from the terrine and slice very carefully. Serve with toast.

29 Smoked haddock beignet

flour	
egg yolks	24 g
lager	100 g
water	150 g
melted butter, tepid	40 g
baker's yeast	10 g
seasoning	
egg whites, whipped	60 g
smoked haddock, diced 2 cm × 2 cm	24 pieces

1. Mix together the flour, egg yolks, lager, water, melted butter and yeast.
2. Allow to prove for 1 hour.
3. Fold in the whipped egg whites.
4. Place the diced smoked haddock in flour, then in the batter.
5. Using a fork, deep fry in hot oil at 170°C until golden brown.

Serve as an appetiser or canapé.

Bigoli with anchovy sauce

Bigoli	4 portions	10 portions
semolina flour	400 g	1 kg
egg	1	3
water	100 ml	250 ml
olive oil		
Anchovy sauce		
olive oil	3 tbsp	200 ml
onion, finely sliced	1	3
anchovy fillets	100 g	250 g
clove of garlic	1	2
fresh parsley, chopped	1 tsp	2 tsp
pepper		

1. To make the pasta dough, combine the flour, egg and water. Mix and knead well, adding extra water if needed, until the dough is smooth and elastic. Turn out onto a lightly floured surface and knead again. Divide the pasta dough into 4 pieces and then knead each piece well.

2. Roll each piece out as thinly as possible, then cut into thin strips and roll them into spaghetti using your fingertips, using more flour if necessary to prevent sticking. Set aside while making the anchovy sauce.

3. Heat the olive oil in a pan. Add the onions and sweat gently before adding the garlic. Cook over a low heat for 10 minutes, stirring occasionally.

4. Add the anchovies to the pan, stir and cook for a further 10 minutes, stirring occasionally until the anchovies have puréed among the onions and created a rich sauce.

5. Meanwhile, bring a large pan of salted water to the boil and cook the pasta for 3–4 minutes or until 'al dente' – cook in batches if necessary.

6. Remove the garlic clove from the pan and add the chopped parsley to finish.

7. Drain the pasta and add it straight into the pan with the sauce: add a couple of tablespoons of the pasta water to loosen. Mix through and season with black pepper. Serve immediately.

 Eel with white wine, horseradish and parsley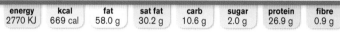

energy	kcal	fat	sat fat	carb	sugar	protein	fibre
2770 KJ	669 cal	58.0 g	30.2 g	10.6 g	2.0 g	26.9 g	0.9 g

	4 portions	10 portions
onion, chopped	50 g	125 g
butter	100 g	250 g
prepared eels	600 g	1½ kg
white wine	125 ml	300 ml
bouquet garni	1	2
potatoes, diced	200 g	500 g
whipping cream	100 ml	250 ml
fresh grated horseradish	1 tsp	3 tsp
parsley, chopped	½ tsp	1 tsp
oil for frying		

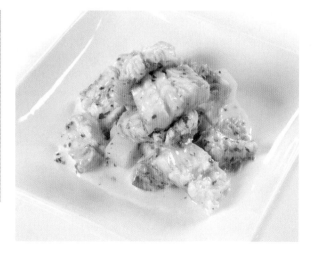

1. Sweat the onions in the butter for 4–5 minutes without colour.

2. Add the eel to the pan and seal well.

3. Add the white wine, bring to the boil adding the bouquet garni and simmer for 15 minutes.

4. Add the potato and cook for a further 20 minutes until the eel is tender.

5. Remove the eel and potatoes and keep warm, pass the stock off into a clean pan and reduce to sauce consistency.

6. Add the cream, horseradish and chopped parsley, and bring to the boil.

7. Check the consistency and seasoning, correct if necessary.
8. Add the cooked eels to the pan of sauce, coat well and place in a serving dish.

 This is a traditional dish but still a classic.

An eel is made up of lateral muscle groups either side of the back bone that work to move the fish around. Eels need a longer cooking time than other fish and shellfish species.

32 Squid

Only fresh squid is suitable for stir-frying, shallow-frying or grilling.

1. Pull the head away from the body together with the innards.
2. Cut off the tentacles just below the eye, and remove the small round cartilage at the base of the tentacles.
3. Discard the head, innards and pieces of cartilage.

4. Taking care not to break the ink bag remove the long transparent blade of cartilage (the back bone or quill).
5. Scrape or peel off the reddish membrane that covers the pouch, rub with salt and wash under cold water.

Squid should either be cooked very quickly or braised for an hour or so.

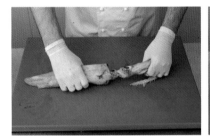
Pull the head away from the body

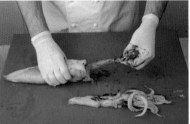
Remove the back bone

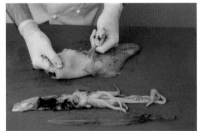
Peel the pouch

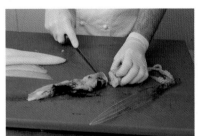
Cut off the tentacles

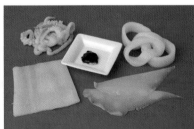
Squid prepared for cooking in a variety of ways

33 Squid with white wine, garlic and chilli

energy	kcal	fat	sat fat	carb	sugar	protein	fibre
1084 KJ	260 cal	17.6 g	2.4 g	2.3 g	0.3 g	23.4 g	0.2 g

	4 portions	10 portions
squid, cleaned	600 g	1½ kg
vegetable oil	60 ml	150 ml
garlic cloves, crushed	2	5
sprigs of parsley, chopped	3–4	7–8
red chilli pepper, seeds removed, finely chopped	1	3
white wine	60 ml	150 ml
fish stock	60 ml	150 ml

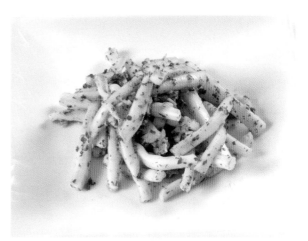

1. Cut the squid in to halves and then into thick strips.
2. Place a pan containing the vegetable oil on the hottest point on the stove.
3. Place the squid in the pan and sauté quickly (this will not take long – the squid will toughen if cooked for too long).
4. Add the garlic, chopped parsley and the chilli. Toss the squid around the pan, working in all the flavours.
5. Add the wine and stock, quickly bring to the boil, check the seasoning and serve.

> *i* The texture of squid is unlike that of other species. The flesh is very high in protein and dense, giving it that 'rubbery' texture when overcooked. Cook quickly and over a high heat.

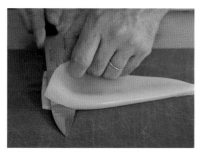

Cut the body of the squid in half

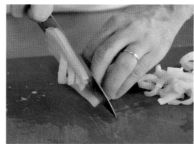

Cut into strips

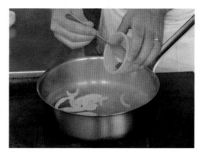

Cook the squid with the other ingredients

34 Bouillabaisse

energy	kcal	fat	sat fat	carb	sugar	protein	fibre
689 KJ	2881 cal	42.3 g	8.5 g	4.8 g	2.1 g	67.6 g	0.5 g

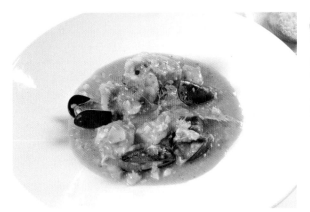

This is a thick, full-bodied fish stew – sometimes served as a soup – for which there are many variations. When made in the south of France, a selection of Mediterranean fish is used. If made in the north of France the following recipe could be typical.

1. Clean, descale and wash the fish. Cut into 2 cm pieces on the bone; the heads may be removed. Clean the mussels if using, and leave in their shells.
2. Place the cut fish, with the mussels and crawfish on top, in a clean pan.
3. Simmer the onion, garlic, wine, water, tomato, saffron and bouquet garni for 20 minutes.
4. Pour on to the fish, add the oil and parsley, bring to the boil and simmer for approximately 15 minutes.
5. Correct the seasoning and thicken with the beurre manié.
6. The liquor may be served first as a soup, followed by the fish accompanied by French bread that has been toasted, left plain or rubbed with garlic.

If using soft fish, e.g. whiting, add it 10 minutes after the other fish.

	4 portions	10 portions
assorted prepared fish, e.g. red mullet, whiting, sole, gurnard, small conger eel, John Dory, crawfish tail	1½ kg	3¾ kg
mussels (optional)	500 ml	1¼ kg
chopped onion or white of leek	75 g	180 g
garlic, crushed	10 g	25 g
white wine	125 ml	300 ml
water	500 ml	1¼ litres
tomatoes, skinned, deseeded, diced or	100 g	250 g
tomato purée	25 g	60 g
pinch of saffron		
bouquet garni (fennel, aniseed, parsley, celery)		
olive oil	125 ml	300 ml
chopped parsley	5 g	12 g
salt and pepper		
butter ⎫ beurre manié	25 g	60 g
flour ⎭	10 g	25 g
French bread		

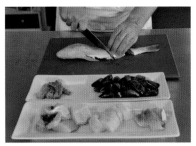

Cut the fish on the bone, into even-sized pieces

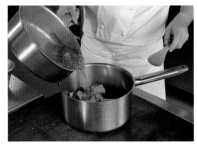

Add the liquid to the fish pieces

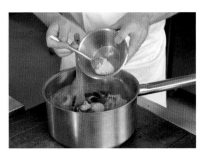

Thicken with beurre manie

Fish soup with rouille

	4 portions	10 portions
olive oil	2 tbsp	5 tbsp
onions, finely chopped	1	3
leeks, sliced	1	3
fennel bulb, chopped	½	1
celery stick, chopped	½	1
garlic cloves, finely chopped	1	2
tomatoes, chopped	200 g	500 g
fennel seeds	2 seeds	¼ tsp
good pinch of saffron stamens		
broad strip of orange rind	1	1
tomato purée	1 tsp	½ tbsp
peppercorns	3	8
fish trimmings and bones, including heads, washed, with the eyes and gills removed	800 g	2 kg
water	1 litre	2.4 litres
fish fillets (e.g. bream, bass, haddock, mullet or gurnard), skinned, cut into chunks	180 g	450 g
grated gruyère and baguette croûtes, to serve		
Rouille		
garlic cloves, chopped	1	3
salt		
egg yolks, pasteurised	1	2
olive oil	60 ml	150 ml
cayenne pepper	¼ tsp	½ tsp
tomato purée	2 tsp	4 tsp
lemon juice	¼ tsp	½ tsp

1. Heat the olive oil in a very large, heavy-bottomed saucepan and add the onion, leek, fennel and celery. Cook over a medium to low heat until the vegetables are soft but not coloured.
2. Add the garlic and tomatoes and cook for about 10 minutes, until the tomatoes are soft.
3. Add the fennel seeds, saffron, orange rind, tomato purée, peppercorns and fish trimmings and cover with the water. Bring to the boil then simmer for about 40 minutes, stirring often.
4. Strain the cooking liquor into another large pan. Press the vegetable mixture to get out as much flavour as possible. Discard the bones and vegetables.
5. Bring the liquor up to simmering point and poach the fish in it for about four minutes. Leave the fish to cool in the liquid a little, then purée in a blender. Taste for seasoning and adjust if necessary.
6. To make the rouille, put the garlic into a pestle and mortar with some salt and grind to a purée. The salt acts as a good abrasive. Transfer to a bowl and mix in the yolks, then start adding the oil drop by drop, beating all the time (use a whisk or a spatula). The mixture should thicken as you add the oil. Stir in the cayenne. Add the tomato purée, then lemon juice to taste. Add more lemon juice or cayenne if you want.
7. Serve the soup hot, offering bowls of gruyère, croûtes and rouille on the side.

Seafood soup

	4 portions	10 portions
olive oil	1 tbsp	2½ tbsp
shallots, finely chopped	2	5
garlic clove, crushed	1	3
fish or chicken stock	800 ml	2 litres
dry white wine	100 ml	250 ml
pinch of saffron		½ tsp
bay leaf	1	3
new potatoes, sliced into ½ cm rounds	250 g	625 g
frozen peas	100 g	250 g
frozen sweetcorn	100 g	250 g
tomatoes, skinned, deseeded, diced	3 (about 300 g in total)	750 g
monkfish fillet, cut into 2.5 cm chunks	200 g	500 g
mussels in the shell, cleaned, de-bearded	340 g	850 g
cooked prawns, defrosted	100 g	250 g

1. Heat the oil in a large pan and fry the shallots and garlic gently for 5–6 minutes, to soften but not brown. Add the wine and reduce by half. Add the stock, saffron and bay leaf and bring to the boil.
2. Add the potatoes to the pan, reduce the heat, cover and simmer gently for about 10 minutes until tender.
3. Increase the heat to high and add the vegetables. Bring back to the boil, then stir in the tomatoes, monkfish, prawns and mussels. Reduce the heat and simmer gently, without stirring, for about 3 minutes until the cod is white and firm and the mussels have opened. Discard any mussels that remain closed. Season to taste, then serve immediately.

Thai fish soup

	4 portions	10 portions
lemon grass	4 sticks	10 sticks
fresh coriander, chopped	1 tsp	3 tsp
green Thai chillies	2	5
fresh root ginger, peeled, finely grated	75 g	180 g
vegetable oil	3 tbsp	8 tbsp
coconut milk	400 ml	1 litre
fish stock	300 ml	750 ml
cornflour	1 tbsp	2½ tbsp
water	3 tbsp	200 ml
Bio Yoghurt	500 g	1¼ litres
mixed fish (e.g. sole, plaice, salmon, cod, scallops, prawns), cut into bite-sized pieces	500 g	1¼ kg
lime juice	1	2
salt and freshly ground white pepper		

1. Finely chop the lemon grass. Deseed the chillies and finely chop them. Finely chop the coriander and reserve. Cook the lemon grass, chillies and ginger in the oil in a frying pan over a low heat for 8 minutes, or until the lemon grass and ginger have softened and the mixture is very fragrant.
2. Add the coconut milk and fish stock, bring to the boil, turn up the heat and reduce by half.
3. Blend the cornflour and water and stir into the yoghurt. Add to the reduced stock, then heat until almost boiling. Add the fish to the pan and poach for 4–5 minutes, until cooked through.
4. At the very last minute add the lime juice and reserved coriander and season to taste with salt and pepper. Serve immediately.

38 Fish forcemeat or farce

	4 portions	10 portions
fish, free from skin and bone	300 g	1 kg
salt, white pepper		
egg whites	1–2	4–5
double cream, ice cold	250–500 ml	600 ml–1¼ litres

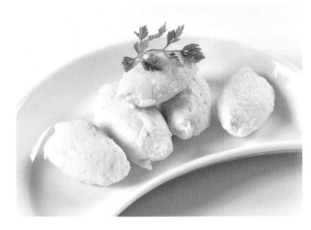

1. Process the fish and seasoning to a fine purée.
2. Continue processing, slowly adding the egg whites until thoroughly absorbed.
3. Pass the mixture through a fine sieve and place into a shallow pan or bowl.
4. Leave on ice or in refrigerator until very cold.
5. Beating the mixture continuously, slowly incorporate the cream.
6. When half the cream is incorporated, test the consistency and seasoning by cooking a teaspoonful in a small pan of simmering water. If the mixture is very firm, a little more cream may be added, then test the mixture again and continue until the mixture is of a mousse consistency.

Mousses, mousselines and quenelles are all made from forcemeat. Salmon, sole, trout, brill, turbot, halibut,

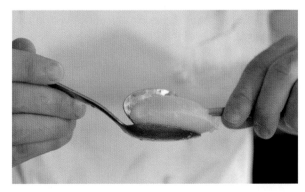

whiting, pike and lobster can all be used for fish forcemeat in the preparation of, for example, mousse of sole, mousselines of salmon, quenelles of turbot, all of which would be served with a suitable sauce (white wine, butter sauce, lobster, shrimp, saffron and mushroom).

Mousses

As mousses are cooked in buttered moulds in a bain-marie in the oven and turned out for service, the mixture should not be made too soft otherwise they will break up.

Mousses are made in buttered moulds, usually 1 per portion, but larger moulds for 2–4 can be made if required. It is sounder practice to use individual moulds because for large moulds the mousse needs to be of a firmer consistency to prevent it collapsing.

They are cooked in a bain-marie in a moderate oven or in a low-pressure steamer.

When making lobster mousse, use raw lobster meat and ideally some raw lobster roe as this gives authentic colour to the mousse when cooked. For scallop mousse use cooked scallops. In order to achieve sufficient bulk it is sometimes necessary to add a little other fish, e.g. whiting, sole, pike.

Mousseline

Mousselines are moulded using two tablespoons, dipping the spoons frequently into boiling water to prevent the mixture sticking.

They are normally moulded into shallow buttered trays, covered with salted water or fish stock, covered with buttered greaseproof paper and gently poached in the oven or steamed. Shellfish mousselines are best cooked in shallow individual moulds because of their looser texture.

Quenelles

Quenelles are made in various shapes and sizes as required:
- Moulded with dessert or teaspoons
- Piped with a small plain tube.

They are cooked in the same way as mousselines.

Fish mousse

Fish mousse will inevitably vary according to the fish used to make the mousse. The recipe below is for the base. The table that follows it gives the quantities of whipping cream.

fish trimmed of bone, skin and scales, cut into 2½ cm dice	150 g
salt	1 tsp
ground pepper	pinch

Fish type	Quantity of whipping cream
monkfish	500 ml
salmon	375 ml
scallops	450 ml
sea bass	500 ml
turbot	300 ml

1. Place the fish in a cold food processor bowl with the blade attachment; blend to a fine mince, stopping twice to ensure that the excess is scraped from the sides of the bowl.
2. Add the salt and pepper, ensuring even distribution. The salt will firm up the mousse, swelling the protein and allowing the cream to be incorporated more easily. Chill the mousse in the refrigerator for 10–15 minutes.
3. Place back in the processor then add the cream in a steady stream, taking about 40 seconds in all – too fast and the cream will whip, too slow and the fat in the cream will be over-worked and split the mousse.
4. Test poach: place a small amount of the mousse in a piece of cling film and seal; poach in simmering water for 1–2 minutes until firm and check for seasoning – add if necessary. Store in the fridge, well covered, for up to 2 days.

 Fish soufflé

	4 portions	10 portions
raw fish, free from skin and bone	300 g	1 kg
butter	50 g	125 g
thick béchamel	250 ml	600 ml
salt and cayenne pepper		
eggs, separated	3	5

Haddock, sole, salmon, turbot, lobster, crab, etc. can all be used for soufflés.
1. Cook the fish in the butter and process to a purée.
2. Mix with the béchamel, pass through a fine sieve and season well.
3. Warm the mixture and beat in the egg yolks.
4. Carefully fold in the stiffly beaten egg whites.
5. Place into individual buttered and floured soufflé moulds.
6. Bake at 220°C for approximately 14 minutes; serve immediately.

A suitable sauce may be offered, e.g. white wine, mushroom, shrimp, saffron, lobster.

If individual moulds are used, less cooking time is required.

The use of an extra beaten egg white will increase the lightness of the soufflé.

A pinch of egg white powder added before whipping will strengthen the foam.

Lobster soufflés can be cooked and served in the cleaned half shells of the lobsters.

Fish *en papillote*

1. The fish should be portioned, free from bones and may or may not be skinned.
2. Garnish with a fine selection of vegetables chosen from carrots, leeks, celery, white mushrooms and wild mushrooms; a small amount of freshly chopped herbs may be added as desired.
3. Moisten with a little dry white wine, then seal the foil parcel and bake for 15–20 minutes (size and fish dependent).
4. Serve with an appropriate sauce (e.g. white wine).

 This method of cookery is fresh-tasting and suitable for most fish or shellfish.

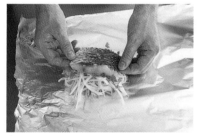
Sea bass en papillote

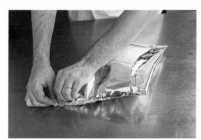
Seal the foil package

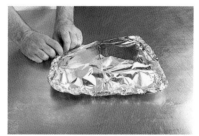
Make sure it is tightly sealed on all sides

Fried fish, Thai style (*pla jian*)

	1 portion
whole fish (e.g. sole, lemon sole, plaice)	1
Marinade	
garlic, chopped	1 tbsp
ginger, grated	1 tbsp
yellow bean sauce	2 tsp
black bean paste	1 tsp
light soy sauce	2 tbsp
fish sauce	2 tbsp
toasted shrimp paste	½ tsp
palm sugar	2 tsp
fish stock	4 tbsp
onion, chopped	2 tbsp
red chilli, finely chopped	1
lemon grass stalk, finely chopped	1

1. To make the marinade, combine all the ingredients. Rub into both sides of the fish, and leave it to stand for at least 1 hour in the chiller.
2. Remove the fish from the marinade, and allow it to drain.
3. Transfer the remaining marinade to a small saucepan. Simmer to reduce to a sauce-like consistency.
4. Heat enough oil to deep fry the fish in a suitable pan over medium heat, and slide the fish into the hot oil. Fry until the fish is cooked through, turning once.
5. Serve on a platter, pouring the reduced sauce over the fish.

43 Steamed fish, Thai style (*pla nergn*)

	1–2 portions
medium-sized fish (e.g. grouper, tilapia)	1
lemon grass stalk, finely sliced	1
bird's eye chillies (*chili padi*), smashed	2
red chillies, finely chopped	2
cloves of garlic, finely chopped	8
lime, zest	1
kaffir lime leaves, finely sliced	2
dried tamarind skin (*asam keping*)	2
oyster sauce	2 tbsp
fish sauce to taste	
lime juice to taste	
sugar to taste	
salt to taste	
spring onions, cut into julienne	15 g
coriander, chopped	15 g
cooking oil	1 tbsp
sesame oil	1 tbsp

i Tamarind is a tropical fruit with an acid taste.

1. Scale the fish and clean it well. Make 2 slanting cuts on each side of the fish.
2. Place the fish in the centre of a baking dish. Place all the ingredients except the coriander, spring onion and oils on top of the fish.
3. Steam the fish on a high heat for about 10–12 minutes.
4. Sprinkle the spring onion and coriander on the fish.
5. Heat up the cooking oil and sesame oil in a frying pan. Spoon the oil mixture over the fish to serve.

44 Fish sausages (*cervelas de poisson*)

As with meat sausages, the variations of fish sausages (also called *boudin*) that can be produced are virtually endless. Almost any type of fish or shellfish can be used, either chopped or minced. The filling can also be a combination of two or more fish, and additional ingredients can be added (e.g. dry duxelle, brunoise of skinned red peppers, a suitable chopped herb such as dill, chervil, parsley and/or a touch of spice).

The selected fish can also be made into a firm mousseline mixture as in the following recipe for pike sausages (*cervelas de brochet*).

	4 portions	10 portions
pike meat	200 g	500 g
egg white	1	3
double cream	½ litre	1.4 litres
salt, white pepper		
sausage skins	100 g	250 g

Note: The number of sausages produced will vary according to the size required.

1. Prepare mousseline mixture as in recipe 38.
2. Place sausage skins in water; then hang up, knot one end.
3. Using a forcing bag, stuff the skins with mousse, being careful not to force it, then knot the other end with a piece of string.
4. Divide sausage into sections by loosely tying with string.

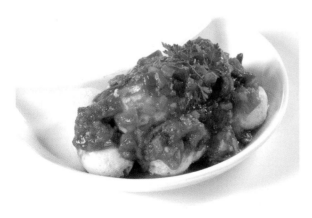

5. Gently poach the sausages in water at 82°C for 15 minutes.
6. Once cooked, carefully remove the sausages and allow to drain for 1–2 minutes.

7. With a sharp knife, remove the sausage skins carefully so as not to spoil the shape, drain well on a clean serviette and serve with a suitable sauce, e.g. tomato, and garnish.

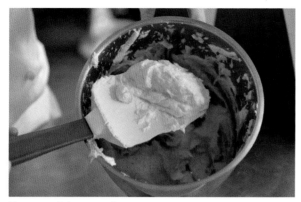
Prepare a fish mousseline

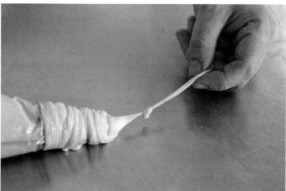
Pipe the mousse into the sausage skin

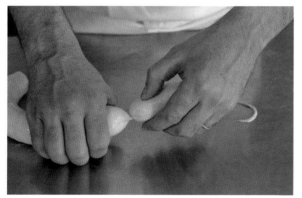
Divide into sections

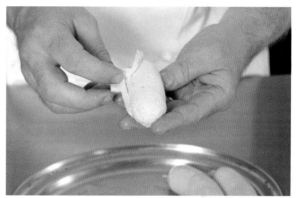
Remove the skin after cooking

45 Russian fish pie (Coulibiac)

energy	kcal	fat	sat fat	carb	sugar	protein	fibre	
3461 KJ	833.63 cal	66.5 g	28.5 g	35.3 g	1.7 g	26.8 g	0.5 g	*

	4 portions	10 portions
brioche or puff paste	200 g	500 g
coarse semolina or rice, cooked in good stock as for pilaff	100 g	250 g
salmon, cut in small thick slices and fried very lightly in butter	400 g	1¼ kg
onion, finely chopped	50 g	125 g
mushrooms, chopped	100 g	250 g
parsley, chopped	1 tbsp	2½ tbsp
hard-boiled egg, chopped	1	2½
fresh vesiga, cooked and roughly chopped	50 g	125 g
melted butter	200 g	500 g

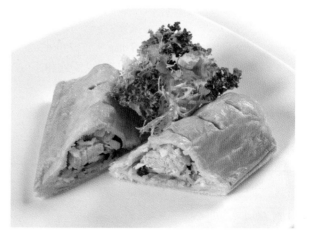

1. Roll out the paste thinly into a rectangle approximately 30 × 18 cm.
2. Place the ingredients in layers one on top of the other along the centre, alternating the layers, and starting and finishing with the semolina or rice.
3. Eggwash the edges of the paste and fold over to enclose the filling completely.
4. Seal the ends and turn over onto a lightly greased baking sheet so that the sealed edges are underneath.
5. If using brioche, allow to prove in a warm place for approximately 30 minutes.
6. Brush all over with melted butter (or eggwash if using puff pastry) and cut two small holes neatly in the top to allow steam to escape.
7. Bake at 190°C for approximately 40 minutes.
8. When removed from the oven, pour some melted butter into the two holes.
9. To serve, cut into thick slices and offer a butter-type sauce, e.g. hollandaise, separately.

Individual coulibiacs can be made using a 20 cm pastry cutter or in the shape shown here.

* The analysis did not include the vesiga.

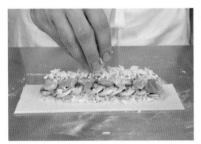
Layer the ingredients

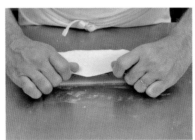
Cover with pastry and seal the edges

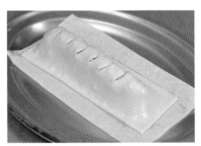
Cut holes in the top

Vesiga is the spinal cord of the sturgeon obtained commercially in the shape of white, semi-transparent dry gelatinous ribbon. It must be soaked in cold water for 4–5 hours when it will swell to 4–5 times the size and the weight will increase six-fold. It is then gently simmered in white stock for 3½–4½ hours. If it is not possible to obtain vesiga, a layer of fish forcemeat may be substituted.

Coulibiac has for many years been a popular dish in high-class restaurants around the world. Other fish may be used to replace the salmon, e.g. haddock, tuna, cod, sea bass, smoked haddock.

If vesiga is unobtainable then use more of all the other ingredients.

With imagination many variations of this dish can be conceived.

46 Creamy smoked fish and coconut kedgeree

	4 portions	10 portions
korma curry paste	3 tbsp	7 tbsp
undyed smoked haddock or cod, cut into large pieces	450 g	1⅛ kg
reduced-fat coconut milk	400 ml	1 litre
bunches of salad onions, thickly sliced	2	5
fresh coriander, chopped	2 tbsp	5 tbsp
frozen peas	100 g	250 g
fresh parsley, chopped	2 tbsp	5 tbsp
basmati rice, cooked	250 g	625 g
lime, cut into 4 wedges	1	2 ½
cream to finish		

1. Fry the korma curry paste for 1–2 minutes in a large saucepan. Add the smoked fish.
2. Stir in the coconut milk, bring to the boil, then reduce to a low heat. Poach for 3–4 minutes, or until the fish is nearly cooked. Add the salad onions, chopped herbs and frozen peas and cook for a further minute.
3. Stir in the basmati rice and simmer for a couple of minutes, until everything is piping hot. Season to taste. Pile on to a serving dish and serve with lime wedges.

47   Smoked fish carbonara

	4 portions	10 portions
smoked cod or haddock fillet, fresh or defrosted, skinned, cubed	400 g	1 kg
smoked pancetta	200 g	500 g
eggs	4	10
egg yolks	4	10
double cream	210 ml	525 ml
wholegrain mustard	2 tbsp	5 tbsp
olive oil	1 tbsp	2½ tbsp
mushrooms, sliced	100 g	250 g
spring onions, chopped	3	7
cherry tomatoes, quartered	4	10
Pecorino cheese, grated	150 g	375 g
fresh tagliatelle	350 g	875 g
black pepper		
fresh parsley, chopped	2 tbsp	5 tbsp

1. Place a large pot of water on the stove and bring to a rolling boil to cook the tagliatelle.
2. While the pasta is cooking, heat a frying pan and fry the pancetta without any extra oil until it is crisp and golden (about 5 minutes). Add the onions and mushrooms and cook for a further 5 minutes. Add the tomatoes and diced fish and stir around the pan for a minute or two (at this point it is only partly cooked).
3. Whisk the eggs, yolks and cream in a bowl and season generously with black pepper, then whisk in the cheese.
4. When the pasta is cooked, drain it quickly in a colander, leaving a little of the moisture still clinging. Quickly return it to the saucepan and add the pancetta, mushroom, onion and fish mix and any oil in the pan, along with the egg and cream mixture and the chopped parsley.
5. Stir very thoroughly, so that everything gets a good coating – what happens is that the liquid egg cooks briefly as it comes into contact with the hot pasta, and the fish will cook through at this point.
6. Serve the pasta on really hot deep plates with some extra grated Pecorino or Parmesan cheese.

48   Crab

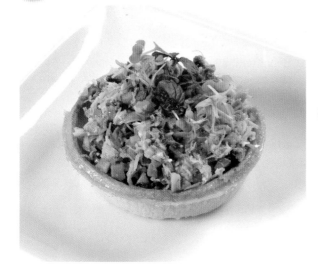

Crab meat can be used in a variety of recipes – for example:

- First courses – on halves of mango or papaya or avocado coated with a mayonnaise or natural yoghurt-based sauce lightly flavoured with tomato ketchup, lemon juice, Worcestershire sauce, etc.
- Sprinkle with fresh white breadcrumbs and melted butter and lightly brown.
- Soup, au gratin, mornay, devilled, curried, soufflé, pancakes, crab cakes or rissoles etc., are obvious other ways of preparing and serving crab.

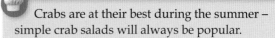
Crabs are at their best during the summer – simple crab salads will always be popular.

Crab tartlets or barquettes

	4 portions	10 portions
shallot, finely chopped, cooked in oil or butter	100 g	250 g
raw mushroom, finely chopped	200 g	500 g
white wine	30 ml	125 ml
crab meat	200 g	500 g
salt and cayenne pepper		

1. Use short, puff or filo pastry. Bake blind.
2. Combine all the ingredients to make the filling.

Crab Malabar (*kekada chat*)

	4 portions	10 portions
cooked crab meat, fresh or frozen and thawed	450 g	1.2 kg
vegetable oil	3 tbsp	7 tbsp
onions, finely chopped	50 g	125 g
cloves of garlic, finely chopped	3	7
paprika	2 tsp	5 tsp
thyme	½ tsp	1 tsp
fennel seeds, crushed	½ tsp	1 tsp
cayenne pepper	½ tsp	1 tsp
fresh tomatoes, blanched, deseeded, diced	200 g	500 g
salt, to taste		
spring onions (both green and white parts), finely chopped	2	5
lettuce leaves and chopped coriander to garnish		

1. Pick over the crab meat and cut into 2 cm pieces.
2. Heat the oil in a large skillet with a lid over a moderate heat and cook the onions, stirring frequently, until golden but not brown. Add the garlic and cook for 1 minute. Add the paprika, thyme, fennel seeds, and cayenne pepper and cook for 2 more minutes. Add one-third of the tomatoes. Lower the heat and simmer covered for 15 minutes.
3. Remove from the heat and gently fold in the crab meat. Cover and refrigerate for 2 to 3 hours.
4. Immediately before serving, add salt to taste and fold in the remaining tomatoes and chopped spring onions.
5. Serve on a bed of lettuce, garnished with the chopped coriander.

 ## Crab and ginger spring roll

	To fill 24–30 spring rolls
bean thread vermicelli noodles	30 g
crab meat, cooked	225 g
white fish fillets (e.g. lemon sole or cod), finely chopped	125 g
cornflour	2 tsp
fresh ginger, finely grated	2 tsp
shallots, finely chopped	4
soy sauce	2 tsp
oyster sauce	2 tsp

To make the spring rolls

i Spring roll wrappers are similar to filo pastry, usually made with rice flour and water.

1. Separate the spring roll wrappers from the pack and cover with a damp paper or cloth to keep them moist.
2. Moisten the edge of a wrapper. Place a little filling at one end. Roll up neatly and tightly, turn in the edges and repeat with the next. Chill.
3. Deep fry, drain and serve immediately.

To make the filling

1. Place the noodles in a bowl. Cover with boiling water and let stand for 5 minutes.
2. Drain and chop the noodles.
3. Combine with the remaining ingredients.

51 Lobster mornay

energy	kcal	fat	sat fat	carb	sugar	protein	fibre
1170 KJ	280.6 cal	18.0 g	10.7 g	7.8 g	3.0 g	22.3 g	0.2 g

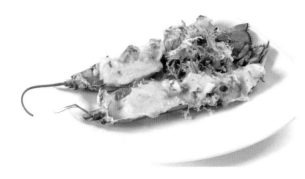

1. Remove the lobsters' claws and legs.
2. Cut lobsters carefully in half lengthwise.
3. Remove all meat. Discard the sac and remove the trail from the tail.
4. Wash shell and drain on a baking sheet upside down.
5. Cut the lobster meat into escalopes.
6. Heat the butter in a thick-bottomed pan, add the lobster and season.
7. Turn two or three times; overcooking will toughen the meat.
8. Meanwhile, finish the mornay sauce.
9. Place a little sauce in the bottom of each shell.
10. Add the lobster, and press down to make a flat surface.
11. Mask completely with sauce, sprinkle with grated cheese, and brown under the salamander. Serve garnished with picked parsley.

	4 portions	10 portions
cooked lobsters (approx. 400 g each)	2	5
butter	25 g	60 g
salt, cayenne		
mornay sauce	250 ml	625 ml
grated cheese (Parmesan)		
parsley (to garnish)		

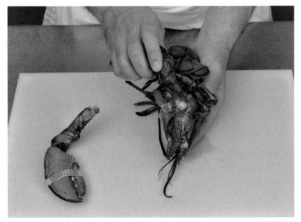

Remove the claws and legs from the lobster

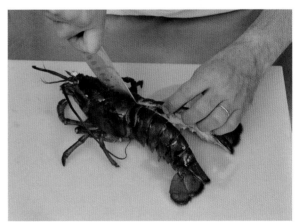

Cut the lobster in half

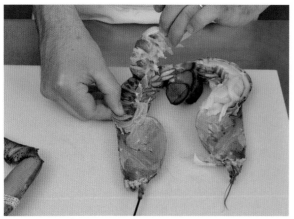

Remove the meat

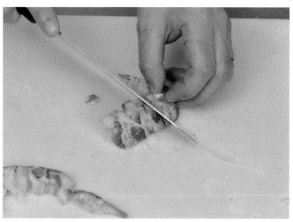

Cut the meat into escalopes

52 Lobster Newburg

energy	kcal	fat	sat fat	carb	sugar	protein	fibre
1556 KJ	375.3 cal	30.7 g	17.5 g	0.6 g	0.6 g	24.1 g	0.0 g

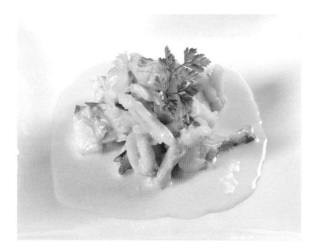

1. Gently reheat the lobster pieces in the butter.
2. Add Madeira and slowly reduce to a glaze.
3. Transfer to a different, cold pan (this reduces the risk of the egg splitting when the liaison is added). With the pan over gentle heat, pour in the liaison and allow to thicken by gentle continuous shaking; do not allow to boil. Correct seasoning, using a touch of cayenne if required.
4. Serve with pilaff rice separately.

Lobster butter

A lobster butter made from the crushed soft lobster shells will improve the colour of the sauce.

1. Sweat the crushed lobster shells in 25–50 g butter over a fierce heat, stirring well.
2. Moisten with stock or water, boil for 10 minutes, strain.
3. Clarify the butter by simmering to evaporate the liquid.

	4 portions	10 portions
cooked lobster meat cut into thickish pieces	400 g	1¼ kg
butter	50 g	125 g
Madeira	60 ml	150 ml
cream ⎫ liaison	120 ml	250 ml
egg yolks ⎭	2	5

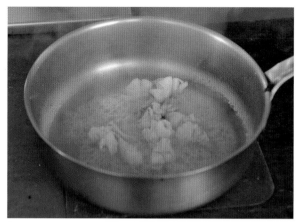

Reduce the Madeira

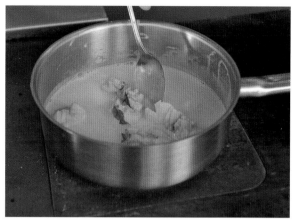

During cooking, shake the pan to help thicken the sauce

53 Lobster tail gratin

energy	kcal	fat	sat fat	carb	sugar	protein	fibre
1751 KJ	421 cal	31.9 g	19.5 g	18.1 g	1.6 g	16.6 g	0.6 g

	4 portions	10 portions
Lobster		
lobster tails (each from a 500–600 g live lobster)	4	10
butter	80 g	200 g
dry sherry	20 ml	50 ml
flour	20 g	50 g
paprika	½ tsp	1 tsp
cream	120 ml	300 ml
seasoning		
Crumb topping		
slices white bread	3	7
cup butter	40 g	100 g
chives, chopped	1 tbsp	2 tbsp
seasoning		

For the lobster

1. Preheat the oven to 190°C.
2. Gently blanch the lobster tails until they are half done, then drain and cool.
3. Remove meat from shells and cut into small pieces, clean and save the shells.
4. Melt butter in a thick-bottomed pan. Stir in sherry and lobster, simmer for 2 minutes.
5. Stir in flour, paprika and cream until thickened, adjust the seasoning then return mixture to shells.
6. Place the filled and topped shells on a baking tray and bake in the oven for 10 minutes.
7. Serve immediately with a green salad or wilted greens.

For the crumb topping

1. Remove crust from bread and place in food processor or grate finely.
2. Melt butter in a pan, add the breadcrumbs and cook until brown.
3. Add the chives and salt and pepper. When the lobster meat is returned to the shell sprinkle over.

Cornish or Scottish (native) lobsters are best for this recipe; their Canadian counterparts may be used but the native varieties will yield a better result.

54 Eggs in cocotte with shrimps, cream and cheese

energy	kcal	fat	sat fat	carb	sugar	protein	fibre
997 KJ	239.9 cal	19.0 g	9.5 g	8.3 g	8.2 g	9.5 g	1.4 g

	4 portions	10 portions
butter or margarine	50 g	125 g
peeled shrimps (potted or fresh)	100 g	250 g
eggs	4	10
cream	4 tbsp	10 tbsp
grated Parmesan cheese	20 g	50 g

1. Butter the cocottes.
2. Add the shrimps.
3. Break the eggs on top.
4. Place in a shallow tray containing 1 cm water.
5. Cook in a steamer or moderate oven until the eggs are lightly set.
6. Pour on the cream, sprinkle with cheese and lightly brown under the salamander.

55 Poached eggs with prawns, sherry and French mustard

energy	kcal	fat	sat fat	carb	sugar	protein	fibre
1271 KJ	305.4 cal	20.1 g	10.0 g	10.9 g	6.1 g	19.1 g	1.0 g

	4 portions	10 portions
eggs	4	10
tomatoes, medium-sized, peeled and sliced	4	10
prawns	100 g	250 g
butter or margarine	25 g	60 g
sherry	2 tbsp	5 tbsp
mornay sauce	250 ml	600 ml
French mustard	½ tsp	1¼ tsp
grated Parmesan cheese	50 g	125 g

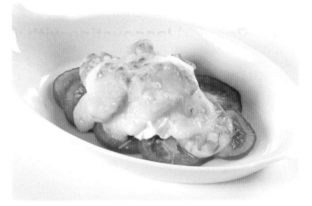

1. Poach the eggs and reserve in a basin of cold water.
2. Divide the tomatoes into individual dishes (e.g. egg dishes) season lightly with salt and pepper. Place on a baking sheet in a moderate oven for approximately 5 minutes.
3. Warm the prawns in the butter and sherry.
4. Reheat the mornay sauce and flavour with the French mustard.
5. Reheat the eggs, drain well. Place on top of the slices of cooked tomato.
6. Sprinkle the prawns over the eggs.
7. Coat with mornay sauce and sprinkle with Parmesan cheese.
8. Glaze under the salamander. Serve immediately.

56 Pork and prawn spring roll filling

	For 24–30 spring rolls
Chinese dried mushrooms	4
uncooked prawns, shelled, finely chopped	250 g
minced pork	150 g
Chinese cabbage leaves, finely shredded	3
peanut oil	2 tsp
clove of garlic finely chopped	1
fresh ginger, finely grated	2 tsp
carrot, finely chopped	70 g
coriander leaves, finely chopped	2 tsp
lemon grass, finely chopped	2 tsp
soy sauce	1 tbsp
oyster sauce	1 tbsp

1. Place the mushrooms in a bowl, cover with boiling water and leave for 20 minutes.
2. Drain the mushrooms and chop finely.
3. Combine all the ingredients together.

57 Roasted langoustine with watercress and balsamic

	4 portions	10 portions
langoustine tails	360 g	900 g
salt to taste		
egg whites, medium	1	4
egg yolks, medium	1	8
double cream	400 ml	1 litre
langoustine tail, diced 1 cm, deglazed	160 g	400 g
cognac	20 ml	50 ml
tarragon, blanched, chopped	½ tsp	1 tsp
chervil, blanched, chopped	½ tsp	1 tsp
cayenne pepper	1 g	2 g

1. In a cold Robo Coup, purée the 900 g of langoustine tails and salt to taste.
2. Add the eggs and one quarter of the cream, blitz and pass through a fine drum sieve.
3. Mix the rest of the cream over ice with the cognac, fried langoustine tails, herbs and seasoning.
4. Cook a tester in cling film and taste.
5. Pipe back into the head of the langoustine and roast in an oven for 8 minutes at 180°C.
6. Serve with wilted watercress and balsamic vinegar.

58 Langoustine and mussel soup

energy	kcal	fat	sat fat	carb	sugar	protein	fibre
2355 KJ	566 cal	36.3 g	20.8 g	21.6 g	5.7 g	39.3 g	1.2 g

	4 portions	10 portions
raw langoustine tails (large), bodies and claws retained for the stock	20	50
mussels, cleaned	400 g	1 kg
fish stock	300 ml	750 ml
butter	80 g	200 g
fresh bay leaves	2	5
dry white wine	50 ml	125 ml
shallots, chopped	1	3
celery sticks, cut into small dice	1	3
rindless dry-cured unsmoked bacon, cut across into short, fat strips	50 g	125 g
potatoes, peeled and cut into small dice	225 g	560 g
plain flour	20 g	50 g
full-cream milk	300 ml	750 ml
whipping cream	120 ml	300 ml
salt		
freshly ground black pepper		

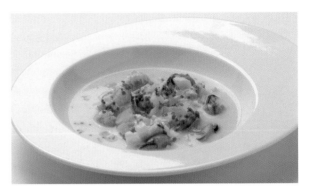

1. If using raw langoustines, put them into the freezer for 30 minutes to kill them painlessly. Then put the langoustines and mussels into a pan and add the stock.
2. Cover, bring to the boil and steam for 2 minutes.
3. Remove from the heat and tip the contents into a colander set over a clean bowl to retain the cooking liquid.
4. Check that all the mussels have opened and discard any that remain closed.
5. Melt about one-third of the butter in a large pan, add the langoustine shells and the bay leaves, cook for 1 minute.
6. Add the wine and the reserved cooking liquor and while it is bubbling away, crush the shells to release all their flavour into the cooking liquid.
7. Cook for 10–12 minutes.
8. Meanwhile, heat the rest of the butter in a pan, add the shallots, celery and bacon, cook gently until the shallots are soft but not coloured.
9. Add the diced potatoes and cook for 1–2 minutes, stir in the flour, then add the milk and cream.
10. Pass the cooking liquor into a clean pan and add to the roux base, stirring continuously to prevent lumps.
11. When all the stock has been added, cook out until the potatoes are soft.
12. Stir in the langoustines and mussels, and adjust the seasoning if necessary.
13. Ladle into warmed soup plates and serve with traditional sour bread.

Proceed with caution when using both mussels and langoustines as they overcook quickly and this will spoil the eating quality.

59 Mussels

When mussels are fresh the shells should be tightly closed. If the shells are open there is the possibility of danger from food poisoning and so the mussels should be discarded.

Preparation for cooking

1. Scrape the shells to remove any barnacles, etc.
2. Wash well and drain in a colander.

To cook

1. Take a thick-bottomed pan with a tight-fitting lid.
2. For 1 litre mussels, place in the pan 25 g chopped shallot or onion.
3. Add the mussels, cover with a lid and cook on a fierce heat for 4–5 minutes until the shells open completely.

Preparation for use

1. Remove mussels from shells, checking carefully for sand, weed and beard.
2. Retain the liquid.

 60 **Mussels in white wine sauce**

energy	kcal	fat	sat fat	carb	sugar	protein	fibre
750 KJ	178 cal	7.9 g	3.6 g	9.4 g	0.9 g	17.7 g	0.4 g

	4 portions	10 portions
shallots, chopped	50 g	125 g
parsley, chopped	1 tbsp	2 tbsp
white wine	60 ml	150 ml
strong fish stock	200 ml	500 ml
mussels	2 kg	5 kg
butter	25 g	60 ml
flour	25 g	60 ml
seasoning		

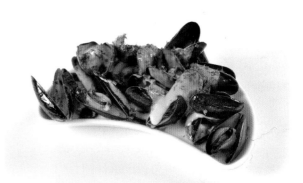

1. Take a thick-bottomed pan and add the shallots, parsley, wine, fish stock and the cleaned mussels.
2. Cover with a tight-fitting lid and cook over a high heat until the shells open.
3. Drain off all the cooking liquor in a colander set over a clean bowl to retain the cooking juices.
4. Carefully check the mussels and discard any that have not opened.
5. Place in a dish and cover to keep warm.
6. Make a roux from the flour and butter; pour over the cooking liquor, ensuring it is free from sand and stirring continuously to avoid lumps.
7. Correct the seasoning and garnish with more chopped parsley.
8. Pour over the mussels and serve.

 61 **Mussels with pasta, turmeric and chervil**

	4 portions	10 portions
olive oil	50 ml	125 ml
chilli, finely chopped	½	1
clove of garlic, finely chopped	1	3
spring onions, chopped	3	8
double cream	3 tbsp	8 tbsp
turmeric	1 tsp	2½ tsp
mussels, cooked	100 g	250 g
spaghetti, cooked	100 g	250 g
fresh chervil, chopped	1 tbsp	2 tbsp
salt and freshly ground black pepper		

1. Heat the oil in a wok and sauté the chilli, garlic and spring onion until soft. Add the turmeric.
2. Add the double cream and mussels and cook until the mussels are heated through and the cream has reduced slightly.
3. Add the spaghetti, season well with salt and freshly ground black pepper and stir together to combine.
4. To serve, transfer to a serving bowl and sprinkle over the chervil.

62 Saffron and curry mussels

	4 portions	10 portions
live mussels	2 kg	5 kg
dry white wine	125 ml	300 ml
small onion, finely chopped	1	2
clove of garlic, finely chopped	1	2
butter	25 g	60 g
plain flour	25 g	60 g
milk	100 ml	250 ml
egg yolk	1	2
mild curry powder	½ tsp	1 tsp
ground saffron	½ tsp	1 tsp
turmeric	½ tsp	1 tsp
double cream	100 ml	250 ml
flat leaf parsley	1 tbsp	2 tbsp

1. Discard any broken mussels, and those that do not close when sharply tapped. Scrub the mussels well, and pull out the beards. Wash them in several changes of water.
2. Bring the white wine, onion and garlic to the boil in a heavy-based frying pan and boil for 1 minute. Add the mussels, cover the pan tightly, and steam for 1 minute, shaking now and then to ensure the mussels cook evenly.
3. Remove the mussels (discarding any that haven't opened) and reserve them in a covered bowl. Strain the mussel cooking broth into a jug and set aside.
4. Melt the butter in a small saucepan, sprinkle over the flour and cook, stirring, for about 3 minutes.
5. Gradually pour in the mussel broth, stirring constantly. Gradually pour in the milk, stirring constantly.
6. Beat the egg yolk, curry powder, saffron, turmeric and cream together, then pour into the sauce, stirring well as you add it. Simmer gently without allowing the sauce to boil.
7. Remove the top shells of about half the mussels, and discard.
8. Pile all the mussels into four warmed shallow bowls and pour the sauce over the top. Scatter with parsley and serve hot.

63 Mussels with cider, cream and chopped apple

	4 portions	10 portions
mussels	2 kg	5 kg
garlic clove, finely chopped	1	3
shallots, finely chopped	2	5
butter	15 g	40 g
bouquet garni (parsley, thyme and bay leaves)	1	2
dry cider or white wine	100 ml	250 ml
double cream	120 ml	300 ml
parsley leaves, coarsely chopped	1 tbsp	2 tbsp
apple, grated	1	2

1. Wash the mussels under plenty of cold, running water. Discard any open ones that won't close when lightly squeezed.
2. Pull out the tough, fibrous beards protruding from between the tightly closed shells and then knock off any barnacles with a large knife. Give the mussels another quick rinse to remove any little pieces of shell.
3. Soften the garlic and shallots in the butter with the bouquet garni, in a large pan big enough to take all the mussels – it should only be half full.
4. Add the mussels and cider, turn up the heat, then cover and steam them open in their own juices for 3–4 minutes. Give the pan a good shake every now and then.
5. Remove the bouquet garni, add the cream and chopped parsley and remove from the heat.
6. Spoon into four large warmed bowls and serve with crusty bread and grated apple.

64 Cockle chowder

energy	kcal	fat	sat fat	carb	sugar	protein	fibre
2223 KJ	536 cal	45.0 g	21.4 g	13.9 g	7.3 g	19.9 g	2.4 g

	4 portions	10 portions
Cockles		
medium shallots, finely diced	2	5
butter	50 g	125 g
cockles, shells tightly closed	2 kg	5 kg
white wine or vermouth	200 ml	500 ml
Chowder		
vegetable oil	50 ml	125 ml
smoked bacon, cut into 1 cm dice	50 g	125 g
medium onion, cut into 1 cm dice	1	3
medium carrot, cut into 1 cm dice	1	3
garlic cloves, finely chopped	2	5
celery sticks, cut into 1 cm dice	1	3
medium potato, peeled and cut into 1 cm dice	1	3
medium yellow pepper, cut into 1 cm dice	1	3
chicken stock	1 litre	2½ litres
whipping cream	100 ml	250 ml
butter	50 g	125 g
salt and pepper		

For the cockles

1. Take a large saucepan with a tight-fitting lid and place over a medium heat, add the shallots and butter and cook for 1 minute without letting the shallots colour.
2. Add the washed cockles, shake the pan, then add the wine and place the lid on the pan immediately. Leave the cockles to steam for 1–2 minutes so that they open and exude an intense liquor.
3. Remove the lid and make sure all the cockles are open. Remove the pan from the heat and discard any with closed shells.

4. Place a colander over a large bowl, and pour the contents of the pan into the colander, reserving the liquor for the chowder.
5. Allow the cockles to cool. Pick out the meat, check carefully for sand and discard the shells. Store the cockle meat in an airtight container in the fridge until you are ready to serve the chowder.

For the chowder

1. In a large saucepan, heat the oil. When hot, add the bacon and cook for about 5 minutes until crisp and brown.
2. Using a perforated spoon, transfer the bacon onto kitchen paper to drain. Add the onion, carrot, garlic, celery and potato to the saucepan, reduce the heat to medium-low and cook the vegetables for 3–4 minutes without colouring.
3. Add the peppers and cook for 5 minutes. Pour in the reserved liquor from the cockles and the chicken stock.
4. Bring to the boil and simmer for 10 minutes or until the volume of liquid has reduced by about half.
5. Add the cooked bacon and cream, then bring to the boil and reduce for a further 2 minutes until the soup thickens slightly.
6. Just before serving, whisk in the butter.

To finish

1. While the chowder is cooking, carefully remove the meat from the shell, checking for sand, and place in a clean pan.
2. Combine the chowder base and the cockle meat together, reheat carefully and serve.

65 Clams

To ensure freshness, the shells of clams should be tightly shut. They can be steamed or poached like mussels.

Clams should be soaked in salt water for a few hours so that the sand in which they exist can be ejected.

Clams can be prepared and served raw (certain types only) or cooked with lemon juice, au gratin (fresh breadcrumbs, chopped garlic, parsley, melted butter), in pasta, stir-fry and fish dishes as garnishes or/and a component of a sea food mixture, and as a soup (clam chowder).

66 Oysters

Oysters are most popular when freshly opened and eaten raw, together with their own natural juice, which should be retained carefully in the deep shell.

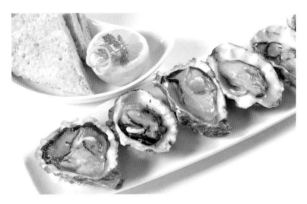

The shells should be tightly shut to indicate freshness.

The oysters should be opened carefully with a special oyster knife so as to avoid scratching the inside shell, then turned and arranged neatly in the deep shell and served on a bed of crushed ice on a plate.

They should not be washed unless gritty and the natural juices should always be left in the deep shell.

Accompaniments: brown bread and butter and lemon. It is usual to serve six oysters as a portion.

Oyster recipes

Oysters can also be cooked in a variety of ways. In all the following recipes they may be initially gently poached for a short time (10–15 seconds) in their own juice and the beards removed (overcooking will toughen them).

- Warm the shells, add a little cheese sauce, place two oysters in each shell, coat with sauce and grated cheese, glaze and serve.
- As previous recipe, dressing the oysters on a bed of leaf spinach.
- Serve on a bed of salt with chopped shallots and red wine vinegar.
- Place two oysters in each shell, coat with white wine sauce, glaze and serve.
- As previous recipe, using champagne in place of white wine.
- Place one oyster on each shell, add a few drops of lemon, barely cover with breadcrumbs lightly fried in butter and gratinate under the salamander or in a very hot oven.
- Pass the well-dried oysters through a light batter, or flour, egg and crumb, deep-fry and serve with quarters of lemon or lime.
- Oysters can also be mixed with any poached fish sauce together with other ingredients if required (e.g. a few lightly poached bean sprouts, button or wild mushrooms), and served in a bouchée, vol-au-vent, or any other shape of puff paste case – square, rectangular or diamond. They may then be served as a first course, fish course or main course, as required.

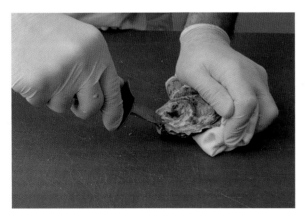

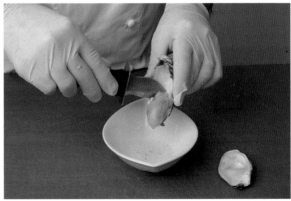

67 Oyster fricassée

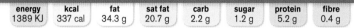

energy	kcal	fat	sat fat	carb	sugar	protein	fibre
1389 KJ	337 cal	34.3 g	20.7 g	2.2 g	1.2 g	5.2 g	0.4 g

	4 portions	10 portions
oysters, shelled and juice retained	24	40
cream	200 ml	500 ml
butter	30 g	75 g
wholegrain mustard	30 g	75 g
parsley, finely chopped	1 tsp	3 tsp
seasoning		
pinch cayenne		

1. Clean the oysters and retain on a clean tray in the refrigerator.

2. Heat the oyster liquor to boiling point, and strain through a double thickness of cheesecloth/muslin.
3. Add oysters to liquor and cook until plump, 1–2 minutes.
4. Remove oysters with a slotted/perforated spoon and place on a clean plate; cover with cling film.
5. Add the cream and butter to liquor and reduce to form a sauce consistency.
6. Add the wholegrain mustard (do not re-boil), seasoning and parsley.
7. Return the oysters to the sauce, gently heat through and serve immediately.

68 Caviar, oyster and vodka sauce

sour cream	150 ml
water	1 tbsp
caviar	50 g
lemon juice	4 g
cayenne pepper	pinch (⅛ tsp)
oyster jus	10 ml
Absolut lemon vodka	20 ml
To finish	
oscietra caviar	1 g
keta caviar	2 g

1. Place all the ingredients except the oyster jus, lemon juice and cayenne pepper into a thermo coupe.

2. Blitz for approximately 1 minute until thoroughly mixed.
3. Place into a suitable bowl.
4. Then add lemon juice, oyster jus and cayenne pepper to taste.
5. Place in a suitable container, cover with cling film and place in the fridge.
6. When required, place the sauce in a pan, warm and add the keta and oscietra caviar.

Lumpfish roe or finely diced cooked mushrooms may be used instead of caviar, to create variations on this recipe.

69 Seared scallop salad with honey-lime dressing

energy	kcal	fat	sat fat	carb	sugar	protein	fibre
829 KJ	198 cal	13.3 g	2.7 g	7.0 g	5.0 g	13.2 g	0.0 g

	4 portions	10 portions
Honey-lime dressing		
limes, juice of	2/3	5/6
honey, or to taste	25 g	60 g
white wine or rice vinegar	1 tbsp	2 tbsp
seasoning		
Seared scallops		
grapeseed or peanut oil	50 ml	125 ml
chopped mangetout, red pepper and courgette cut into thin strips	500 g	1250 g
mixed greens (such as pea shoots, watercress, baby spinach or escarole)	400 g	1 kg
large scallops (roe removed)	12	30

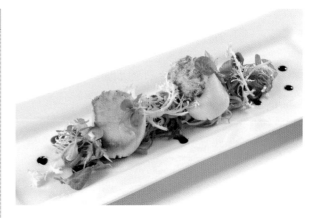

For the dressing

1. In a non-reactive bowl whisk together the lime juice, honey, vinegar and salt until the honey is completely incorporated. Taste and adjust accordingly. Set aside.

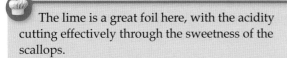

The lime is a great foil here, with the acidity cutting effectively through the sweetness of the scallops.

For the seared scallops

1. Heat oil in a large cast-iron or non-stick pan over medium-high heat.
2. Place the vegetable strips into pan and quickly sauté
3. Arrange on the plate and top with the salad leaves.
4. Clean the pan and add a little more butter, and sear the scallops very quickly until golden.

In this chapter you have learned to:

1. prepare fish and shellfish dishes
2. prepare associated products and garnishes.

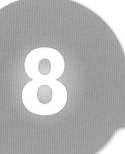

Fermented dough and batter products

This chapter covers Unit 308: Produce Fermented Dough and Batter Products.

In this unit, you will learn:

1. about the key commodities used in pastry and bakery work of all kinds

2. how to produce and finish fermented dough and batter products.

The first section of this chapter (pages 281–292) provides an introduction to bakery and pastry work of all kinds.

Preparation and materials

All baking times and temperatures stated are approximate, as a pastry cook learns through experience how raw materials bake differently in various types of oven. When using forced air convection ovens it is often necessary to reduce the stated temperatures in accordance with manufacturers' recommendations. Also, certain ovens produce severe bottom heat and to counteract this the use of double baking sheets (one sheet on top of another) is necessary.

Modern techniques and equipment

In the modern pastry department there are a variety of new techniques and equipment that can help the pastry cook to achieve better-quality products, improve presentation and reduce time. For example, there are a wide variety of commercial basic mixes, pastes and fonds, and the range of specialist small equipment increases all the time, especially the various types of moulds available, like florentine moulds (including the comb chocolate finish, dockers and trellis cutters) widely used in production.

Techniques are being developed all the time: the use of silicone paper has been revolutionary in baking. Many pastry chefs pin out pastry on a silicone-lined baking sheet, cutting the shape required then removing the excess paste. This gives a better shape with no chance of the paste sticking to the sheet.

The fundamental ingredients

Flour

Flour is one of the most important ingredients in patisserie, if not *the* most important.

There are a great variety of high-quality flours made from cereals, nuts or legumes, such as chestnut flour, cornflour, and so on. They have been used in patisserie, baking, dessert cuisine and savoury cuisine in all countries throughout history. The king of all of them is without doubt wheat flour.

The composition of wheat flour

Wheat flour is basically composed of starch, gluten, sugar, fats, water and minerals.

Starch is the main component of flour. Another important element is gluten, which is elastic and impermeable. Found mainly in wheat, this is what makes wheat flour the most common flour used in bread making.

The quantity of sugar in wheat is very small and it plays a very important role in fermentation. Wheat contains only a maximum of 16 per cent water, but its presence is important. The mineral matter (ash), which is found mainly in the husk of the wheat grain and not in the kernel, determines the purity and quality of the flour.

From the ear to the final product – flour – wheat goes through several distinct processes. These are carried out in modern industrial plants, where wheat is subjected to the various treatments and phases necessary for the production of different types of flour. These arrive in perfect condition to our workplaces and are made into preparations like sponge cakes, yeast dough, puff pastries, cookies and pastries.

What you need to know about flour

- Flour is a particularly delicate material, and it must be used and stored with special care. It must always be in the best condition, which is why storing large quantities is not recommended.
- It must be kept in a clean, dry, aerated storeroom.
- Warm and humid places must absolutely be avoided.

Types of flour in pastry work

- **White flour** is heavily milled and sieved to remove the outer skins and germ. It will store better without the germ, which contains fat and enzymes. About 70 per cent of the wheat is extracted to produce white flour. It is usually fortified by added calcium, iron, vitamin B1 and nicotinic acid.
- **Wholemeal flour** is the whole grain crushed into flour. (The bran is not digested by humans – this acts as roughage.) Stoneground flour is ground by stones, and is said to have a superior flavour.
- **Germ flour** (Hovis-type flour) is a mixture of 75 per cent white flour plus 25 per cent cooked germ. The germ is cooked to delay the onset of rancidity in the fat. Cooking gives a malted flavour.
- **Starch-reduced flour** is prepared for commercial products. Much of the starch is washed out, leaving the gluten and other proteins.
- **Self-raising flour** is white flour, usually of medium to soft strength, with the correct proportion of raising agent to give sufficient raising action for cake making.
- **High-ratio flour** is flour that has been finely milled in order that it is able to absorb more liquid and sugar.
- **Rye flour** is milled from rye, a grass grown as a grain. It is closely related to barley and wheat and is used to produce rye bread, including pumpernickel. Rye bread is a commonly eaten food in Northern and Eastern Europe. Rye flour has a lower gluten content than wheat flour and contains a higher proportion of soluble fibre.
- **Gluten-free flour** can be eaten by those with a gluten intolerance. Such people cannot consume foods containing wheat, barley or oats as they cause intestinal and other problems. Increased awareness of gluten sensitivity has led to the increase of grain products made with gluten-free flour. Rice flour is the most common ingredient in gluten-free pasta, bread and crackers. Many products are also made with soy flour, cornflour,

potato flour or buckwheat flour (note that buckwheat is not actually wheat). Other gluten-free flours include chickpea, fava bean and almond flours.

There are also these grades of flours:

- **Strong flours** are milled from a mixture of wheat, in which spring wheat predominates, and contains 10–16 per cent strong glutens used for bread, yeast doughs and puff pastry.
- **Medium general purpose flour** contains less strong and elastic gluten; it is used for plain cakes, scones and rich-yeast mixtures.
- **Soft flour (cake flour)** contains a small percentage of gluten to give a soft structure to a cake. Uses include sponge cakes and biscuits.

Eggs

The egg is one of the principal ingredients in cookery. Its great versatility and extraordinary properties as a thickener, emulsifier and stabiliser make its presence important in various creations in patisserie: sauces, creams, sponge cakes, custards and ice creams. Although it is not often the main ingredient, it plays specific and determining roles in terms of texture, taste and aroma, among other things. The egg is fundamental in preparations such as brioches, crèmes anglaise, sponge cakes and crèmes pâtissière. The extent to which eggs are used (or not) makes an enormous difference to the quality of the product.

A good custard cannot be made without eggs, for they cause the required coagulation and give it the desired consistency and finesse.

Eggs are also an important ingredient in ice cream, where their yolks act as an emulsifier thanks to the lecithin they contain, which aids the emulsion of fats.

What you need to know about eggs

- Eggs act as a texture agent in, for example, patisseries and ice creams.
- They intensify the aroma of pastries like brioche.
- They enhance flavours.
- They give volume to whisked sponges and batters.
- They strengthen the structure of preparations such as sponge cakes.
- They act as a thickening agent – in crème anglaise, for example.
- They act as an emulsifier in preparations such as mayonnaise and ice cream.
- They act as a stabiliser – in ice cream, for example.
- A fresh egg should have a small, shallow air pocket inside it.
- The yolks of fresh eggs should be bulbous, firm and bright.
- The fresher the egg, the larger the proportion of thick white to thin.
- Eggs should be stored far from strong odours as the shell is porous and the odours can be easily absorbed.
- In a whole 60 g egg, the yolk weighs about 20 g, the white 30 g and the shell 10 g.
- Eggs are available in four grades: small (48 g); medium (58 g); large (68 g); very large (76 g).

Eggs in pastry work

Egg albumen (protein) is soluble in cold liquid; it begins to coagulate immediately on application of heat, becoming opaque and firm. The degree of firmness depends on the degree of heat and length of cooking time. Egg yolk does not harden to the same extent or as quickly as the white, due to the high percentage of fat. If egg is overcooked or added too quickly to hot liquid, curdling will result.

- **Thickening.** The coagulation of protein on heating to 68°C is responsible for the thickening properties.
- **Lightening.** By means of whisking either egg white or whole egg, air is entangled and lightness given to a mixture. This enables eggs to:
  - act as a raising agent in cakes
  - produce light dishes, e.g. soufflés and meringues.
- **Glazing.** Beaten egg used as a glaze (eggwash).
- **Binding.** The coagulating properties of the egg will give cohesiveness to a mixture containing dry ingredients.
- **Emulsifying.** The lecithin contained in the yolk will assist in the emulsification (mixing) of products.
- **Coating.** Beaten egg forms a protective coating for foods.
- **Enriching.** The addition of whole eggs or yolks to a mixture is a means of adding protein and fat. Eggs improve nutritive value and flavour.

When beating egg whites to form a foam a little egg white powder may be added to strengthen the mixture.

Salt

Where salt is found

Salt (chemical name 'sodium chloride') is one of the most important ingredients. It is well known that salt is a necessary part of the human diet, present in small or large proportions in many natural foods. We generally associate it with seasoning of foods to improve their flavour, but it is also necessary in the making of many sweet dishes.

Characteristics and advantages of using salt in yeast dough

Salt can enhance flavour in savoury and some sweet products.

It is a good idea to add a pinch of salt to all sweet preparations, nougats, chocolate bonbons and cakes to intensify flavours.

Salt softens sugar and butter, activates the taste buds and enhances all aromas.

What you need to know about salt

- Salt gives us the possibility of many combinations. At times, these may seem normal (like a terrine of foie gras and coarse salt), others surprising (like praline with coarse salt).
- From a healthy-eating perspective chefs should take extra care when using excessive amounts of salt as over-consumption is a major cause of hypertension (high blood pressure).

Sea and rock salt

- Sea salt is obtained by the evaporation of seawater. Its mineral content gives it a different taste from table salt, which is pure sodium chloride, usually refined from mined rock salt (halite). Generally more expensive than table salt, it is commonly used in gourmet cooking due to its enhanced flavour.

Fats

Fats and oils are composed of fatty acids and glycerine. Fatty acids may be saturated or unsaturated.

- **Saturated fatty acids.** A saturated fat has each carbon atom in the fatty acids combined with two hydrogen atoms. Saturated fats are solid at room temperature and predominate in fats of animal origin, e.g. butter, cream, hard cheese, egg yolks, lard and suet. They are also present in hard margarines.

- **Unsaturated fatty acids**
  - (a) *Monounsaturated fatty acids*. These have an adjacent pair of carbon atoms, each with only one hydrogen atom attached, so they are capable of taking up more hydrogen atoms. Monounsaturated fats are soft at room temperature but will solidify when in the coolest part of the refrigerator. They are present in many animal and vegetable fats. Oleic acid, found in olive oil, is an example of a monounsaturated fatty acid.
  - (b) *Polyunsaturated fatty acids*. These have two or more pairs of carbon atoms, which are capable of taking up more hydrogen atoms. Polyunsaturated fats are very soft or oily at room temperature and will not solidify even in a refrigerator. They are present in soya bean, corn and sunflower seed oils.

Atom structures of monounsaturated and polyunsaturated fatty acids

- **Butter** is composed of the fat of milk, traces of curd (casein) and milk sugar lactose, water and mineral matter, which includes salt added to improve flavour and help preservation. A good butter improves the flavour of cakes, biscuits and pastry.
- **Lard** is derived from pig fat. Good lard is a pure white fat. It is a tough, plastic fat, with no creaming properties but excellent shortening properties.
- **Suet** is obtained from around the kidneys of beef cattle. It is a hard fat and cannot be rubbed into flour or creamed. It is added by chopping or shredding finely into the mixture. Suet is used to make suet pastry, which is usually steamed. Baking gives a hard, dry result. Commercial suet is purified fat that has been shredded and mixed with wheat or rice flour to stop the pieces of fat sticking together.
- **Vegetarian suet** is produced from fat such as

palm oil combined with rice flour. It resembles shredded beef suet and is used as a vegetarian substitute in recipes.

- **Vegetable fats and oils.** Soya beans, sunflower seeds, cotton seeds, groundnuts, sesame seeds, coconuts, palm kernels and olives all yield oils that are used in cooking fats and oils, margarine and creams.
- **Margarine**
  (a) *Cake margarine*. This is developed to have good creaming properties.
  (b) *Pastry margarine*. This is blended to produce a tough plastic margarine that has a fairly high melting point. It may contain a high percentage of stearin (a type of fat) or may be hydrogenated to harden it.
- **High-ratio fat** is hydrogenated edible oil, to which a quantity of a very pure and refined emulsifying agent has been added, e.g. glyceryl monostearate (GMS), although other emulsifiers may be used. By the use of such special fats, cakes can be made containing higher than normal quantities of liquid. Combining the use of this special type of emulsifying shortening with high-ratio flour, it is possible to successfully make cakes with abnormal percentages of both sugar and liquid; high-ratio cakes are so called because of their high percentages of sugar and liquid.
- **Compound fats and oils** are practically 100 per cent salt free and have no flavour. They are made by refining extracted vegetable oils. The blend of oils is hydrogenated to produce the consistency desired, processed by creaming and chilling, and then packed.

Creaming properties

Fats for some types of pastry work must cream well. To do this they must possess a 'plastic', waxy consistency and have a good flavour. Fats may be purchased that have had their chemistry altered so that they cream well. These are known as plasticised or pre-creamed fats.

Butter

An indispensable fat

Butter is the symbol of perfection in fats. It brings flowery smoothness, perfumes and aromas, and impeccable textures to our preparations. It is a point of reference for good gastronomy. Butter has a very long history, but its origin is unknown. Many books have been written about it, but we can only conclude that it was probably discovered by accident.

Butter is an emulsion – the perfect symbiosis of water and fat. It is composed of a minimum of 82 per cent fat, a maximum of 16 per cent water and 2 per cent dry extracts.

What you need to know about butter

- It is a very delicate ingredient that can quickly spoil if a series of basic rules are not followed in its use.
- It has the property of absorbing odours very easily. It should always be stored far from anything that produces strong odours and it should be kept well covered.
- It should not be kept beyond its sell-by-date.
- Good butter has a stable texture, pleasing taste, fresh odour, homogeneous colour and, most important, it must melt perfectly in your mouth.
- It enriches preparations like cookies, petits fours and cakes and keeps products like sponge cakes soft.
- Butter enhances flavour – as in brioches, for example.
- The melting point of butter is between 30°C and 35°C approximately.

In summary, butter brings many qualities for cookery processes.

Sweeteners

Chemical properties of sucrose (common sugar)

Common sugar, or sucrose, consists of carbon (C_{12}), hydrogen (H_{22}) and oxygen (O_{11}), and is composed of two bonded molecules (in equal parts): glucose and fructose.

Inverted sugar

Inverted sugar is, after sucrose, one of the most commonly used sugars, thanks to its properties. It is a molecularly equal mix of the products obtained in the hydrolysis of sucrose (fructose and glucose) and is made from the hydrolysis of sugar in the presence of an enzyme.

Inverted sugar syrup

This is a white, sticky paste and has no particular odour. It consists of no less than 62 per cent dry matter and more than 50 per cent inverted sugar. It is what we most frequently use. With equal proportions of dry matter and sucrose, its sweetening capacity is 25–30 per cent greater.

It melts at 35°C and cannot withstand more than 75°C, unless moisture (liquid) is added; otherwise, it loses its properties. It has a constant moisture percentage – that is, it has hygroscopic properties.

Liquid inverted sugar

This is a yellowish liquid with no less than 62 per cent dry matter. It contains more than 3 per cent inverted sugar, but less than 50 per cent.

Applications of inverted sugar

- It improves the aroma of products.
- It improves the texture of doughs.
- It prevents the dehydration of frozen products.
- It reduces or stops crystallisation.
- It is essential in ice cream making – it greatly improves its quality and lowers its freezing point.

Glucose

Glucose takes on various forms:

- the characteristics of a viscous syrup, called crystal glucose
- its natural state, in fruit and honey
- a dehydrated white paste (used mainly in the commercial food industry, but also used in our profession)
- 'dehydrated glucose' (atomised glucose) – a glucose syrup from which the water is evaporated; this is used in patisserie, but mainly in the commercial food industry.

Characteristics and properties of glucose syrup

- It is a transparent, viscous paste.
- It prevents the crystallisation of boiled sugars, jams and preserves.
- It delays the drying of a product.
- It adds plasticity and creaminess to ice cream and the fillings of chocolate bonbons.
- It prevents the crystallisation of ice cream.

Honey

Honey, a sweet composite that bees make with the nectar extracted from flowers, is without doubt the oldest known sugar. It has the property of lowering the freezing point of ice cream.

It can be used like inverted sugar, but it is important to take into account that honey, unlike inverted sugar, will give flavour to the preparation. Also, it is inadequate for preparations that require long storage, since honey re-crystallises after some time.

Isomalt

Isomalt sugar is a sweetener that is still little known in the patisserie world, but it has been used for some time. It has properties distinct from those of the sweeteners already mentioned. It is produced through the hydrolysis of sugar, followed by hydrogenation (the addition of hydrogen). Produced through these industrial processes, this sugar has been used for many years in large industries, in candy and chewing gum production, and is now earning a place in gastronomy.

One of its most notable characteristics is that it can melt without the addition of water or another liquid. This is a very interesting property for making artistic decorations in caramel. Its appearance is like that of confectioners' sugar: a glossy powder. Its sweetening strength is half that of sucrose and it is much less soluble than sugar, which means that it melts less easily in the mouth.

Isomalt's main claim in gastronomy over the past five or six years has been the replacement of normal sugar or sucrose when making sugar decorations, blown sugar, pulled sugar or spun sugar as the hydroscopic properties are lower than normal sugar, therefore it will be less affected by atmospheric variance.

Isomalt was originally developed for diabetics (it is twice as sweet as sucrose) but has the unfortunate side effect of being a laxative.

Milk

Milk is a basic and fundamental element of our diets throughout our lives. It is composed of water, sugar and a minimum of 3.5 per cent fat.

Whole milk

Natural whole milk is milk with nothing added or removed. *Whole standardised milk* is whole milk standardised to a minimum fat content of 3.5 per cent.

Semi-skimmed milk

Semi-skimmed milk is the most popular type of milk in the UK with a fat content of 1.7 per cent, compared to 4 per cent in whole milk and 0.3 per cent in skimmed milk.

Skimmed milk

Skimmed milk has a fat content of between 0.1 and 0.3 per cent. Skimmed milk therefore has nearly all the fat removed.

Milk is essential in a large number of preparations from ice creams, yeast doughs, mousses and custards to certain ganaches, cookies and muffins. Yeast dough will change considerably in texture, taste and colour if made with milk instead of water.

Milk has a lightly sweet taste and little odour. Two distinct processes are used to conserve it:

1 **pasteurisation** – the milk is heated to between 73°C and 85°C for a few seconds, then cooled quickly to 4°C

2 **sterilisation (UHT)** – the milk is heated to 140–150°C for 2 seconds, then cooled quickly. In this situation the sugar caramelises.

Milk is homogenised to evenly disperse the fat, since the fat has a tendency to rise to the surface (see 'Cream', below).

What you need to know about milk

- Pasteurised milk has better taste and aroma than UHT milk.
- Milk is a useful agent in the development of flavour in sauces and creams.
- Because of its lactic ferments, it facilitates the maturation of doughs and creams.
- There are other types of milk, such as sheep's/ewe's, goat's and rice milk. All are very interesting to use in dessert recipes.

Cream

Cream is another of the most frequently used dairy products. It is used in many recipes because of its high fat content and great versatility.

Cream is obtained from milk when it is left to sit. A film forms on the surface because of the difference in density between fat and liquid. This process is accelerated mechanically in large industries through heat and centrifuge.

There are two main methods for conserving cream:

1 **pasteurisation** – the cream is heated to 85–90°C for a few seconds and then cooled quickly; this cream retains all its flavour properties

2 **sterilisation (UHT)** – this consists of heating the cream to 140–150°C for 2 seconds; cream treated this way has a different flavour, but it keeps longer.

What you need to know about cream

- Cream whips with the addition of air, thanks to its fat content. This retains air bubbles formed during beating.
- Cream is an agent that adds texture.
- All cream, once boiled and cooled, can be whipped again with no problem.
- To whip cream well, it must be cold (around 4°C).
- Infusions with cream can be hot or cold. If cold, this requires an infusion time of at least 12 hours.
- The properties of creams are largely down to the fat content.
- There are many different types of cream, with varying consistencies and tastes.

Channel Island extra thick double cream

A rich, thick cream that is made with milk from Guernsey and Jersey cows, it can be used straight from the tub. It has a fat content of 48 per cent.

- **Uses:** spoon over puddings or fruit or add to sauces for a rich, creamy taste. Also ideal for using to fill sponge cakes or gâteaux.
- **To store:** keep in the fridge for up to 5 days, once opened use within 3 days and consume by the use-by-date.

Clotted cream

Clotted cream is the thickest and richest type of cream available and is traditionally made in Devon or Cornwall. The cream is gently scalded to produce its golden crust. It has a spoonable consistency and does not need to be whipped before serving. It has a fat content of 55 per cent and is not recommended for cooking because it tends to separate on heating.

- **Uses:** traditionally served on scones with jam, also good on fresh fruit and ice cream.
- **To store:** keep in the fridge for up to 2 weeks and consume by the use-by-date. It can be frozen for up to 1 month.

Crème fraîche

This is fresh cream which is treated with a bacteria culture that thickens it and gives it a slightly sour taste. It is suitable for spooning, is widely used in French cookery and is becoming increasingly popular in Britain. It has a fat content of 39 per cent and cannot be whipped. For a healthier alternative choose the half-fat version.

- **Uses:** crème fraîche is ideal for serving with fruit and puddings. It can also be used for making salad dressings and dips. It can be used in cooking to add a creamy taste to curries, sauces and casseroles.

- **To store:** keep in the fridge for up to 5 days, once opened use within 3 days and consume by the use-by-date. It cannot be frozen.

Double cream

This is the most versatile type of fresh cream, it can be used as it is or whipped. Double cream contains 48 per cent fat.

- **Uses:** it can be used as a pouring cream over fruit and puddings, used in cooking or whipped and incorporated into dishes or served separately. Whipped double cream can be spooned or piped on to desserts and cakes.
- **To store:** keep in the fridge for up to 5 days, once opened use within 3 days and consume by the use-by-date. It can be frozen for up to 2 months when lightly whipped.

Extra thick single cream

This has the same fat content as single cream (18 per cent) but it has been homogenised to produce a thick spoonable consistency similar to double cream: it cannot be whipped.

- **Uses:** serve with fruit and desserts.
- **To store:** keep in the fridge for up to 5 days, once opened use within 3 days and consume by the use-by-date. It is unsuitable for freezing.

Flavoured creams

Available at Christmas, brandy cream and Calvados and cinnamon cream are made from a combination of double cream, sugar and alcohol.

- **Uses:** serve with Christmas pudding, apple tart or any chocolate or nut pudding. Spoon over warm mince pies or use to fill brandy snaps. A spoonful of flavoured cream in hot chocolate is delicious.
- **To store:** keep in the fridge and consume by the use-by-date. Once opened use within 3 days.

Goat's milk double cream

Made from pasteurised goat's milk from St Helen's Farm in Yorkshire, goat's milk double cream has an ice white appearance and tastes smooth and mild. Goat's milk double cream is suitable for cow's milk-free and vegetarian diets.

- **Uses:** it can be used for whipping, pouring or simply spooning on to desserts.
- **To store:** keep in the fridge for up to 5 days, once opened use within 3 days and consume by the use-by-date. It can be frozen for up to 2 months when lightly whipped.

Organic extra thick cream

Organic thick cream is made from milk produced on farms practising organic farming methods to Soil Association standards.

- **Uses:** spoon on to fruit, puddings and cakes or add to soups and sauces for a rich creamy taste.
- **To store:** keep in the fridge for up to 5 days, once opened use within 3 days and consume by the use-by-date. It is unsuitable for freezing.

Reduced fat extra thick cream

With 50 per cent less fat than standard thick double cream but all the delicious flavour, this cream contains 24 per cent fat. It is not suitable for whipping or boiling.

- **Uses:** serve with fruit or puddings or use in cooking for a rich, creamy flavour.
- **To store:** keep in the fridge for up to 5 days, once opened use within 3 days and consume by the use-by-date. It is unsuitable for freezing.

Reduced fat single cream

With 25 per cent less fat than standard single cream (it has 12 per cent fat) this is an ideal low fat alternative. It is not suitable for whipping or boiling.

- **Uses:** in sauces, soups and dressings and coffee and to pour over fruit.
- **To store:** keep in the fridge for up to 5 days, once opened use within 3 days and consume by the use-by-date. It is unsuitable for freezing.

Single cream

Single cream is a thin cream traditionally used for pouring and for enriching cooked dishes. It contains 18 per cent fat.

- **Uses:** for pouring over fruit and puddings and in cooking, especially in soups and sauces although it should never be allowed to boil. It is not suitable for whipping.
- **To store:** keep in the fridge for up to 5 days, once opened use within 3 days and consume by the use-by-date. It cannot be frozen unless it is incorporated into a cooked dish.

Soured cream

This is a tangy cream made from fresh single cream. It has a thick texture and a mildly acidic taste. It is commercially soured by adding a culture – similar to that used in the production of yogurt. It has a fat content of 18 per cent and cannot be whipped.

- **Uses:** it can be used in savoury dishes such as

beef stroganoff and soups and as a base for savoury dips.

- **To store:** keep in the fridge for up to 5 days, once opened use within 3 days and consume by the use-by-date. It cannot be frozen.

Whipping cream

This cream will whip to double its original volume, which makes it perfect for adding to dishes where a light, creamy result is needed. Whipping cream contains 38 per cent fat.

- **Uses:** perfect for mousses and soufflés, filling cakes and gâteaux, decorating trifles and topping fruit and ice cream. Float whipped cream on coffee or hot chocolate. Once whipped the cream does not hold its volume for long so it should be used straight away.
- **To store:** keep in the fridge for up to 5 days, once opened use within 3 days and consume by the use-by-date. Whipping cream can be frozen for up to 2 months when lightly whipped.

Fruit
Quality requirements of fruit

Fresh fruit used for desserts and in pastry work should be:

- Whole and of fresh appearance. For maximum flavour the fruit must be ripe but not overripe.
- Firm, according to the type and variety.
- Clean, to remove traces of pesticides and fungicides, by washing before use.
- Free from external moisture.
- Free from any unpleasant smell or taste.
- Free from pests or disease.
- Sufficiently mature. It must be capable of being handled and travelling without damage.
- Preferably free of any defects characteristic of the variety in shape, size and colour if using for final presentation (e.g. a poached peach), although there is much promotion supporting the ethics of using second and third class fruits (e.g. misshapen but retaining all other qualities).
- Free of bruising or damage.

Working with dough

Why does dough ferment?

In order to understand why yeast dough rises, we must note that the main ingredients of natural leavening are water, air and, most importantly, sugar, which is transformed into carbon dioxide and causes the leavening. This carbon dioxide forms bubbles inside the dough and makes it rise. Fermentation is a transformation undergone by organic matter (sugars).

Yeast goods

Yeast is a living organism – it is a plant of the fungi group. Yeast produces the gas carbon dioxide by fermentation. This occurs when it is given food in the form of sugar, warmth (25–29°C) and moisture, water or milk.

Types of yeast

- **Compressed/fresh yeast** is the most widely used. It is a very pure form of yeast packed and sold in cakes. It crumbles easily and will keep in a cold place for 2–3 days. Fresh yeast has a characteristic smell, is a putty colour and will cream readily.
- **Dried yeast** can be stored indefinitely if kept dry

and well sealed. It takes longer to cream and is more concentrated.

Conditions for the fermentation of yeast

Yeast requires food, warmth and moisture. Yeast is destroyed at temperatures higher than those given above, and its activity is retarded at lower temperatures. Yeast can be destroyed during the mixing or rising processes if it is put in a very hot place.

Flying starter/Polish

This is a method where some of the flour from the recipe is removed (approximately 30 per cent) and mixed with the liquids from the bread recipe a couple of hours before you make the dough.

The time span of 2 hours is the absolute maximum – obviously, this is temperature dependent – but the main principle for adopting this method is that a good proportion of the flour has already been fermented and ripened.

It also prevents what bakers term 'green dough'. This is when the bread loaf or roll sits very flat and a cross-section is almost a semi-circle with a very flat edge. A good, well-fermented dough, when sliced, will yield a very thin foot that the roll loaf will sit on and offer almost a full circle when sliced laterally – the approximate percentage of loaf roll to sit on the floor of the deck oven is between 5 and 10 per cent, and not 30 per cent as in some cases when a green dough occurs.

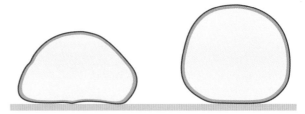

The shape of a loaf made with a green dough (left) and one made with a well-fermented dough (right)

Advanced methods of dough production

There are several advanced methods of dough production that are used in the bakery industry and to a much lesser extent in the hospitality industry. These are:

- the bulk fermentation process
- the mechanical dough development process
- the activated dough development process
- the sponge and dough process.

The bulk fermentation process

This process was used before the introduction of high speed mixing and dough conditioners which both eliminate the need for bulk fermentation time. Some bakers still prefer this bread making process because of the fine flavour produced during fermentation and evident in the final product. Hotels and restaurants producing bread products for their menus probably still use this method.

Basic principles of the method

1. Sieve together the dry ingredients.
2. Add the fat content and rub through the dry ingredients.
3. Disperse the yeast into tempered water and add to the above ingredients.
4. Form a dough.
5. Check consistency.
6. Mix until a smooth clear dough is obtained and the gluten-forming proteins are developed.
7. Cover the dough and keep warm during the bulk fermentation time.

Bulk fermentation time (BFT)

This term is used to describe the length of time that the dough is allowed to ferment in bulk and can be from one to six hours, during which time the dough is kept covered to prevent 'skinning' and the temperature is monitored to control the rate of fermentation.

Changes that occur during fermentation

1. The yeast produces large quantities of carbon dioxide and a small amount of alcohol.
2. Action by enzymes ripens the gluten-forming proteins.
3. The gluten-forming proteins become extensible and develop the ability to retain carbon dioxide.
4. The ripening process of the gluten produces flavour.

Advantages of bulk fermentation

1. The mixing is completed in one operation with no need for special machinery.
2. The dough has a greater tolerance of fermentation.
3. The baked product has a finer flavour.

Disadvantages of bulk fermentation

1. Expensive flours are required.
2. Fermentation and production time is increased and needs more attention.
3. The fermenting dough requires space.
4. It may be necessary to start production early.

The mechanical dough development process

This process revolutionised the bakery and bread industry. The process relies on the use of ascorbic acid being used along with increased water and high energy. Using this process the dough only needs to be mixed once (no BFT, knocking back or second proving needed). The process is mostly used in bakeries and large-scale production of bread and other dough products.

Basic principles of the method

1. Place the ingredients into the mixing chamber in the following order:
   - cold water
   - dry ingredients
   - fat and yeast.
2. Mix to the required energy input.
3. The dough is now ready to be scaled and processed.

Advantages of mechanical dough development

1. The mixing time is considerably reduced from up to 20 minutes to 3–4 minutes and the bulk fermentation period is eliminated which:
   - saves production time
   - removes the need for fermentation space
   - saves labour time allowing for better organisation of workload and working hours.
2. An increased yield and consistent results are obtained because of:
   - the increased water level
   - reduced fermentation losses.

Disadvantages of mechanical dough development

1. A special high speed mixer is required for this process.
2. Costs are increased because of the need to add ascorbic acid.
3. There is some loss in the flavour due to shorter fermentation period.

The activated dough development process (ADD)

This is another process where no bulk fermentation is needed, instead dough conditioners are used to give the required results. ADD does not need special mixing machines; the mixing machines frequently available in kitchen areas are sufficient. This means that a kitchen wanting to produce dough products can do so more quickly and use less space than is needed for bulk fermentation methods.

It may also be used in large scale production and bakeries.

Basic principles of the method

1. Sieve together the dry ingredients including the dough conditioner.
2. Add the fat content and rub through the dry ingredients.
3. Disperse the yeast into tempered water and add to the above ingredients.
4. Form a dough, check consistency.
5. Mix until a smooth and clear dough is obtained and the gluten-forming proteins are fully developed.
6. The dough is now ready to be scaled and processed.

Advantages of the activated dough development process

These are similar to those listed for mechanical dough development but with the added advantage that no specialist machinery is needed.

Disadvantages of the activated dough development process

These are also similar to those listed for mechanical dough development but the addition of dough conditioners is an added expense.

The sponge and dough process

This is a two-stage process which has been used for many years to produce bread and fermented products and also eliminates the need for dough conditioners.

It is possible to add the sponge to many bread and fermented products. It can also be added to dough which is made using the mechanical dough development process, or the activated dough development process.

The sponge

A sponge is a basic dough made from the four main ingredients; flour, salt, yeast and water. The sponge is then allowed to ferment for 12–16 hours in bulk, and the rate of fermentation is controlled by:
- the level of yeast
- the level of salt
- the water temperature and final dough temperature
- the use of strong bread flour to sustain the long fermentation period.

Basic principles of the method

Stage one – the sponge

1. Sieve together the dry ingredients.
2. Disperse the yeast into tempered water and add to the dry ingredients.
3. Form a dough, check consistency.
4. Mix until a smooth, clear dough is obtained and gluten-forming proteins are fully developed.
5. Cover the dough and maintain the dough temperature.
6. After completion of the fermentation time, the sponge is ready to be added to the freshly made dough.

Stage two – the dough

1. Mix all of the ingredients together for 2 minutes and form a dough.
2. Break the sponge into pieces and add them to the dough.
3. Mix until a smooth and clear dough is obtained and the gluten-forming proteins are fully developed.
4. Cover the dough and keep warm during the BFT.
5. The dough is now ready to be scaled and processed.

Advantages of the sponge and dough process

1. There is no need for a special mixing machine.
2. There is no need to use a dough conditioner at the dough stage.
3. The BFT is significantly reduced after the dough stage.
4. The addition of sponge gives a better flavour and improved crumb structure.

Disadvantages of the sponge and dough process

1. Extra time and planning of production is required as the sponge must be made the day before and will need allocated space.
2. The sponge requires more attention by staff – for example, temperature control.

These advanced methods of dough production are adapted from P Connelly and M Pittam, *Practical Bakery* (Hodder Arnold, 1997).

1 Baguette

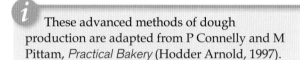

Dough starter	Makes 6–8
fresh yeast	5g
cold water	135ml
strong white bread flour, preferably organic	100g
rye flour	100g
Dough	
water	680ml
traditional white bread flour, preferably organic, plus extra for dusting	1.7kg
fine sea salt	15g
fresh yeast	22g

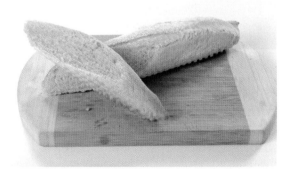

1. For the dough starter, whisk the yeast into the water until dispersed.
2. Mix the white and rye flours in a separate bowl until well combined.
3. Pour the yeast mixture over the flours, whisking well to form a thick paste. Cover the bowl with a damp tea towel and set aside to ferment for at least 6 hours.
4. For the dough, line two large baking sheets with greaseproof paper.
5. Add the water to the fermented dough starter and mix well to combine.

6. Place the flour into a mixing machine, set with the dough hook. Add the salt to one side of the bowl of the food processor, then add the yeast to the other side, being careful not to let the salt and yeast touch at this stage as the salt will attack the yeast and damage its ability to ferment.

7. Add the starter dough mixture to the mixing machine and mix on a low speed for 5 minutes. The slow mixing process will give the flour the opportunity to fully absorb the water.

8. Scrape the dough from the sides of the bowl of the food processor and from the dough hook, then continue to mix on a medium speed for a further 5–7 minutes, or until the dough is smooth and elastic. The faster speed will warm the gluten in the flour making the dough elastic and creating the right environment for the fermentation to happen.

9. Prove until doubled in size.

10. Scale into a 350g piece roll as required. Prove until doubled. Score with a sharp knife.

11. Bake with steam at 250°C for 20 minute. Tap at the bottom – if it sounds hollow it is cooked.

> To bake with steam, use a combination oven with steam *or* place a bowl or tray of water in a conventional oven during baking.

2 Ciabatta

	Makes 4 rolls
Dough starter (sour)	
water	180g
strong flour	350g
fresh yeast	½tsp
Dough	
strong flour	450g
yeast	10g
water	340g
salt	20g
extra virgin olive oil	50g
coarse semolina, for dusting	

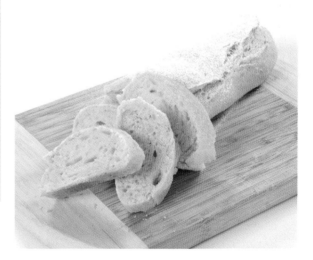

1. To make the starter, mix the ingredients by hand into a rough dough. Cover with cling film and leave for 17 to 24 hours. Continue with the rest of the dough recipe after this time.

2. Place the flour in a mixing bowl. Rub in the yeast.

3. Add the starter dough, water, salt and oil. Mix well until the ingredients are combined.

4. Mix in a mixing machine on low speed for 2–5 minutes.

5. Place in an oiled bowl and rest for 1 hour.

6. Knock back the dough on a floured surface. Divide it into 4 pieces shaped like slippers.

7. Dust the baking sheets with coarse semolina. Place the 4 ciabattas on the baking sheets, brush with water and sprinkle with more semolina.

8. Prove for approximately 30 minutes.

9. Bake at 230°C for 18 to 20 minutes.

3 Focaccia

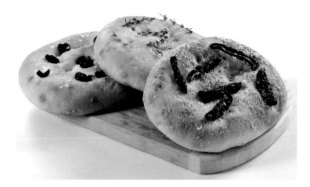

	Makes 4 loaves
Sponge batter	
fresh yeast	40 g
warm water	180 ml
sugar	15 g
strong flour	225 g
Focaccia dough	
strong flour	855 g
sugar	30 g
salt	20 g
warm water, at 40°C	480 ml
olive oil	180 ml
garnish (see below)	
Salamoia	
water, at 20°C	260 g
extra virgin olive oil	260 g
salt	50 g

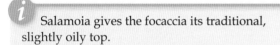
i Salamoia gives the focaccia its traditional, slightly oily top.

1. To make the sponge batter, disperse the yeast in the water. Add the sugar and flour. Mix well, cover and leave to ferment.
2. For the dough, sieve together the flour, sugar and salt. Add this mixture and the warm water to the fermented sponge batter.
3. Start to mix in a mixing machine. Feed in the olive oil while mixing.
4. Knead to a smooth dough.
5. Prove until the dough has doubled in size.
6. Brush a baking sheet with oil. Place the dough on the sheet. Push it out and push dimples into it with your fingers.

7. Brush with olive oil and sprinkle with a garnish (see below).
8. Prove until the dough has doubled in size.
9. Bake at 220°C for approximately 20 minutes.
10. To make the salamoia, whisk all the ingredients together so that they emulsify and the colour changes to light green.
11. Brush the focaccia with the salamoia as soon as it is removed from the oven.

Whisk the salamoia well immediately before use, so that the salt is dispersed throughout.

Garnishes

Possible garnishes for focaccia include:

- rosemary and rock salt
- olives and sunblush tomatoes
- garlic jam
- aromatic tomato paste
- pesto.

4 Tomato and basil rolls

	Makes 35 rolls
strong flour	1 kg
yeast	30 g
water, at 37°C	300 ml
milk powder	22 g
salt	20 g
caster sugar	10 g
sunflower oil	50 g
tomato juice	300 ml
sun-dried tomatoes, finely chopped	75 g
dried basil	1 tsp
eggwash	

1. Sieve the flour onto paper.
2. Disperse the yeast in the water.
3. Mix the milk powder, salt, sugar and oil into the tomato juice.
4. Place the flour in the mixing bowl. Add both the liquids at once.
5. Mix on a slow speed in a food processor for 5 minutes, until a smooth dough forms.
6. Cover with cling film and bulk ferment for 1 hour.
7. Knock back the dough.
8. Add the tomatoes and basil to the dough.
9. Divide the dough into rolls. Place on a silicone-lined baking sheet in neatly spaced, staggered rows.
10. Prove until the dough doubles in size.
11. Egg wash the rolls carefully. Bake at 243°C for 8 to 10 minutes with steam.

5 Walnut and olive rolls

	Makes 35 rolls
strong flour	1 kg
yeast	30 g
water, at 37°C	600 ml
milk powder	22 g
salt	20 g
caster sugar	10 g
olive oil	50 g
walnuts, chopped	50 g
olives, sliced	50 g
eggwash	

1. Sieve the flour onto paper.
2. Dissolve the yeast in half of the water.
3. Mix the milk powder, salt, sugar and oil into the other half of the water.
4. Place the flour in the mixing bowl. Add both the liquids at once.
5. Mix on a slow speed for 5 minutes in a food processor, until a smooth dough forms.
6. Cover with cling film and bulk ferment for 1 hour.
7. Knock back the dough.
8. Add the chopped walnuts and sliced olives to the dough.
9. Divide the dough into rolls. Place on a silicone-lined baking sheet in neatly spaced, staggered rows.
10. Prove until the dough doubles in size.
11. Egg wash the rolls carefully. Bake at 243°C for 8 to 10 minutes with steam.

6 Pain de campagne

	Makes 2 loaves
Dough starter	
strong flour	400 g
dark rye flour	100 g
yeast	10 g
water	350 g
salt	10 g
Pain de campagne	
starter dough	half of the batch
strong flour	500 g
dark rye flour	100 g
yeast	5 g
water	400 ml
salt	15 g

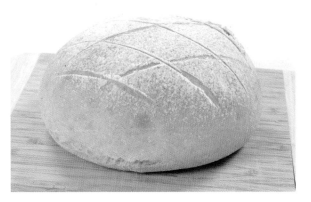

1. To make the starter dough, mix the two flours together and rub in the yeast. Add the water and salt and mix until smooth. Place in a bowl, cover and refrigerate overnight.
2. Take out half of the batch of starter dough and bring to room temperature.
3. Add the flours and yeast to the starter and rub in.
4. Add the water and mix to a dough.
5. Add the salt and mix for 7 minutes in a food mixer with a dough hook.
6. Allow to ferment for 1 hour.
7. Knock back the dough and shape into 2 round loaves.
8. Dust the tops with flour. Prove until the loaves have doubled in size.
9. Bake at 220°C for approximately 30 minutes.

 Pumpernickel is a traditional German rye bread which also uses rye flour.

7 Rye bread

	Makes 1 medium-sized loaf
fresh yeast (or dried yeast may be used)	15 g
water, at 37°C	60 ml (4 tbsp)
black treacle	15 ml (1 tbsp)
vegetable oil	15 ml (1 tbsp)
caraway seeds (optional)	15 g
salt	15 g
lager	250 ml
rye flour	250 g
unbleached bread flour	175 g
polenta	1 tbsp
eggwash	

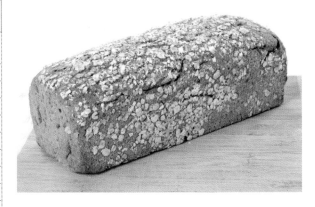

1. Disperse the yeast in the warm water.
2. In a bowl mix the black treacle, oil, two-thirds of the caraway seeds (if required) and the salt. Add the lager. Add the yeast mixture and mix in the sieved rye flour. Mix well.
3. Gradually add the bread flour. Continue to add the flour until the dough is formed and it is soft and slightly sticky.

4. Turn the dough onto a lightly floured surface and knead well.

5. Knead the dough until it is smooth and elastic.

6. Place the kneaded dough into a suitable bowl that has been brushed with oil.

7. Cover with a damp cloth and allow the dough to prove in a warm place until it has doubled in size. This will take about 1½–2 hours.

8. Turn the dough onto a lightly floured work surface, knock back the dough to original size. Cover and allow to rest for approximately 5–10 minutes.

9. Shape the dough into an oval approximately 25 cm long.

10. Place onto a baking sheet lightly sprinkled with polenta.

11. Allow the dough to prove in a warm place, preferably in a prover, until double in size (approximately 45 minutes to 1 hour).

12. Lightly brush the loaf with eggwash, sprinkle with the remaining caraway seeds (if required).

13. Using a small, sharp knife, make three diagonal slashes, approximately 5 mm deep, into the top of the loaf.

14. Bake at 190°C for approximately 50–55 minutes.

15. When cooked, turn out. The bread should sound hollow when tapped and the sides should feel crisp.

> Only a little salt is necessary to 'control' the yeast. Many people will prefer less salty bread.

8   Wholemeal and black treacle soda bread

	Makes 1 loaf
strong white flour	330 g
wholemeal flour	330 g
baking powder	15 g
bicarbonate of soda	15 g
salt	15 g
black treacle	2¼ tbsp
buttermilk	300 ml
vegetable oil	75 ml
water	225 ml

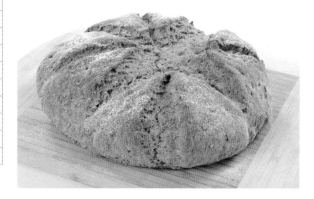

1. Sieve all the dry ingredients together.

2. Mix together the treacle, buttermilk and oil.

3. Make a well in the dry mixture and add the treacle mixture and the water.

4. Mix lightly to a scone consistency – the mixture should feel tacky.

5. Shape into a round loaf. Cut a cross in the top and dust with flour.

6. Place in an oven preheated to 220°C. Reduce the heat to 180°C and bake for about 25 minutes.

9 *Brioche à tête*

	Makes 20, or 2 loaves
strong flour	500 g
fresh yeast	15 g
warm milk	70 ml
eggs	4
salt	15 g
sugar	30 g
butter, softened	250 g
eggwash	

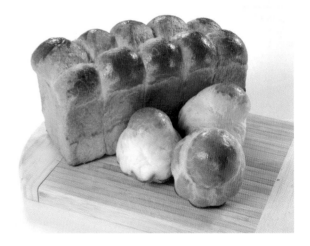

1. Sieve the flour and place it into a mixing machine with a dough hook.
2. Dissolve the yeast in the warm milk.
3. Beat together the eggs, salt and sugar.
4. Add the yeast and egg mixtures to the flour and mix on a slow speed with a hook attachment. Mix to a smooth dough (this will take about 5 minutes).
5. Stop the machine and change to a beater attachment. Mix on a slow speed while adding the butter in small pieces. As the dough softens, increase the speed.
6. Once all the butter has been added, continue mixing for at least five minutes, until the dough is smooth, glossy and elastic.
7. Cover and rest at room temperature for 30 minutes.
8. Brush the moulds with soft (**not** melted) butter.
9. Turn out the dough onto a lightly floured surface. Knead until smooth.
10. Divide into 50 g pieces and cover with cling film.
11. Uncover one piece at a time, place it into a mould and lightly egg wash the top.
12. Prove until the dough reaches the top of each mould (approximately doubled in size).
13. Bake at 220°C for 10–12 minutes.
14. Remove from the moulds immediately after baking and place on a wire rack to cool.

i *Brioche à tête* is prepared in small, moulded rolls. Brioche may also be made in large loaves (brioche Nanterre).

Different brioche recipes use a different proportion of butter to flour. In this recipe there is 50 per cent as much butter. To make brioche commune, use 25 per cent; for brioche mousseline, 75 per cent; for brioche surfine, 100 per cent, i.e. the same amount of butter as of flour.

10 **Panettone**

	Makes 1 cake
strong flour	400 g
salt	½ tsp
yeast	15 g
warm milk, at 37°C	120 ml
eggs	2
pasteurised egg yolk	40 g
caster sugar	75 g
butter, softened	150 g
mixed peel	115 g
raisins	75 g
eggwash and nibbed sugar to glaze	

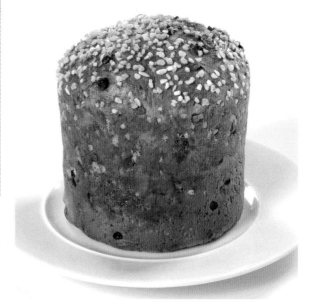

1. Use a cake tin approx. 18 cm in diameter. Line your tin using a double layer of greaseproof paper, making sure the paper comes about 7 cm above the top of the cake tin.
2. Sieve the flour and salt together into a bowl and make a well in the centre.
3. Mix the yeast and warm milk and pour into the centre of the flour, add the whole eggs and mix.
4. Add the egg yolks and sugar and work in the softened butter. Allow to prove.
5. Mix in the peel and raisins, place into the prepared tin, egg wash and sprinkle with nibbed sugar. Allow to double in size.
6. Bake in a preheated oven at 190°C for 20 minutes turning down to 170–180°C for a further 25–30 minutes.
7. Allow to cool in the tin for ten minutes and then place onto a wire rack to cool.

 This is an Italian cake served at Christmas.

11 Savarin paste

energy	kcal	fat	sat fat	carb	sugar	protein	fibre
700 KJ	167 cal	7.4 g	3.9 g	21.5 g	2.5 g	4.9 g	0.8 g

*

	8 portions	20 portions
strong flour	200 g	500 g
yeast	5 g	12 g
warm milk	125 ml	300 ml
eggs	2	5
butter, softened	50 g	125 g
sugar	10 g	25 g
salt	pinch	large pinch
savarin syrup (see below)		
apricot glaze		

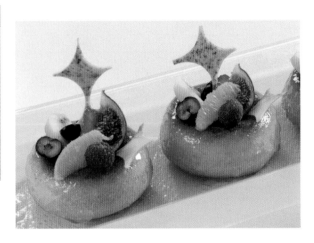

1. Sieve the flour in a bowl and warm.
2. Cream the yeast with a little of the warm milk in a bowl.
3. Make a well in the centre of the flour and add the dissolved yeast.
4. Sprinkle with a little of the flour from the sides, cover with a cloth and leave in a warm place until it ferments.
5. Add the remainder of the warm milk and the beaten eggs, remove from the bowl and knead well to a smooth elastic dough.
6. Put back in the bowl, add the butter in small pieces, cover with a cloth and allow to prove in a warm place.
7. Add the sugar and salt, mix well until absorbed.
8. Half fill a greased savarin mould or individual moulds, and prove.
9. Bake at 220°C for about 30 minutes.
10. Turn out when cooked, cool slightly.
11. Soak carefully in hot syrup (see recipe below).
12. Brush over with apricot glaze.

Syrup for savarin

	4 babas	10 babas
sugar	100 g	250 g
bay leaf	1	2–3
rind and juice of lemon	1	2–3
water	¼ litre	600 ml
coriander seeds	2–3	6–7
small cinnamon stick	½	1–1½

1. Boil all the ingredients together and strain.
2. Use as required.

* Using syrup, 1 portion of complete savarin provides: 967 kJ/229 kcal energy; 7.4 g fat; 3.9 g sat. fat; 38.2 g carbohydrate; 19.1 g sugar; 5.0 g protein; 0.8 g fibre.

12 Blinis

	Makes approx. 15
buckwheat flour	225 g
plain flour	225 g
salt	
eggs	3
fresh yeast	45 g
sugar	10 ml/2 tsp
warm milk	720 ml
butter, melted	1 tbsp

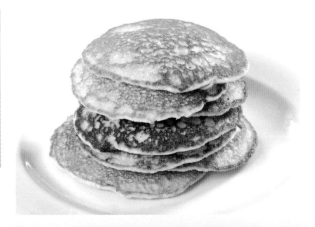

1. Sift the flours into a bowl and add the salt.
2. Make a well in the centre and drop in 2 whole eggs and 1 egg yolk.
3. Cream the yeast with the sugar and add the milk. Mix well.
4. Pour the yeast mix gradually into the flours and mix to a smooth batter. Add the melted butter.
5. Cover with a sheet of greased cling film or a cloth and leave in a warm place for 1 hour.
6. Just before cooking, whisk the remaining egg white and fold it into the mixture.

7. Grease a heavy frying pan lightly with oil. Heat it gently over a steady heat. When the frying pan is hot, pour enough of the batter on to the surface to make blinis 5 cm in diameter. When bubbles rise, turn the blinis over and cook the other side to a light brown.
8. Keep the blinis warm in a cool oven between sheets of greaseproof paper.

13 Crumpets

	Makes 10 to 12
strong white flour	125 g
caster sugar	15 g (2 tsp)
fresh yeast, crumbled	7 g (1 tsp)
fine sea salt	3 g (½ tsp)
warm water, at 32°C	50 g
lukewarm milk	100 g
bicarbonate of soda, dissolved in 1 tsp boiling water	5 g (¾ tsp)

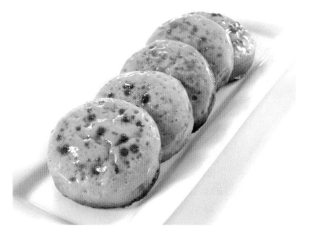

1. Combine the flour, sugar, yeast, salt, water and milk in a bowl and beat together with a spoon to make a very smooth batter. Leave in a warm place for 45 minutes or until the batter has begun to bubble.
2. Lightly grease a large heavy-based frying pan or griddle. If you have 8–10 cm diameter metal rings, grease these too and place them on the pan to heat. When both pan and rings are smoking hot, reduce the heat and place a heat diffusing pad under the pan (or turn the heat very low). Leave for a minute to cool down slightly.
3. Pour the batter into a jug and stir in the dissolved bicarbonate of soda, stirring well to make sure that it is evenly combined. Pour a little of the batter into each of the rings to a depth of 1 cm. If not using rings, pour the batter directly onto the hot pan in discs of 8–10 cm in diameter.
4. Leave the crumpets to cook for 3 minutes, or until the surface is full of holes and the batter almost set. Flip the crumpets over and cook on

the other side until lightly coloured. (This is when you can tell if the heat is right – the bottom of the crumpets should be dark brown but not burnt; if burnt then reduce the heat.)

5. The crumpets may pop out of the rings on their own. If they do not, run a sharp knife around the inside of the rings to loosen them. Place the cooked crumpets on a wire rack to cool, then oil the rings once more and put back on the pan to heat. When the rings are hot, make another batch of crumpets.

To make crumpets that stand tall, use greased metal rings (like egg rings). If you do not have rings, just pour the batter directly onto the griddle. They will be thinner but just as good.

9 Petits fours

This chapter covers Unit 309: Produce Petits Fours.

In this unit, you will learn to:

1. produce and finish petits fours
2. produce sugar and chocolate décor.

For information about the key commodities used in many of these dishes, refer to Chapter 8.

Chocolate

Chocolate is produced from the cocoa bean with the addition of sugar and sometimes milk and other flavourings.

Chocolate must be treated with great care. If chocolate is overheated it will taste strong and burnt. Water will change the characteristics of chocolate, caus-ing it to thicken, and affecting the texture, taste and appearance.

Main characteristics of the cacao tree and its fruit (cocoa beans):

- The majority of the world's cacao trees are concentrated around the equator.

- The cacao tree needs a hot, humid and rainy climate – the tropics are ideal for it.
- High levels of wind and sun can be damaging to the cacao tree and it must be protected from both.
- A productive tree can measure between 5 and 10 m in height, depending on its age.
- The fruit, or 'cocoa pod', measures between 15 and 30 cm.
- Each cocoa pod holds approximately 30–40 seeds (cocoa beans).

What you need to know about cocoa

- **Cocoa bean:** once called 'cocoa almond' or 'cocoa grain', this is the seed that is found in the pods of cacao trees. After being treated, it is packed and sent to be sold on the international market. It is from this bean that cocoa butter, chocolate liquor, cocoa powder and cocoa nibs are extracted.
- **Cocoa nibs:** these are roasted, shelled cocoa beans broken into small pieces. This is a very interesting product with an intense flavour – 100 per cent cocoa. It gives aroma, flavour and texture to many preparations, like sponge cakes, chocolate bonbons, pound cakes, muffins, ice creams, cookies and cake decorations. Care should be taken not to use excess quantities so that the balance with the other ingredients is not upset.
- **Chocolate liquor:** this is a smooth, liquid paste. In addition to being the base for other cocoa derivatives, such as cocoa butter or cocoa powder, it can be used in all types of desserts and cakes, and items such as toffee. One of its main characteristics is that it contains no sugar, which gives it a slightly bitter flavour in its pure state.
- **Cocoa butter:** once obtained, chocolate liquor is pressed to extract the fat (cocoa butter) and separate it from the dry extract. Cocoa butter is the 'spine' of chocolate, since its proper crystallisation determines whether chocolates (couvertures) have adequate densities and melting points. We would recommend melting cocoa butter at 55°C (it begins melting at 35°C) to achieve proper de-crystallisation. Cocoa butter is used to coat with a spray gun – mixed with chocolate in greater or lesser quantity – chocolate bonbon moulds, desserts, cakes and artistic pieces, or in pure form for moulds and marzipan figurines.
- **Cocoa powder:** two products are extracted from pressed chocolate liquor: cocoa butter in liquid form, and dry matter, which is ground and refined to make cocoa powder. The quality of cocoa powder depends on its finesse, its fat content, the quantity of impurities it contains, its colour and its flavour. It is very important to store it in a dry place and in an airtight container.

Types of chocolate

- **Cooking chocolate** is very often a chocolate substitute and is unsuitable for moulding and for luxury chocolate work.
- **Real chocolate** is produced from cocoa beans, roasted and ground to produce a cocoa mass. Cocoa butter and chocolate liquor form the basis of all chocolate products; the higher the percentage of cocoa solids contained in the chocolate, the richer the chocolate.
- **Couverture** is very high in cocoa butter and requires careful handling.
- **Compound chocolate** is sold by specialist suppliers – it gives a crisp, hard coat.

Chocolate is available in bars, buttons or drops. Buttons and drops have the advantage that they melt quickly and easily.

Preparing and using chocolate

Equipment for working with chocolate

- thermometer
- double boiler or porringer
- dipping fork and ring
- moulds, preferably plastic
- pastry brushes.

Melting chocolate

Chop the chocolate into small pieces and melt slowly in a bowl standing in hot water.

Microwave melting

Break the chocolate into small pieces and place into a non-metallic bowl. Put the microwave on full power for about 20 seconds. After each 20 seconds, stir the chocolate. Do not allow too long before stirring, otherwise hot-spots develop in the bowl, resulting in burnt chocolate.

Tempering chocolate

As already mentioned, cocoa butter is a vital component of chocolate, since the final result depends on its crystallisation. It determines good hardness, balance, texture and shine, and it prevents excessive hardening, whitening and the formation of beads of oil on the surface.

When we melt chocolate, the cocoa butter melts and its particles separate. To achieve a perfect result we must re-bond them by cooling the chocolate, i.e. re-crystallising the cocoa butter.

Tempering allows us to manipulate chocolate and combine it with other ingredients or make artistic pieces that, when re-crystallised, regain the texture and consistency of the chocolate before it was melted.

It is essential that a thermometer is used for this process. Tempering is necessary because of the high proportion of cocoa butter and other fats in the chocolate. This stabilises the fats in the chocolate to give a crisp, glossy finish when dry.

A recipe for tempered chocolate is provided later in this chapter (recipe 22).

Moulding chocolate

Many different types of moulds are available for use in making confectionery. Moulds must always be scrupulously clean. Several days before you intend to use the moulds, they should be washed thoroughly, rinsed well and dried. Keep in a dry place. Immediately before use, polish the inside with cotton wool. Do not touch the inside with your fingers as this may tend to leave a mark on the finished item. Even the smallest amount of oil from the skin may cause problems when removing the chocolate from the mould. It is not necessary to wash the mould after each use, but you must not touch the inside of the mould between fillings.

Protect finished goods from damp and humidity. It is advisable when decorating moulded items to wear cotton gloves to avoid marking the surface.

A recipe for moulded chocolate décor is provided later in this chapter (recipe 23).

Chocolate marbling

Using tempered chocolate and white chocolate, a marbled or combed effect may be created by spreading the chocolate on to acetate or polythene sheets. The flexibility of the acetate or polythene allows you to 'shape' the chocolate as it sets.

What you need to know about chocolate

- Its main enemies are humidity, water and quick changes in temperature.
- The ideal room temperature for working with chocolate is 18°C with 30 per cent humidity.
- Chocolate products should be stored in dry places at 15–16°C and 20 per cent humidity.
- Chocolate absorbs all odours and should therefore be stored well covered.
- The higher its fat content, the faster it melts in your mouth.
- Good chocolate is characterised by its good flavour, smoothness and snap.
- In tempering, it is essential to check temperature with a thermometer and to perform the 'paper test'. This is done by dipping a piece of paper into the tempered chocolate. The tempering is optimal if, in about 2 minutes, it has crystallised with a flawless, uniform shine and without stains or fat drops on the surface.
- A glossy surface is a sign of good tempering.

Chocolate can also be used for finishing other foods. Chocolate coats are used for decorating cakes and gâteaux. Chocolate shapes cut with specialised cutters add impressive finishing touches to sweet dishes.

Ingredient additions to chocolate

- **Butter.** Always use unsalted butter as salt can affect the taste and therefore produce an inferior product.
- **Sugar.** Generally caster and icing sugars are used.
- **Milk.** Use whole milk rather than skimmed or semi-skimmed, as this gives more body to finished sweets.
- **Glucose.** Liquid glucose is easier to measure if you warm the syrup. Use warm spoons and knives to measure and scrape with.

Making chocolate confectionery

There are several recipes for chocolate confectionery in this chapter (recipes 9 to 11). The following advice is useful for any chocolate confectionery work.

Dipping chocolates

In order to dip centres in chocolate successfully it is important that sufficient chocolate is melted to cover them completely when dipped. It is easier to dip chocolates if you have a set of dipping forks. As you become proficient at dipping centres, you will soon develop the skills to make and decorate finished chocolate with the dipping tools.

Dipping hard centres

1. Drop the sweet into the chocolate and turn it over using a fork. When completely covered, lift out of the chocolate with the fork.

2. Tap the fork on the side of the bowl so that the excess chocolate falls away, then draw the bottom of the fork across the lip of the bowl to remove any accumulation underneath the sweet.

3. Place the dipped chocolate on to a sheet of parchment paper to dry. If the chocolate is difficult to remove, gently ease it off using a flat-bladed knife.

4. For round sweets, use a dipping ring. This metal ring is usually thicker than the prongs of the dipping fork

5. Leave the dipped chocolates in a cool, dry place for several hours to set completely.

Finishing chocolates and truffles

As in all forms of food preparation the finishing of chocolates and truffles is very important. The finish can sometimes help to identify the flavour or content of the chocolate. They may be finished by piping designs on each chocolate or dipping in a different type of chocolate to the filling using a contrast of flavours and finishes (i.e. white, dark or milk). Chocolates may also be personalised by using logos and emblems. Tiny chocolate or sugar flowers may be used. Crystallised or glacé fruits may be used alongside marzipan flowers and fruits. Rose and crystallised violet petals are sometimes used.

Sugar work

Boiled sugar

Sugar is boiled for a number of purposes – in pastry work, bakery and sweet-making.

The soaked sugar (approximately 125 ml water per 250 g sugar) is boiled steadily without being stirred. Any impurities on the surface should be carefully removed, otherwise the sugar is liable to granulate. Once the water has evaporated the sugar begins to cook and it will be noticed that the bubbling in the pan will get slower. It is now necessary to keep the sides of the pan free from crystallised sugar; this can be done either with the fingers or a clean, wet pastry brush. In either case the fingers or brush should be dipped in ice water or cold water, rubbed round the inside of the pan and then quickly dipped back into the water.

The cooking of the sugar then passes through several stages, which may be tested with a sugar thermometer or by the fingers (dip the fingers into ice water, then into the sugar and quickly back into the ice water).

Note: to prevent the granulation of sugar a tablespoon of glucose may be added before boiling. If using cream of tartar it is advisable to add this to the sugar three-quarters of the way through the cooking. The addition of lemon juice (citric acid) will make the sugar elastic.

Degrees of cooking sugar

- **Small thread (104°C).** When a drop of sugar held between thumb and forefinger forms small threads when the finger and thumb are drawn apart.

- **Large thread (110°C).** When proceeding as for small thread the threads are more numerous and stronger. Used for crystallising fruits, fruit liqueur making and some icings.

- **Soft ball (116°C).** Proceeding as above, the sugar rolls into a soft ball. Used in the production of fondant, fudge, pralines, pâté â bombe, Italian meringue, peppermint creams and classic buttercreams.

- **Hard ball (121°C).** As for soft ball, but the sugar rolls into a firmer ball, used for products such as nougat and marshmallows.

- **Soft crack (140°C).** The sugar lying on the finger peels off in the form of a thin pliable film, which sticks to the teeth when chewed.

- **Hard crack (153°C).** The sugar taken from the end of the fingers, when chewed, breaks clean in between the teeth, like glass. Used for dipping fruits and the production of butterscotch and toffee.

- **Caramel (176°C).** Cooking is continued until the sugar is a golden-brown colour. Used for cream caramels.

Points to note

1. Never attempt to cook sugar in a damp atmosphere, when the humidity is high. The sugar will absorb water from the air and this will render it impossible to handle.

2. Work in clean conditions as any dirt or grease can adversely affect the sugar.

3. The choice of equipment is also important – copper sugar boilers are ideal as these conduct heat rapidly.

4. Never use wooden implements for working with or stirring the sugar. Wood absorbs grease, which can in turn ruin the sugar.

5. The sugar is cooked to temperature according to the specific purpose of the product being made.

6. If you are colouring the sugar, it is advisable to use powdered food colourings as these tend to be brighter. Before using, dilute with a few drops of 90 per cent-proof alcohol. Add the colourings to the boiling sugar when the sugar reaches 140°C. For poured sugar, if you want a transparent effect, add the colour while the sugar is cooking.

7. Once the sugar is poured on to marble and it becomes pliable, it should be transferred to a special, very thick and heat-resistant plastic sheet.

8. To keep the sugar pliable, it should be kept under infrared or radiant heat lamps.

9. For a good result with poured sugar, use a small gas jet to eliminate any air bubbles while you pour it.

10. Ten per cent calcium carbonate (chalk) may be added to sugar for pouring to give an opaque effect and to improve its shelf life. This should be added at a premixed ratio of 2 parts water to 1 part chalk at 140°C.

11. To keep completed sugar work, place in airtight containers, the bottom of which should be lined with a dehydrating compound, such as silica gel, carbide or quicklime.

12. If you are using a weak acid, such as lemon juice or cream of tartar, to prevent crystal formation, it is advisable to add the small amount of acid towards the end of the cooking. Too much acid will over-invert the sugar, producing a sticky, unworkable product.

Sugar boiling: pulled, blown, poured

There are now available on the market a range of commercial products that greatly assist the pastry chef in the production of specialised sugar work – isomalt, for example. This product is *not* hygroscopic, enabling finished goods to be stored relatively easily. It can be used several times over and has a long shelf life. These commercial products are simple to use, quick and labour saving.

❶ Poppy seed tuiles

	Makes 80 tuiles
glucose	50 g
granulated sugar	500 g
water	200 g
soft flour	150 g
butter, melted	250 g
almonds, nibbed	250 g
poppy seeds	250 g

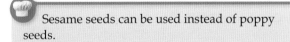

Sesame seeds can be used instead of poppy seeds.

1. Add the glucose and sugar to the water. Bring to the boil.

2. Remove from the heat. Stir in the flour and allow to stand for a few minutes.

3. Add the rest of the ingredients and mix well.

4. Place ½ teaspoon portions of the mixture onto a silicone mat, with space between them. Batten out with a fork.

5. Bake at 180°C for 3–4 minutes. Remove from the oven and invert immediately into tuile moulds.

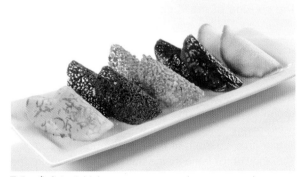

Tuiles (left to right: banana, poppy seed, sesame seed, chocolate, coconut)

2   Coconut tuiles

	Makes 50 tuiles
icing sugar	300 g
flour	100 g
desiccated coconut	100 g
egg whites	250 g
butter, melted, not hot	200 g
vanilla essence	

1. Mix the dry ingredients together well in a food processor.
2. Mixing on a slow speed, gradually add the egg whites, then the melted butter and vanilla essence.
3. Pipe onto silicone mats, in bulbs about 2½ cm in size.
4. Tap the tray to flatten the bulbs.
5. Bake at 205–220°C.
6. Mould inside a tuile plaque.

3   Fruit tuiles

	Makes 25 tuiles
Fruit coulis	
berries (cranberries, blueberries, raspberries, strawberries)	225 g
icing sugar	225 g
Tuiles	
fruit coulis	100 g
icing sugar	200 g
plain flour	50 g
butter, melted	80 g

1. To make the fruit coulis, macerate the berries and sugar together until the fruit starts to leak. Liquidise, then pass.
2. To make the tuiles, beat all the ingredients together.
3. Chill the mixture for 1 hour, then spread on a silicone mat.
4. Bake at 180°C for 6–8 minutes, until translucent.

4   Chocolate tuiles

	Makes 60 tuiles
cocoa powder	30 g
sugar	450 g
water	250 g
pectin	10 g
chocolate paste, made with 100% cocoa chocolate	150 g
unsalted butter	150 g

1. Place the cocoa powder and 360 g of the sugar in the water. Bring to the boil.
2. Whisk in the pectin and the remaining sugar.
3. Simmer on a medium heat for 10 minutes.
4. Remove from the heat and add the chocolate paste and butter. Mix together.
5. Place ¼ teaspoon portions of the mixture onto silicone mats, well spaced apart.
6. Bake at 200°C for 9–10 minutes, until they start to bubble. To check that they are done, place one onto marble and test that it snaps when broken.
7. Mould in a tuile plaque.

5 Macaroons

	Makes 60 macaroon pairs
icing sugar	225 g
ground almonds	125 g
egg whites	4
caster sugar	25 g
flavouring (see below)	

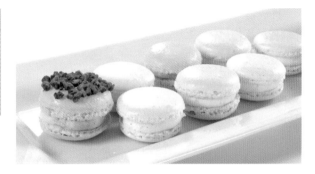

1. Sieve the icing sugar and ground almonds together.
2. In a separate bowl, whisk the egg whites and caster sugar together until the mixture forms soft peaks.
3. Combine all the ingredients together, including the flavouring (see below). Keep folding the mixture until it reaches the correct consistency – when lifted up, it should fall back slowly.
4. Pipe the macaroons. Allow to rest for 30 minutes.
5. Preheat the oven to 165°C with the damper out.
6. Bake the macaroons for 20 minutes.
7. Once cooled, sandwich the macaroons with flavoured buttercream, ganache or fondant.

Possible flavourings for macaroons

Possible flavourings include:

- vanilla essence
- raspberry essence
- various compounds.

To make chocolate macaroons, use the same recipe but use 205 g of icing sugar and 20 g of cocoa powder.

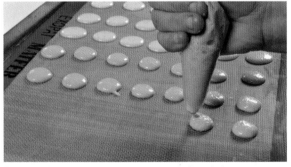

Pipe out the mixture into macaroons ready to bake

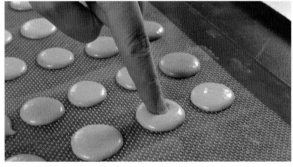

A skin will form over each macaroon

6 Florentines

	Makes 150
sweet paste or sablé paste	400 g
cream	300 ml
butter, cut into pieces	225 g
granulated sugar	450 g
honey	225 g
flaked almonds	340 g
ground almonds	120 g
strong flour, sieved	120 g
glacé fruits, chopped	450 g

1. Roll the paste out to ½ cm thick. Butter a baking sheet and line it with the paste. (You may need more than one sheet, depending on size.)
2. Dock the paste well.
3. Bake at 205°C for 10–15 minutes, until three-quarters cooked.
4. Place the cream into a thick-bottomed saucepan. Add the butter, then the sugar, then the honey. Boil to soft ball (118°C).
5. Remove from the heat. Add the flaked and ground almonds, flour and fruit. Mix well.

6. Spread this mixture evenly over the paste.
7. Return to the oven and cook until the surface begins to bubble.
8. Allow to cool for at least 4 hours.
9. Cut into 2 cm squares.

 This is a variation on the traditional recipe for chocolate-backed florentines.

7 Malakoff

	Makes 100 pieces
milk chocolate couverture	500 g
hazelnut praline paste	500 g
pistachio nuts, whole, roasted	100 g
almonds, flaked, roasted	200 g
Chocolate glacage	
unsalted butter	125 g
dark chocolate couverture	250 g
walnut oil	60 g

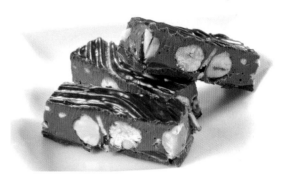

1. To make the Malakoff, melt the milk chocolate.
2. Whisk in the praline paste. Add the roasted nuts and mix well.
3. Pour into a tray lined with silicone paper, to a depth of 1½ cm.
4. Refrigerate until it has set firm.
5. Make the glacage by melting and combining the ingredients.
6. When the Malakoff has set, cover the top with the glacage. When the glacage is on the point of setting, comb scrape it to make a pattern. Leave to set.

 To store Malakoff, wrap it in cling film and keep it in a cool place. Do not refrigerate it.

 Chocolate glacage is a glaze or topping used on pastries and desserts.

8 White chocolate fudge

	Makes 100 pieces
single cream	426 ml
caster sugar	680 g
glucose	340 g
butter	113 g
white chocolate, broken into pieces	225 g

1. Bring the cream, sugar and glucose to the boil slowly.
2. Add the butter. Cook until the mixture forms a firm, soft ball.
3. Remove from the heat. Add the unmelted chocolate pieces and stir through.
4. Leave to stand in the pan for 10 minutes.
5. Pour out and leave to set.

9 Chocolate truffles

	Makes 60 pieces
double cream	150 ml
unsalted butter	25 g
spirit/liqueur (optional)	20 ml
dark chocolate couverture	150 g
milk chocolate couverture	200 g
chocolate couverture, melted, tempered (for dipping)	200 g (approx.)
finish (see below)	

1. Bring the cream and butter to the boil.
2. Pour it over the dark and milk chocolate couverture. Whisk together.
3. Add liqueur if required (see below).
4. Stir in a bowl over ice, until the mixture is firm enough to pipe.
5. Cover a tray with paper. Pipe the mixture onto the paper in evenly sized bulbs. Place in the fridge to set.
6. Once the truffles have set, roll them again to make them smooth.
7. Dip the truffles in melted, tempered chocolate couverture and then in the chosen finish (see below).
8. Allow to set.
9. To store, layer the truffles between sheets of paper and seal the container. Keep refrigerated.

Flavourings and finishes

Spirit or liqueurs that may be used to flavour the truffles include:

- rum
- brandy
- Grand Marnier
- sherry.

To finish, the truffles may be rolled in one of the following:

- grated chocolate
- cocoa powder
- icing sugar
- cinnamon sugar.

Alternatively, they can be left plain.

10 Caramels

	Makes 120
granulated sugar	360 g
cream, 35 per cent fat	600 g
glucose	240 g
vanilla pod	1
milk chocolate couverture	35 g
unsalted butter, cold	150 g
milk chocolate shells	60

1. Heat the sugar to 175°C to make a dry caramel.
2. Heat the cream, glucose and vanilla together. Add them gradually to the caramel.
3. Melt the chocolate couverture and add it gradually to the mixture to form an emulsion.
4. Leave to cool to 35°C.
5. Take the butter from the fridge and add it gradually to the mixture.
6. Place the cooled mixture into the chocolate shells. Allow it to set, then seal and decorate the shells.

Suggestions for decoration

- Spin half the shell with dark chocolate.
- Stick on pieces of moulded chocolate.
- Dip the top quarter of the shell in melted chocolate and then in grated chocolate.

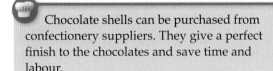

Chocolate shells can be purchased from confectionery suppliers. They give a perfect finish to the chocolates and save time and labour.

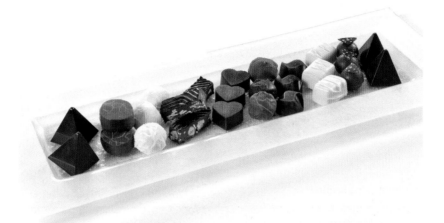

Chocolates (left to right: pyramids filled with ganache, pralines, white truffles, Malakoff, raspberry ganache, milk/dark truffles, honey ganache, Cointreau truffles, caramels, more pyramids)

11 Caramel truffles

	Makes 1585 g, 120 portions
whipping or double cream	500 g
Trimoline	100 g
caster sugar	325 g
plain chocolate	575 g
milk chocolate	75 g
butter	10 g
chocolate spheres	120

1. Place the sugar and Trimoline together in a pan and take to a caramel, being mindful that it will turn from caramel to burnt quickly.
2. Remove from the heat and slowly add the cream. Return to the heat to dissolve the set caramel.
3. Once dissolved, add the chocolate and emulsify.
4. Add the butter.

5. Remove and allow to chill naturally.
6. Once it has reached room temperature place in a disposable piping bag.
7. Snip off the end of the bag and carefully pipe the mix into the desired chocolate spheres.
8. Allow to set and carefully close the top of each sphere with melted chocolate.
9. Once set, roll in desired chocolate, allow to set and then serve.

i Chocolate spheres can be purchased from good provision distributors in milk, dark and white; all the major confectioner's suppliers make the product.

Trimoline is an inverted sugar syrup.

12 Pralines

	Makes 80
milk chocolate couverture	600 g
double cream	200 ml
unsalted butter	50 g
praline, coarsely crushed (see recipe 21)	to taste
baker's chocolate or couverture	200 g

1. Melt the couverture.
2. Heat the cream and butter together.
3. Using a dry, heatproof spatula, emulsify the hot cream into the melted chocolate.
4. Stir in the crushed praline.
5. Pour into a stainless steel tray lined with silicone paper.
6. Cover and leave overnight to set.
7. Melt the baker's chocolate and very quickly spread a thin layer over the praline ganache.
8. Remove from the tray and cut into 12 mm squares or rectangles.
9. Using chocolate forks, dip the pieces into tempered couverture and then mark them with the fork. Leave on silicone paper to set.

13 Nougat Montelimar

	Makes approx. 50–60 pieces
granulated sugar	350 g
water	100 g
honey	100 g
glucose	100 g
egg white	35 g
glacé cherries	50 g
pistachio nuts	50 g
nibbed almonds	25 g
flaked almonds or flaked hazelnuts	25 g

1. Place the sugar and water into a suitable pan, bring to the boil and cook to 107 °C.
2. When the temperature has been reached, add the honey and glucose and cook to 137 °C.
3. Meanwhile, whisk the egg whites to full peak in a machine, then add the syrup at 137 °C slowly, while whisking on full speed.
4. Reduce speed, add the glacé cherries cut into quarters, chopped pistachio nuts, and the nibbed and flaked almonds.
5. Turn out onto a lightly oiled tray or rice paper and mark into pieces while still warm.
6. When cold, cut into pieces and place into paper cases to serve.

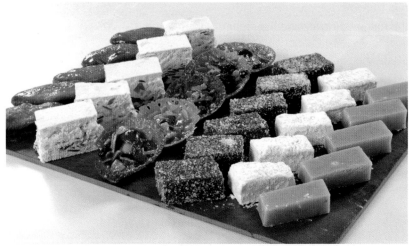

Petit fours (left to right: financiers, nougat, florentines, cassis pâté des fruits, marshmallows, fudge)

14 Marshmallows

	Makes approx. 50 pieces
granulated or cube sugar	600 g
egg whites	3
leaf gelatine, soaked in cold water	35 g

1. Place sugar in a suitable saucepan with 125 ml water and boil to soft ball stage, 140°C.
2. When sugar is nearly ready whisk the egg whites to a firm peak.
3. Pour in boiling water and continue to whisk.
4. Squeeze the water from the gelatine and add.
5. Add colour and flavour if desired.
6. Turn out onto a tray dusted with cornflour and dust with more cornflour.
7. Cut into sections and roll in a mixture of 5 tablespoons of icing sugar and 2 tablespoons of cornflour.

15 Turkish delight

	Makes 50 pieces
water	500 ml
caster sugar	450 g
icing sugar	100 g
lemon juice	1 tbsp
cornflour	150 g
cream of tartar	1 tsp
rose water	1 tbsp
Grenadine	1 tbsp
To finish	
cornflour	2 tbsp
icing sugar	5 tbsp

1. Dust a baking tray measuring 20 × 25 cm with cornflour. Pour half of the water into a heavy-based saucepan and add the sugars and lemon juice. Heat until the sugar has dissolved and then bring to the boil.
2. Reduce the heat and simmer until the mixture reaches 115°C on a sugar thermometer (soft ball stage). Remove from the heat.
3. In a separate saucepan, mix the cornflour and cream of tartar together with the remaining water until the mixture is smooth. Cook over a medium heat until the mixture thickens.
4. Gradually pour the hot sugar syrup into the cornflour paste, stirring continuously. Return the mixture to the heat and simmer for about one hour, until the mixture is pale and feels stringy when a little of the cold mixture is pulled between the fingers. Stir in the rose water and Grenadine.
5. Pour the mixture into the prepared baking tin and leave to set overnight.
6. Cut into squares. Mix the cornflour and icing sugar together and toss the Turkish delight in it. Store in an airtight container, between layers of greaseproof paper.

16 *Cassis pâté des fruits* (blackcurrant jellies)

	Makes 60
blackcurrant pulp	400 g
caster sugar	360 g
granulated sugar	100 g
Pectin mixture	
pectin	30 g
caster sugar	40 g

1. Heat the blackcurrant pulp to 50°C.
2. Add the caster sugar and then bring to the boil and skim.
3. Add the pectin mixture and cook to 105°C.
4. Remove from the heat and leave to settle for 10 seconds.
5. Pour the mixture into a prepared tray. Wrap in cling film.
6. Leave to set for 4 hours.
7. Just before serving, cut into 2 cm cubes. Roll the pieces in the granulated sugar and place into petit four cases.

These jellies should **not** be stored in the fridge.

Use other varieties of fruit purée (pulp) for different flavours of jelly.

17 Chocolate lollipops

	Makes 10
chocolate couverture	200 g

1. Pour circles of tempered chocolate couverture (see recipe 22) onto a very clean non-stick mat.
2. As the couverture begins to thicken, carefully place a lollipop stick in the centre of the chocolate, leaving enough for a handle.
3. Sprinkle with any additional ingredients/ decoration, e.g. chopped nuts, dried fruits (sultanas, raisins, chopped dried raspberries), nibbed sugar, space dust, etc.

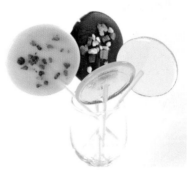

Sugar and chocolate lollipops

18 Sugar lollipops

	Makes 25
water	200 ml
sugar	500 g
glucose	100 g

1. Cook all the ingredients to 155°C.
2. Flavour with concentrated flavour compounds.
3. Once the sugar begins to thicken, proceed as per the chocolate lollipops omitting any garnishes.

19 Dried fruit

water	500 ml
granulated sugar	300 g
glucose	50 g
fruit (lemons, limes, oranges, apples, pears)	

1. Boil the water, sugar and glucose together to make a syrup.
2. Prepare the fruit. Leave the skin on. Remove the core from apples and pears. Slice the fruit very thinly using a meat slicer. Brush slices of apple or pear with lemon juice to prevent browning.
3. Pass each slice through the hot syrup. Lay them on silicone mats.
4. Leave to dry in the oven overnight.

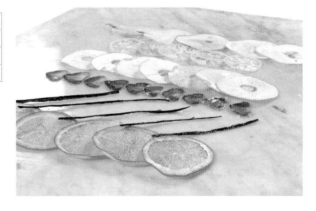

20 Nougatine

	Makes 1 kg
granulated sugar	500 g
water	200 ml
glucose	100 g
flaked almonds	375 g

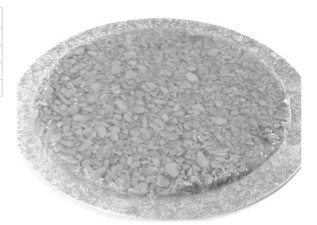

1. Boil the sugar, water and glucose to a light caramel.
2. Remove from the heat and immediately stir in the almonds.
3. Roll out between silicone mats on a baking sheet.
4. Cut out into shapes as required.

21 Praline

	Makes 875 g
flaked almonds, hazelnuts and pecans (any combination)	375 g
granulated sugar	500 g

1. Place the nuts on a baking sheet and toast until evenly coloured.
2. Place the sugar in a large, heavy stainless steel saucepan. Set the pan over a low heat and allow the sugar to caramelise. Do not over-stir, but do not allow the sugar to burn.
3. When the sugar is evenly coloured and reaches a temperature of 170°C, remove from the heat and stir in the nuts.
4. Immediately deposit the mixture onto a Silpat mat. Place another mat over the top and roll as thinly as possible.
5. Allow to go completely cold. Break up and store in an airtight container.

22 Tempered chocolate

Chocolate that is to be moulded or used in decoration needs to be tempered. Methods are provided below for tempering large or small quantities.

The marble method for large quantities

1. Melt carefully to between 45°C and 50°C for dark couverture avoiding steam and moisture and never melting over direct heat (refer to manufacturer's instructions as temperatures can vary between different producers).
2. Once the couverture has reached the melting temperature, remove from the heat source.
3. Pour 70 per cent of it onto a very clean and dry marble surface/slab. Work continuously by spreading outwards and pulling back to the centre until the couverture reaches 26°C to 27°C.
4. Quickly add the couverture back to the remaining 30 per cent, stirring continuously until it reaches its working temperature of 31°C to 32°C.

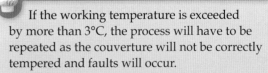

If the working temperature is exceeded by more than 3°C, the process will have to be repeated as the couverture will not be correctly tempered and faults will occur.

Always check the manufacturer's recommended melting temperature as this differs for some types of chocolate.

The seeding method for small quantities

1. Finely chop 30 per cent of the total weight of the couverture being tempered.
2. Melt the remaining 70 per cent of the couverture following stages 1 and 2 of the marble method.
3. Add all the finely chopped chocolate to the melted couverture, stirring continuously until the mass comes down to 31°C to 32°C.

Milk and white chocolate couverture

The instructions given above relate to dark chocolate couverture. For milk or white chocolate couverture, follow the same instructions, but using lower temperatures:

- Melting temperature, 40°C to 45°C.
- Cooling temperature, 26°C.
- Working temperature, 28°C to 29°C.

23 Moulded chocolate decorations

Before moulding chocolate, it needs to be tempered (see recipe 22).

Copeaux, cigarettes (pencils) and shavings

1. Thinly spread a small quantity of tempered couverture onto a marble surface/slab into a rectangular shape.
2. Work the chocolate until it sets, then immediately slice with a large clean chopping knife. The blade needs to be at a 45° angle and the slice action needs to be quick, pushing away at a 45° angle.

Ribbons

1. Thinly spread tempered couverture onto acetate strips and immediately run down the length of the acetate with a comb scraper to create chocolate stripes. (It is recommended that you use A4 size acetate, cut into strips lengthways.)
2. Allow to set before spreading over with a different coloured tempered couverture, working quickly.
3. Cut into short lengths and bend to form loops and secure in place with a paper clip.

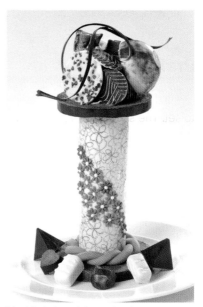

Moulded chocolate centrepiece

4. When completely set, carefully remove the paper clips and acetate and the loops can be assembled to form a bow using tempered couverture

24 Spraying chocolate

| cocoa butter | 100g |
| chocolate (60–70 per cent) | 300g |

i Spraying chocolate is used for glazing and to create special effects on desserts and pastries.

1. Melt together the cocoa butter and chocolate over a bain-marie, ensuring that there are no lumps.
2. Place in a lightly warmed chocolate spraying machine and spray.

25 | **Bubble sugar**

	Makes 750 g
water	100 ml
fondant	450 g
glucose	300 g
unsalted butter	20 g
colouring	

1. Cook the water, fondant and glucose to 150°C.
2. Remove the thermometer. Add the butter and colouring. Swirl to mix the ingredients.
3. Pour onto a silicone mat and leave to set.
4. Break into pieces. The pieces can then be stored in an airtight container until needed.
5. Blitz the pieces of sugar in a food processor.
6. Sieve them over a silicone mat in a slightly uneven layer.
7. Melt in the oven at 165°C.
8. Allow to set. The sugar sets very thin, with bubbles throughout.
9. Store in an airtight container and keep dry. Use to decorate sweet dishes.

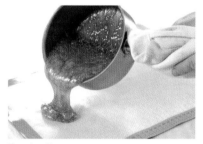
Pouring the sugar

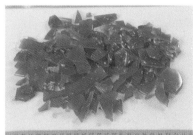
The set sugar, broken into pieces

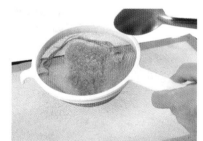
Sifting the sugar after it has been blitzed

26 Poured sugar centrepiece

water	500 ml
granulated cane sugar	1 kg
glucose	200 g
soluble strong powdered colours, pre-mixed (if required)	a few drops
For opaque sugar (if required)	
calcium carbonate (chalk-heavy precipitate)	30 g
water	60 g

1. Clean out a copper sugar boiler with salt and lemon. Rinse but do **not** wipe dry.
2. Place the water in the pan, then the granulated sugar, then the glucose.
3. Bring to the boil slowly. Stir carefully – do not scrape the bottom or sides.
4. Skim off impurities.
5. Cook on a fast boil. Place a thermometer in the pan.
6. If opaque sugar is required, dissolve the calcium carbonate in water. When the temperature of the sugar reaches 130°C, add the calcium solution.
7. If coloured sugar is required, when the temperature of the sugar reaches 150°C, add a few drops of colour solution.
8. Cook until the temperature reaches between

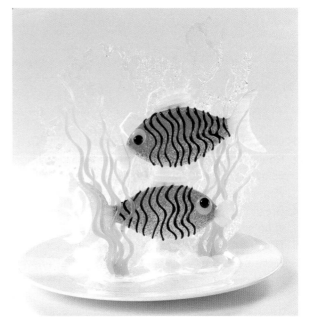

155 and 160°C. Remove from the heat and allow to stand.

9. Pour the sugar out into moulds. Always pour into the centre of the mould, and pour in a steady stream.

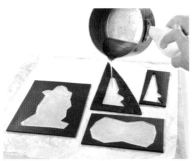

Pouring

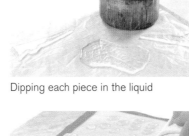

Dipping each piece in the liquid

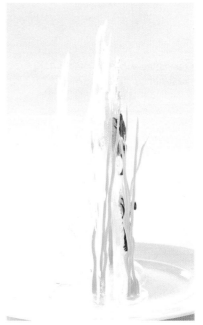

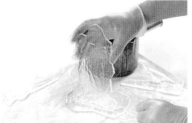

Sticking in place

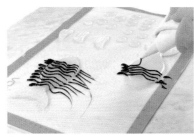

Piping

A side view of the completed centrepiece, showing how the pieces are structured

10. Allow to set completely before trying to move or touch the sugar.
11. To assemble a shape from moulded pieces, heat the edge of each piece with a spirit burner to melt the sugar slightly. Hold it in place and it will harden, welding the two pieces together.
12. To finish, blast with cold air from a hairdryer to quickly set the joins.

27 Piped sugar spirals

	Makes approx. 50
water	100 ml
fondant	500 g

1. Place the water in a copper sugar boiler. Add the fondant.
2. Cook until a pale caramel forms.
3. Allow to stand for 5 minutes.
4. Pipe onto a silicone mat in spirals.
5. Allow to set.
6. Warm the spirals and pull them up to the desired height.

28 Pulled sugar

isomalt	1 kg

1. Bring the isomalt to the boil. Whisk to make sure that the isomalt dissolves completely.
2. Cook until the temperature reaches 165°C (for not more than 20 minutes, or it will get too hot).
3. Plunge into ice to arrest the cooking.
4. Pour out and allow to set.
5. Place the sugar on a board under a lamp and allow it to reheat slowly. When it starts to run, turn it. When the sugar becomes pliable, it is ready to be pulled.
6. Pull and fold the sugar evenly, 20 to 30 times, until it is completely opaque. Use the lamp to keep it at the right consistency.
7. After this point, if the sugar gets cold and hard, it can be brought back by microwaving on a low heat setting in 8- to 10-second bursts.
8. Form into shapes as required.

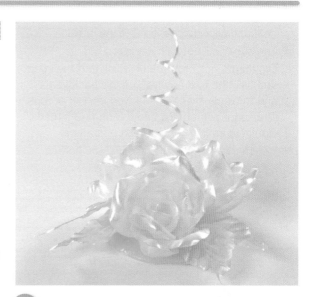

Add a few drops of an acid such as lemon juice to the isomalt. This will make the sugar more pliable and easier to work with.

Isomalt is sugar rearranged with hydrogen. It is less susceptible to moisture than sugar.

It was developed as a sweetener for diabetics, but unfortunately it acts as a laxative. For this reason, it is only used as an ingredient for decorations like pulled sugar.

29 Spun sugar

water	180 ml
granulated sugar	500 g
glucose	125 g
pure peanut oil for greasing	

1. Place the water into a pan, add the sugar, stir gently with a metal spoon.
2. Place over a gentle heat, stir until the sugar begins to boil.
3. Once the sugar starts to foam, skim off the white foam.
4. Clean around the inside of the pan with a clean brush dipped in clean water. This will help to prevent crystallisation.
5. Add the glucose, cook over a high heat.
6. When the sugar reaches 152°C, take off the heat and allow to cool for 2–5 minutes.
7. The sugar will not spin if it is too hot.
8. Dip the prongs of a fork or whisk into the sugar and flick the fork or whisk rapidly backwards and forwards over an oiled wooden rod or rods. The sugar will run down and form fine threads. Continue until a web or mesh of sugar is formed.

9. Carefully collect the spun sugar, place on a tray of silicone paper.
10. Use as required.

Making sugar flowers

Spun sugar is also used to make the stamens of sugar flowers. Gently roll a handful into an oblong shape approximately 2 cm diameter and with a heated knife cut off about 3–4 cm, taking care that the other end remains open. Dip the opened end into crystallised sugar tinted with colour.

30 Pastillage

	Makes 500 g
gelatine	2½ sheets
lemon juice	25 g
icing sugar	450 g

1. Separate the gelatine leaves and soak them in iced water.
2. Sieve the icing sugar onto paper twice.
3. Drain the gelatine and squeeze out the water. Add the gelatine to the lemon juice and warm to dissolve.
4. Place approximately half the icing sugar in a clean bowl, make a well in the centre and add the dissolved gelatine and lemon juice. Mix to a smooth paste.
5. Gradually add the rest of the icing sugar and work/knead to obtain a smooth firm paste.

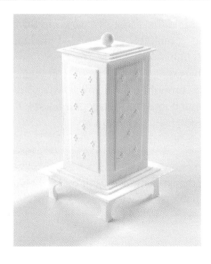

6. Place the paste in a clean plastic bag and cover with a damp cloth.
7. Allow to rest for 20 minutes before using.

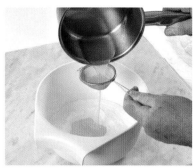

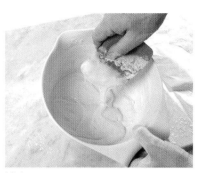

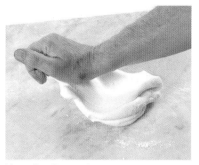

Pouring the dissolved gelatine into the sugar

Mixing

Kneading the paste

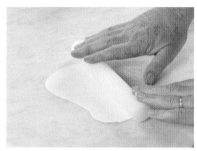

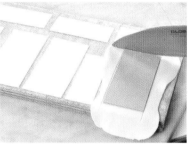

Rolling

Cutting out shapes as required

10 Paste products

This chapter covers Unit 310: Produce Paste Products.

In this unit, you will learn:

1. how to produce paste products
2. how to finish paste products.

For information about the key commodities used in many of these dishes, refer to Chapter 8.

1 Short paste (*pâte à foncer*)

energy	kcal	fat	sat fat	carb	sugar	protein	fibre
6269 KJ	1493 cal	92.6 g	38.0 g	155.5 g	3.1 g	18.9 g	7.2 g	*

	5–8 portions	10–16 portions
soft flour	200 g	500 g
salt	pinch	large pinch
lard or vegetable fat	50 g	125 g
butter or margarine	50 g	125 g
water	2–3 tbsp	5–8 tbsp

1. Sieve the flour and salt together into an appropriate size bowl.
2. Now rub in the fat to achieve a sandy texture.
3. Make a well in the centre and add sufficient water to make a fairly firm paste.
4. Handle as little and as lightly as possible.

The amount of water used varies according to:
- the type of flour (a very fine soft flour is more absorbent)
- the degree of heat (e.g. prolonged contact with hot hands, and warm weather conditions).

Wholemeal short paste

For wholemeal short pastry use half to three-quarters wholemeal flour in place of white flour.

* Using half lard and half hard margarine for 5–8 portions

2 Lining paste

	Makes 500 g, 3 × 15 cm tarts
flour	250 g
sugar	10 g
salt	5 g
butter	125 g
water	40 ml
egg	1

1. Combine the dry ingredients together; rub in the butter. Add the water and egg to gently form a dough.
2. Cling film and leave to rest in the refrigerator for several hours before using.

 Lining paste may be used in place of sweet paste, as it is less rich.

3 Sweet paste (*pâte à sucre*)

energy	kcal	fat	sat fat	carb	sugar	protein	fibre
7864 KJ	1872 cal	109.2 g	46.4 g	208 g	55.6 g	25.7 g	7.2 g	*

	5–8 portions	10–16 portions
egg	1	2–3
sugar	50 g	125 g
margarine or butter	125 g	300 g
soft flour	200 g	500 g
salt	pinch	large pinch

Method 1

1. Taking care not to over-soften, cream the egg and sugar.
2. Add the margarine or butter, and mix for a few seconds.
3. Gradually incorporate the sieved flour and salt. Mix lightly until smooth.
4. Allow to rest in a cool place before using.

Method 2

1. Sieve the flour and salt. Lightly rub in the margarine to achieve a sandy texture.
2. Make a well in the centre. Add the sugar and beaten egg.
3. Mix the sugar and egg until dissolved.
4. Gradually incorporate the flour and margarine, and lightly mix to a smooth paste. Allow to rest before using.

* Using hard margarine for 5–8 portions

50 per cent, 70 per cent or 100 per cent wholemeal flour may be used; the butter may be reduced from 125 to 100 g.

4 Sablé paste

	? portions
egg	1
caster sugar	75 g
butter or margarine	150 g
soft flour	200 g
salt	pinch
ground almonds	75 g

1. Lightly cream the egg and sugar without over-softening.
2. Lightly mix in the butter; do not over-soften.
3. Incorporate sieved flour, salt and the ground almonds.
4. Mix lightly to a smooth paste.
5. Rest in refrigerator before use.

 Alternatively, 50 per cent wholemeal and 50 per cent white flour may be used, or 70 per cent wholemeal and 30 per cent white flour.

Sablé paste may be used for petits fours, pastries and as a base for other desserts.

5 Puff paste

Puff pastry is one of the most interesting creations of our profession. It brings many tastes and textures to our products. It is a dough with a centuries old origin. Basically, it consists of making layers by folding a flour paste and a fat of the same texture.

Its applications are versatile, as much in patisserie as in cooking. Its texture is light and crisp, and it is buttery and crunchy to the palate. It can be combined with all types of food in sweet and savoury dishes. One of the differences in making it is in the fat used. There is no comparison between the taste and texture of a puff pastry made with butter and one made with any other fat.

When the flour paste and the fat are laid in successive folds and rolled between each turn, rather than kneaded, the two elements do not bind completely. The fat forms a separating layer which, when cooked, retains the steam generated by the water in the dough and produces the layer separation effect. The flour paste, which includes part of the fat, becomes crunchy and takes on a nice golden tone rather than becoming hard and dry.

	5–8 portions	10–16 portions
strong flour	200 g	500 g
salt		
margarine or butter	200 g	500 g
water, ice-cold	125 ml	300 ml
few drops of lemon juice or ascorbic or tartaric acid		

1. Sieve the flour and salt
2. Rub in one-quarter of the butter or margarine.
3. Make a well in the centre.
4. Add the water and lemon juice or acid (to make the gluten more elastic), and knead well into a smooth dough in the shape of a ball.
5. Relax the dough in a cool place for 30 minutes.
6. Cut a cross halfway through the dough and pull out the corners to form a star shape.
7. Roll out the points of the star square, leaving the centre thick.
8. Knead the remaining butter or margarine to the same texture as the dough. This is most important; if the fat is too soft it will melt and ooze out, if too hard it will break through the paste when being rolled.
9. Place the butter or margarine on the centre square, which is four times thicker than the flaps.
10. Fold over the flaps.
11. Roll out to 30 × 15 cm, cover with a cloth or plastic and rest for 5–10 minutes in a cool place.
12. Roll out to 60 × 20 cm, fold both the ends to the centre, fold in half again to form a square. This is one double turn.
13. Allow to rest in a cool place for 20 minutes.
14. Half-turn the paste to the right or the left.
15. Give one more double turn; allow to rest for 20 minutes.
16. Give two more double turns, allowing to rest between each.
17. Allow to rest before using.

The lightness of the puff pastry is mainly due to the air that is trapped when folding the pastry during preparation.

The addition of lemon juice (acid) is to strengthen the gluten in the flour, thus helping to make a stronger dough so that there is less likelihood of the fat oozing out; 3 g (7½ g for 10 portions) ascorbic or tartaric acid may be used in place of lemon juice.

The rise is caused by the fat separating layers of paste and air during rolling. When heat is applied by the oven, steam is produced causing the layers to rise and give the characteristic flaky formation.

Care must be taken when rolling out the paste to keep the ends and sides square.

6 Choux paste (*pâte à choux*)

energy	kcal	fat	sat fat	carb	sugar	protein	fibre
6248 KJ	1488 cal	106.6 g	43.3 g	99.3 g	4.1 g	38.9 g	4.5 g *

	5–8 portions	10–16 portions
water	250 ml	625 ml
sugar	pinch	large pinch
salt	pinch	large pinch
butter, margarine or oil	100 g	250 g
strong flour	125 g	300 g
eggs	4	10

1. Bring the water, sugar, salt and fat to the boil in a saucepan. Remove from the heat.
2. Add the sieved flour and mix in with a wooden spoon.
3. Return to a moderate heat and stir continuously until the mixture leaves the sides of the pan.
4. Remove from the heat and allow to cool.
5. Gradually add the beaten eggs, beating well. Do not add all the eggs at once – check the consistency as you go. The mixture may not take all the egg. It should just flow back when moved in one direction.

50 per cent, 70 per cent or 100 per cent wholemeal flour may be used.

Possible reasons for faults in choux paste

- Greasy and heavy:
  - basic mixture over-cooked.
- Soft, not aerated:
  - flour insufficiently cooked
  - eggs insufficiently beaten in the mixture
  - oven too cool
  - under-baked.

* Using hard margarine for 5–8 portions

7   Strudel paste

	32 portions
strong flour	680 g
eggs, whole	3
egg yolks	3
oil	3 tbsp
salt	7 g
water, cold	to make up to 575 ml

1. Sift the flour and place into a mixer.
2. Place the eggs, egg yolks, oil and salt into a measuring jug. Add cold water to the 575 ml mark.
3. Add the liquid to the flour and mix with a hook attachment, to make a smooth dough. If the dough is very sticky, add more flour.
4. Divide the dough into 4 equal pieces. Wrap each piece in cling film and leave to rest in a cool area.
5. Cover a free-standing table, away from the wall, with a large, clean cloth. Dust the cloth with flour.
6. Roll out the paste as far as possible across the table with a rolling pin.
7. Stretch and pull the paste out by hand.

 Make sure you have all the ingredients and equipment needed for the strudel before you start rolling out the paste, because the finely rolled paste will dry out quickly and may crack.

 8   Hot water paste

	4 portions	10 portions
strong plain flour	250 g	625 g
salt		
lard or margarine	125 g	300 g
water	125 ml	312 ml

1. Sift the flour and salt into a basin.
2. Make a well in the centre.
3. Boil the fat with the water and pour immediately into the centre of the flour.
4. Mix with a wooden spoon until cool.
5. Mix to a smooth paste and use while still warm.

You can use 4 parts lard to 1 part butter or margarine.

Some pies are not cooked in moulds. Instead they are hand raised using a hot water pastry.

 9   Biscuits for cheese

	Makes 80–100
strong flour	625 g
paprika	3 g
salt	½ tsp
sesame seeds	20 g
olive oil	65 g
water	250 ml

1. Put all of the dry ingredients into a mixing bowl.
2. Add the oil and water and mix to form a dough – be careful though, it may not take all of the water.
3. Wrap in cling film and rest for 30 minutes.
4. Roll out the dough as thinly as possible, cut and bake at 180°C until golden on both sides.
5. Store in an airtight container until needed.

10　Pastry cream (*crème pâtissière*)

	Makes 14 litres
vanilla pod (can be replaced with a few drops of vanilla arome)	1
milk	1 litre
eggs	4
caster sugar	200 g
flour	100 g
custard powder	30 g

1. Split open the vanilla pod and scrape out the seeds. Place pod and seeds in a heavy stainless steel pan, add the milk and place on the heat.
2. Whisk the eggs and sugar together.
3. Sieve the flour and custard powder onto paper and then add to the egg and sugar mixture. Whisk them all together to form a liaison.
4. When the milk has boiled, pour about one-third into the liaison and whisk in.
5. Bring the rest of the milk back to the boil, then pour in the liaison. Whisk hard until the mixture comes back to the boil again.
6. Simmer gently for 5 minutes.
7. Pour into a sterilised tray and stand on a wire rack. Stir occasionally to help the mixture cool quickly.
8. When cold, store in a plastic container in the fridge. Use within 3 days.

Variations

For these creams, make up pastry cream according to the recipe above, then add the additional ingredient:

- **Crème mousseline:** beat in 100 g of soft butter. The butter content is usually about 20 per cent, but can be as high as 50 per cent depending on its intended use.
- **Crème diplomat:** when the pastry cream is chilled, fold in an equal quantity of whipped double cream.

 Vanilla arome is a high-quality natural vanilla essence.

11　Almond cream (*frangipane*)

	8 portions
butter	100 g
caster sugar	100 g
eggs	2
ground almonds	100 g
flour	10 g

1. Cream the butter and sugar.
2. Gradually beat in the eggs.
3. Mix in the almonds and flour (mix lightly).
4. Use as required.

12　Swiss apple flan

	Makes a 20 cm flan
sweet paste (recipe 3)	250 g
apricot jam	20 g
almond cream	200 g
dessert apples, small	5
apricot glaze	100 ml
flaked almonds, roasted	50 g
neige-decor or icing sugar, for dusting	

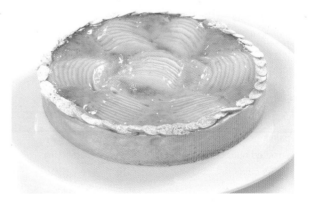

1. Make up the sweet paste (see recipe 3 for instructions) and place a 20 cm flan ring on a baking tray. Line it with the sweet paste. Dock the pastry base.

2. Beat the jam until smooth. Spread a very thin layer over the flan base, using the back of a spoon.

3. Spread the almond cream inside the pastry case: the case should be no more than half full.

4. Peel and core the apples. Cut them in half and score them. Place them onto the flan, evenly spaced. The ideal arrangement is 8 halves around the edge and 1 in the centre.

5. Bake at 165°C for 25–35 minutes.

6. Allow to cool. Brush with boiling apricot glaze. Place flaked almonds around the edge of the flan and dust the almonds with neige-decor.

> *i* Neige-decor is made from dextrose, wheat starch and vegetable fat. It is used to finish and decorate pastries and desserts. Unlike icing sugar, it does not melt easily and will stay where it is placed.

13 Pear flan bourdaloue

	Makes a 20 cm flan
sablé paste (recipe 4)	250 g
pear halves	8
crème mousseline (recipe 10)	500 g
strip almonds	50 g
apricot glaze	100 ml
neige-décor or icing sugar, for dusting	

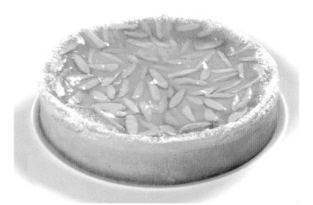

1. Make up the sablé paste (see recipe 4 for instructions) and place a 20 cm flan ring on a baking tray. Line it with the sablé paste. Dock the pastry base. Chill for 20–30 minutes.

2. If the pears are fresh, poach them. If they are tinned, drain and dry them.

3. Beat the crème mousseline until smooth. Spread a very thin layer on the flan base.

4. Score the pears and flatten them slightly. Arrange them in the flan so that they cover the base completely. The pears should **not** be higher than the sides of the flan.

5. Fill the flan with the rest of the crème, completely covering the pears and level with the edge of the pastry.

6. Sprinkle liberally with almonds. Bake at 180°C for approximately 25 minutes.

7. Allow to cool. Brush with boiling apricot glaze. Dust the edge with neige-decor.

14 Plum and soured cream tart

	Makes 1	Makes 3
Sweet paste		
soft flour	170 g	500 g
unsalted butter	85 g	250 g
icing sugar	45 g	125 g
eggs	1	2
Filling		
eggs, beaten	1	4
plums	6	18
unsalted butter	45 g	130 g
caster sugar	60 g	180 g
grated nutmeg	small pinch	pinch

	Makes 1	Makes 3
soured cream	140 ml	400 ml
semolina	15 g	50 g
zest and juice of lemon	½	1
Topping		
soft flour	75 g	200 g
butter	50 g	150 g
demerara sugar	25 g	70 g

1. Line 20 cm flan rings with the pastry and chill in the fridge.

2. Bake blind at 190°C for 15 minutes until golden brown. Egg wash the tart cases and cook for 2 minutes then lower the oven to 150°C.

3. Cut the plums in half, remove the stones, and arrange them cut side up over the base of the tart. Cream the butter and the sugar together until light and fluffy.

4. Gradually beat in the remaining egg, and then stir in the nutmeg, soured cream, semolina, lemon zest and juice. Pour the mixture over the plums and bake for 25 minutes until lightly set.

5. Meanwhile, for the topping, rub the flour and butter together until it resembles fine breadcrumbs, stir in the demerara sugar.

6. After 25 minutes sprinkle the crumble mixture over the top of the tart and bake for another 25 minutes.

7. Decorate with sliced plums.

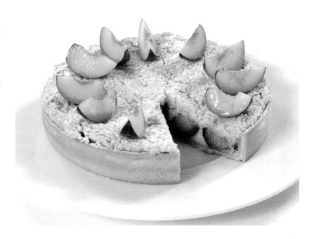

15 Baked blueberry cheesecake

	Makes 1 (6 portions)
digestive biscuits	150 g
butter, melted	50 g
full-fat cream cheese	350 g
caster sugar	150 g
eggs	4
vanilla essence	5 ml
zest and juice of lemon	1
blueberries	125 g
soured cream	350 ml

1. Blitz the biscuits in a food processor. Stir in the melted butter. Press the mixture into the bottom of a lightly greased cake tin with a removable collar.

2. Whisk together the cheese, sugar, eggs, vanilla essence and lemon zest and juice, until smooth.

3. Stir in the blueberries, then pour the mixture over the biscuit base.

4. Bake at 160°C for approximately 30 minutes.

5. Remove from the oven and leave to cool slightly for 10–15 minutes.

6. Spread the soured cream over the top and return to the oven for 10 minutes.

7. Remove and allow to cool and set. Chill until needed.

16 Baked chocolate tart (aero tart)

	Makes a 20 cm flan
sweet paste (recipe 3)	approx. 200 g
Filling	
eggs	3
egg yolks	3
caster sugar	60 g
butter	200 g
chocolate pistoles (55% cocoa, unsweetened)	300 g

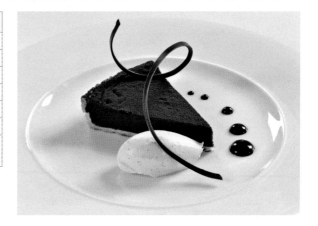

1. Roll out the sweet paste and line a 20 cm flan ring. Bake the flan case blind.

2. For the filling, whisk the eggs, yolks and sugar together.

3. Bring the butter to the boil, remove and mix in the chocolate pistoles until they are all melted.
4. Once the sabayon is light and fluffy, fold in the chocolate and butter mixture, mixing very carefully so as not to beat out the air.
5. Pour into the cooked flan case and place in

a deck oven at 150°C until the edge crusts (approximately 5 minutes). Chill to set.
6. Once set, remove from fridge and then serve at room temperature.

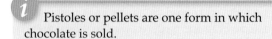

> *i* Pistoles or pellets are one form in which chocolate is sold.

17 Pecan tart

	Makes a 25 cm flan
sweet or lining paste	250 g
eggs	4
light brown sugar	185 g
golden syrup	85 g
salt	2 g
vanilla extract	½ tsp
whiskey	30 ml
unsalted butter, melted	40 g
pecan nuts	285 g
apricot glaze	
chocolate for piping	

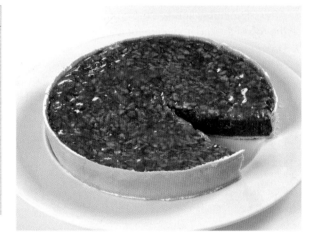

1. Make up the paste (see recipes 2 or 3 for instructions) and place a 20 cm flan ring on a baking tray. Line it with the paste and bake the flan case blind.
2. Whisk the eggs a little, to break them up.
3. Mix in the sugar, syrup, salt, vanilla and whiskey.
4. Stir in the butter and pecan nuts.
5. Dock the flan case. Pour the pecan mixture into the case.
6. Bake at 180°C for approximately 30 minutes, until firm.
7. Allow to cool completely. Brush with apricot glaze. Remove from the flan ring.

18 Croissants

	Makes 14–16
strong white flour	500 g
yeast	23 g
salt	10 g
caster sugar	50 g
egg	1 (or 55 g)
milk, cold	125 g
water	125 g
butter	200 g
eggwash	

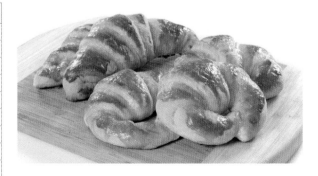

1. Put the flour into a mixing bowl and rub in the yeast, then add the salt and sugar.
2. Add the egg, milk and water and mix together using a scraper and turn out onto a work surface.
3. Work the dough for 3–4 mins.
4. Form the dough into a ball. Cut a cross with a knife (as for puff pastry – see recipe 5), put into a plastic bag and rest the dough in the fridge for 1 hour.

5. Lightly flour a work surface, take the dough out and, starting at the centre where the cross was made, roll out the four corners of the dough.

6. Flatten the butter and make into a square and place in the middle of the dough. Wrap the butter with the dough.

7. Give the paste a turn followed by a 30 minute rest. Repeat the process two more times.

8. After the paste has rested, roll the paste 30 x 75 mm and 4 mm thick. Cut the dough into 2 strips and cut each strip into 6–7 triangles. Roll each triangle up into a croissant shape. Place on a baking tray and prove very slowly for 1 hour then egg wash. Bake at 220 °C for 18–20 minutes.

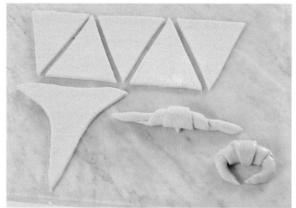

Folding croissants

Pain aux raisins

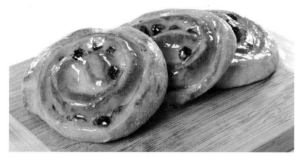

Prepare croissant dough and roll it out to the same thickness as for croissants. Spread the dough with crème pâtissière and sprinkle with raisins (soaked in rum). Roll up. Cut into 1 cm slices and prove and cook as for crossiants.

Pain au chocolate

Prepare croissant dough and roll it out to the same thickness as for croissants. Cut the dough into rectangles and place a strip of chocolate down the centre and roll up.

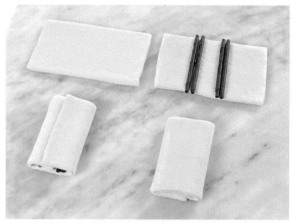

Filling and folding pain au chocolate

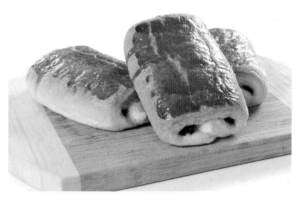

19 Danish pastries

	Makes 40
strong flour	900 g
fresh yeast	40 g
milk, cold	400 ml
eggs	4
caster sugar	140 g
oil	100 ml
salt	pinch
unsalted butter	500 g
fillings (see below)	
eggwash	
apricot glaze	
water icing	

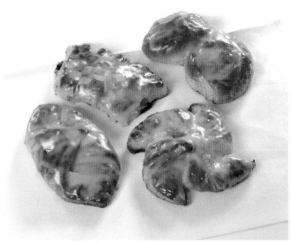

A selection of Danish pastries

1. Sift the flour.
2. Dissolve the yeast in the milk.
3. Whisk the eggs with the caster sugar, oil and salt.
4. Combine all the ingredients **except** the butter, and mix them on a slow speed in a food processor until the liquid is absorbed and the dough is smooth.
5. Line a tray with cling film. Roll the dough into a rectangle to fit the tray. Lay it on the tray and cover with cling film. Rest in the fridge for 30 minutes.
6. Bat out the butter to soften it. Place it between layers of cling film and roll it out to a rectangle two-thirds the size of the dough.
7. Prepare deep trays of ice and put them to one side. Cover a marble slab with cling film and lightly dust it with flour.
8. Lay the dough onto the slab. Place the butter on top so it neatly covers two-thirds of the dough, starting at one end.
9. Fold the dough over in thirds (this is turn 1).
10. Roll the paste out in the opposite direction to which it was first rolled. Use the ice to keep the rolling pin cool. Fold it in thirds (turn 2).
11. Wrap the dough in cling film and rest in the fridge for 30 minutes.
12. Prepare everything again as at step 7. Repeat step 10 (this is turn 3).
13. The dough is now ready for use. If it is to be stored, roll it out and cut it in half. Wrap each piece in two layers of cling film. Refrigerate or freeze.

14. To make up the pastries, prepare a marble as for step 7. Roll out the dough into a rectangle, approximately 6 mm thick.
15. Cut, fill and shape the dough as required (see below for suggested shapes and fillings).
16. Place the pastries on baking sheets, spaced well apart, and egg wash.
17. Prove until the pastries have doubled in size.
18. Bake at 205°C for 12–15 minutes.
19. Brush with apricot glaze and then with water icing.

1 kg of paste will yield about 20 individual pastries.

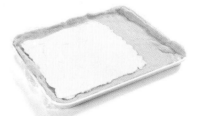

Covering the paste with the butter

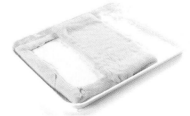

Folding the paste

Apple envelopes

1. Divide the paste into 10 cm squares.
2. Pipe a small amount of frangipane (see recipe 11) or pastry cream (see recipe 10) diagonally across each square. Lay cooking apple slices coated with cinnamon sugar on top.
3. Fold over the corners and seal well.

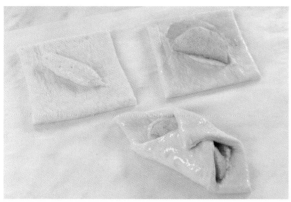

Folding the envelopes

Plum windmills

1. Divide the paste into 8–10 cm squares. Make a cut in each corner of the square.
2. Pipe a small bulb of frangipane (see recipe 11) or pastry cream (see recipe 10) in the centre of the square. Place half a plum on top (apricots can be used instead of plums here).
3. Fold over alternate corners and seal well.

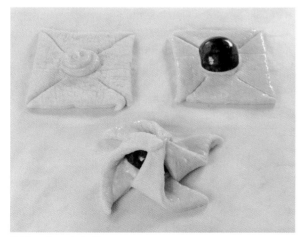

Folding the windmills

Sultana roulade

| Frangipane (almond cream) |
| Sultanas soaked in rum |

1. Spread the paste evenly with frangipane (see recipe 11). Spread the cream so that it is 3 mm thick.
2. Sprinkle with sultanas soaked in rum.
3. Egg wash the top edge of the dough and roll it up.
4. Cut into 2 cm slices.

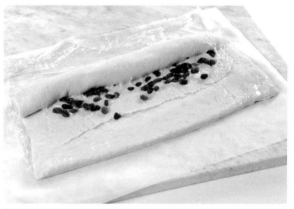

Folding the sultana roulade

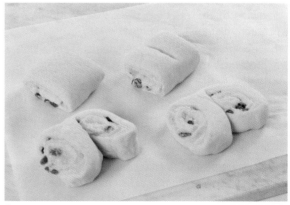

Shaping the sultana roulade

Cockscombs

1. Cut the paste into 2 large strips.
2. Pipe frangipane (see recipe 11) or pastry cream (see recipe 10) down the centre of each strip. Place blueberries on top if desired.
3. Egg wash the edge of the strip, fold over and seal. Make a series of 1½ cm cuts along the edge.
4. Cut into 8 cm lengths and bend each one.
5. Sprinkle with flaked almonds before proving.

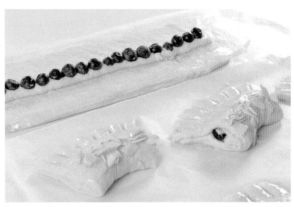

Shaping the cockscombs

20 Gâteau pithivier

	Makes 2
puff paste	1 kg
pastry cream	60 g
almond cream (frangipane – recipe 11)	600 g
eggwash (yolks only)	
granulated sugar	

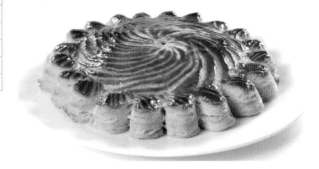

1. Divide the paste into four equal pieces (see recipe 5). Roll out each piece in a circle with a 22 cm diameter, 4 mm thick.
2. Rest in the fridge between sheets of cling film, preferably overnight.
3. Lightly butter two baking trays and splash with water. Lay one circle of paste onto each tray and dock them.
4. Mark a 16 cm diameter circle in the centre of each.
5. Beat the pastry cream (see recipe 10), if desired, and mix it with the almond cream (see recipe 11).
6. Spread the cream over the inner circles, making them slightly domed.
7. Egg wash the outer edges of the paste. Lay one of the remaining pieces over the top of each one, smooth over and press down hard.
8. Mark the edges with a round cutter. Cut out a scallop pattern with a knife.
9. Egg wash twice. Mark the top of both with a spiral pattern using a knife.
10. Bake at 220°C for 10 minutes. Remove from the oven and sprinkle with granulated sugar. Turn the oven down to 190°C and bake for a further 20 to 25 minutes.
11. Glaze under a salamander.

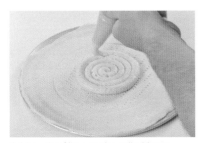

Adding the filling to the rolled base

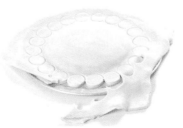

Trimming the edge

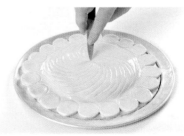

Marking the top

21 Strawberry soleil

	Makes 1 (8 portions)
puff pastry	250 g
pastry cream	400 g
slice of sponge, approx. 20 cm diameter	1
Grand Marnier or rum	20 ml
strawberries, hulled (or raspberries)	2 punnets
redcurrant glaze	200 ml

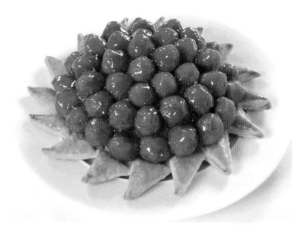

1. Roll the pastry (see recipe 5). Rest it, then cut and fold it into a soleil (sun) shape. Dock the central area, egg wash the points and press down.
2. Bake blind at 205°C for about 15 minutes. Dock the base again at least once during cooking.
3. Beat the pastry cream until smooth (see recipe 10). Spread it in the centre of the pastry to within 2 cm of the inside edge. Spread it in a cone shape.
4. Cut a slice of sponge to fit and lay it on top of the cream. Sprinkle with the Grand Marnier.
5. Spread a little more pastry cream on top of the sponge.

6. Arrange whole strawberries all over the sponge, pointing outwards. Brush with boiling redcurrant glaze, making sure any gaps are filled in.

> To cut the pastry into a sun shape, use a metal or cardboard template.

22 Walnut and apricot jalousie

	20 portions
puff pastry	1 kg
apricot halves	16–20
eggwash	
apricot glaze	
neige-decor	
Walnut frangipane	
butter	150 g
caster sugar	150 g
eggs	2–3
soft flour	50 g
ground almonds	75 g
ground walnuts	85 g

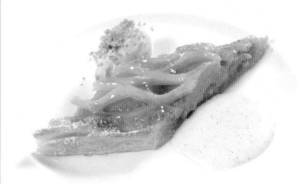

1. To make the frangipane, cream together the butter and sugar until the butter has turned white and fluffy.
2. Gradually add the eggs to the butter mixture.
3. Sieve the flour and ground almonds, and fold them into the mixture. Then fold in the ground walnuts.

4. Roll out half the puff pastry in a rectangle that is 5 cm wider than the apricot halves. Dock well.
5. Pipe the walnut frangipane in one straight line down the centre of the paste.
6. Place the apricots onto the frangipane, overlapping at the wide end.
7. Roll out the rest of the pastry to the same length as the first piece, but half the width. Cut this piece with a trellis cutter.

8. Egg wash the sides of the base piece. Place the trellis piece over the top and seal at each side.
9. Crimp the edges. Egg wash the top.
10. Bake for 20 to 25 minutes at 210°C.
11. Brush with boiling apricot glaze. Allow to cool slightly, then dust the edges with neige-decor.

> If using tinned apricots, make sure that they are well drained and dried before use.

23 Mille-feuilles Napoleon

	10 portions
puff paste (recipe 5)	600 g
pastry cream	400 ml
strawberries, small or halves	225 g
icing sugar	20 g
Crème diplomat	
double cream, whipped	300 ml
pastry cream	300 ml

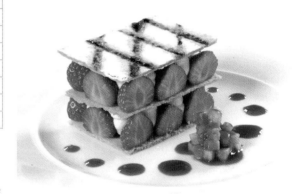

1. Roll out the puff paste in a very thin sheet (see recipe 5). Dock well. Rest the pastry with a clean baking sheet on top to prevent it from rising. Bake at 205 to 220°C.
2. Prepare the crème diplomat by folding the whipped double cream into the chilled pastry cream.
3. Cut the puff paste neatly into rectangles, approx. 9 cm × 5 cm. Allow 3 pieces per portion.
4. Take one rectangle of paste and pipe on swirls of crème diplomat, with strawberry halves between the swirls.
5. Place a second rectangle on top and layer with crème and strawberries as before.
6. Dust the third rectangle of paste with icing sugar and sear in diagonal lines with a hot poker. Place gently on top of the dessert.
7. Serve with a cordon of strawberry coulis or crème anglais.

24 Gâteau St Honoré

	8 portions
choux paste (recipe 6)	500 g
puff paste disc (recipe 5)	16 cm
pastry cream	300 ml
kirsch	30 ml
double cream, whipped	300 ml
caramel	1 kg

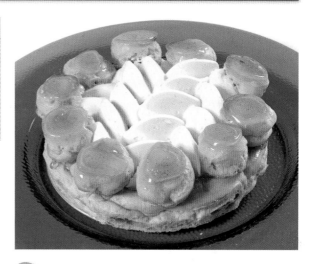

1. Pipe the choux paste in a ring around the edge of the puff paste disc, and also pipe a set of profiteroles.
2. Bake at 220°C for 10 minutes, then at 165°C for 15 to 20 minutes.
3. Beat the pastry cream (see recipe 10). Flavour it with kirsch and fold in the whipped double cream.
4. Fill the profiteroles with the cream.
5. Dip the profiteroles in caramel and then stick them to the ring of choux paste on the base.
6. Fill the centre with quenelles of the cream.

i Traditionally, this gâteau is filled with *crème chibouste (crème St Honoré)*: pastry cream with leaf gelatine added (6 g per 250 ml) while hot, made into a meringue by carefully folding in sugar and 5 beaten egg whites.

25 Petit religieuse

	8 portions
choux paste (recipe 6)	500 g
puff paste (recipe 1)	6 cm discs
fondant (chocolate, coffee or other flavour)	1 kg
pastry cream	300 ml
kirsch or chocolate	30 ml
double cream, whipped	300 ml

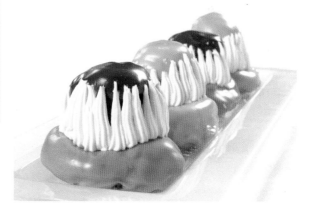

1. Pipe the choux paste into 8 cm rings and 4 cm buns – make an equal number of each (see recipe 6 for choux paste).
2. Bake at 220°C for 10 minutes, then at 165°C for 15 to 20 minutes.
3. Place each choux paste ring onto a puff paste base. Glaze the pastry with fondant and allow to set.
4. Beat the pastry cream (see recipe 10). Flavour it with kirsch or chocolate and fold in the whipped double cream.
5. Fill the centre of each ring with cream and place a bun on top.
6. Pipe a crown of chantilly cream onto each.

26 Croquembouche

water	400 ml
granulated sugar	1 kg
glucose	200 g
profiteroles, piped and baked	
crème diplomat	
nougatine	

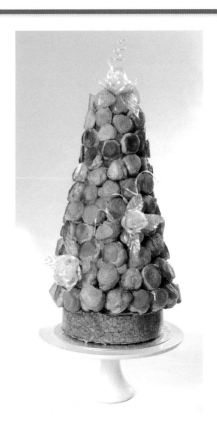

Quantities required depend on the size of croquembouche required.

1. Boil the water, sugar and glucose to make a caramel.
2. Dip each profiterole in caramel and allow to cool.
3. When cool, fill with crème diplomat (see recipe 10).
4. Using caramel as glue, assemble the profiteroles in a cone-shaped mould.
5. Assemble the nougatine (see page 315) in shapes to form a base.
6. Once the caramel has set, turn the profiteroles out of the mould onto the nougatine base.
7. Decorate with cut-out nougatine shapes and pulled sugar (see page 319).

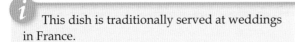

i   This dish is traditionally served at weddings in France.

11 Desserts

This chapter covers Unit 311: Produce Hot, Cold and Frozen Desserts.

In this unit, you will learn to:

1. produce and finish hot desserts
2. produce and finish cold and frozen desserts.

For information about the key commodities used in many of these dishes, refer to Chapter 8.

	Chocolate and pecan nut brownies	371		Roulade sponge	366
	Melon soup	120		Savarin paste	300

Soufflés

As long as you follow the key principles of soufflé making, you should be able to make soufflés successfully, from whatever flavourings you prefer, without using a recipe; however, this is not to be recommended until you have grasped the basic foundation.

When whipping the egg whites, the bowl and whisk must be free from fat or grease. Indeed, you should avoid all fats when making soufflés as they inhibit the egg proteins and burst the air bubbles. The egg whites and sugar should be whisked to a smooth, stiff peak with small air bubbles – the smaller the air bubbles, the bigger the lift. The purée used to flavour the soufflé should be reasonably thick as this will help support the soufflé while it is cooking.

The mould must be well greased to ensure that the proteins in the egg do not stick to the glaze on the porcelain. Make sure you clean off the excess soufflé mixture from around the rim of the dish as this could cause the soufflé to stick and prevent it from rising evenly. Soufflés should always be placed directly into a pre-heated, hot, oven.

Ice cream

Regulations governing ice cream making

Any ice cream sold must comply with the following compositional standards.

- It must contain not less than 5 per cent fat and not less than 2.5 per cent milk protein.
- It must conform to the Dairy Product Regulations 1995.

For further information contact the Ice Cream Alliance (see www.ice-cream.org).

After heat treatment according to the Dairy Product Regulations, the mixture is reduced to 7.1°C within 1½ hours and kept at this temperature until the freezing process begins. Ice cream needs this treatment so as to kill harmful bacteria. Freezing without correct heat treatment does not kill bacteria; it allows them to remain dormant. The storage temperature for ice cream should not exceed −12°C.

The ice cream making process

1. **Weighing:** weighing is an essential process to ensure consistent results.
2. **Pasteurisation:** without a doubt this is a vital stage in making ice cream. Its primary function is to minimise bacterial contamination by heating the mixture of ingredients to 85°C, then quickly cooling it to 4°C.
3. **Homogenisation:** high pressure is applied to cause the explosion of fats. This process makes ice cream more homogenous, creamier, smoother and much lighter. It is not usually done for home-made ice cream.
4. **Ripening:** this basic but optional stage refines flavour, further develops delicate aromas and improves texture. This occurs during a rest period (4–24 hours), which gives the stabilisers and proteins time to act, improving the overall structure of the ice cream. This has the same effect on a crème anglaise, which is much better the day after it is made than it is on the same day.
5. **Churning:** here, the mixture is frozen while air is simultaneously incorporated.

Functions and approximate percentages of the main components of ice cream

- Sucrose (common sugar) not only sweetens ice cream, but its solids also give it body. An ice cream that contains only sucrose (not recommended) has a higher freezing point.
- The optimum sugar percentage of ice cream is between 15 and 20 per cent.
- Ice cream that contains dextrose has a lower freezing point, and better taste and texture.

- As much as 50 per cent of the sucrose can be substituted with other sweeteners, but the recommended amount is 25 per cent.
- Glucose improves smoothness and prevents the crystallisation of sucrose.
- The quantity of glucose used should be between 25 and 30 per cent of the sucrose (by weight).
- The quantity of dextrose used should be between 6 and 25 per cent of the substituted sucrose (by weight).
- If we use inverted sugar in ice cream, it lowers the freezing point.
- Inverted sugar improves texture and delays crystallisation.
- The quantity of inverted sugar used should be a maximum of 33 per cent of the sucrose (by weight). It has a high sweetening coefficient and gives the mix a low freezing point.
- The purpose of cream in ice cream is to improve creaminess and taste.
- Egg yolks act as stabilisers for ice cream due to the lecithin they contain – that is, they facilitate the emulsion of fats in water.
- Egg yolks improve the texture and viscosity of ice cream.
- The purpose of stabilisers is to prevent crystal formation by absorbing the water contained in ice cream and making a stable gel.
- The quantity of stabilisers in ice cream should be between 3 and 5 g per kg of mix, with a maximum of 10 g.
- Stabilisers promote air absorption.

What you need to know about ice cream

- Maintaining hygiene with respect to materials, personnel, the kitchen and the pastry section is essential while making ice cream.
- An excess of stabilisers in ice cream will make it sticky.
- Stabilisers should always be mixed with sugar before adding, to avoid lumps.
- Stabilisers should be added at 45°C, which is when they begin to act.
- Cold stabilisers have no effect on the mix, so the temperature must be raised to 85°C.
- Ice cream should be cooled quickly to 4°C, because rapid microorganism proliferation occurs between 20°C and 55°C.

Sugar syrups

For many pastry dishes – for example, sorbets – sugar syrups of a definite density are required. This density is measured by a hydrometer known as a saccharometer. The saccharometer is a device that measures the density of stock syrups. This is measured in either brix or degrees baumé. The instrument is a hollow glass tube sealed at each end. One end is weighted with lead shot so that when it is placed in the solution it floats upright. The scale marked in either brix or baumé indicates the depth at which the tube floats. This is influenced by the density of the sugar, which in turn is controlled by the ratio of sugar to water used for the solution. The instrument thus measures the amount of sugar in the solution.

BAUMÉ	DENSITY	BAUMÉ	DENSITY	BAUMÉ	DENSITY	BAUMÉ	DENSITY
5	= 1.0359	13	= 1.0989	21	= 1.1699	29	5 1.2515
6	= 1.0434	14	= 1.1074	22	= 1.1799	30	5 1.2624
7	= 1.0509	15	= 1.1159	23	= 1.1896	31	5 1.2736
8	= 1.0587	16	= 1.1247	24	= 1.1995	32	5 1.2850
9	= 1.0665	17	= 1.1335	25	= 1.2095	33	5 1.2964
10	= 1.0745	18	= 1.1425	26	= 1.2197	34	5 1.3082
11	= 1.0825	19	= 1.1515	27	= 1.2301	35	5 1.3199
12	= 1.0907	20	= 1.1609	28	= 1.2407	36	5 1.3319

Sorbets

Sorbets belong to the ice cream family; they are a mixture of water, sucrose, atomised glucose, stabiliser and fruit juice, fruit pulp or liqueurs.

What you need to know about sorbet

- Sorbet is always more refreshing and easier to digest than ice cream.
- Fruit for sorbets must always be of a high quality and perfectly ripe.
- The percentage of fruit used in sorbet varies according to the type of fruit, its acidity and the quality desired.
- The percentage of sugar depends on the type of fruit used.
- The minimum sugar content in sorbet is about 13 per cent.
- As far as ripening is concerned, the syrup should be left to rest for 4–24 hours and never mixed with the fruit because its acidity will damage the stabiliser. (See the section on 'Sugar syrups'.)
- Stabiliser is added in the same way as for ice cream.
- Sorbets are not to be confused with granitas, which are semi-solid.

Stabilisers

For what do we use gelling substances?

Within the realm of stabilisers are gelling substances, thickeners and emulsifiers. These are products we use regularly, each with its own specific function; but their main purpose is to retain water to make a gel. The case of ice cream is the most obvious, in which they are used to prevent ice crystal formation. They are also used to stabilise the emulsion, increase the viscosity of the mix and to give us a smoother product that is more resistant to melting. There are many stabilising substances, both natural and artificial.

Edible gelatine

Edible gelatine is extracted from animals' bones (pork and veal). Sold in sheets of approximately 2 g, leaves of gelatine are soaked in liquid to soften then drained before use.

Gelatine sheets melt at 40°C and should be melted in a little of the liquid from the recipe before being added to the base preparation.

Pectin

Pectin is another commonly used gelling substance because of its great absorption capacity. It comes from citrus peel (orange, lemon, etc.), though all fruits contain some pectin in their peel.

It is essential to mix pectin with sugar before adding it to the rest of the ingredients.

Agar-agar

Agar-agar is a gelatinous marine algae found in Asia. It is sold in whole or powdered form and has a great absorption capacity. It dissolves very easily and, in addition to gelling, adds elasticity and resists heat (a reversible property). Suitable for vegetarian diets.

Other stabilisers

- **Carob gum** comes from the seeds of the carob tree, makes sorbets creamier and acts as a stabiliser.
- **Guar gum** and **carrageen** are, like agar-agar, extracted from marine algae and are alternatives to using gelatine, which is a meat product.

Sauces

Sauces in pastry have changed dramatically over the past 15 years and have gone from the classic anglaise, Chantilly and coulis preparations to what we see in modern restaurants today, such as foams and oils.

One key factor that cements both modern and classic approaches is that both need to work with the principle ingredient. The sauce is an integral part of the dish whether it be pastry or savoury, and must be treated as such and not added to the dish for aesthetic reasons alone. Essentially, the sauce must complement the dish.

E'spumas and foams

The word e'spuma directly translates from Spanish into foam or bubbles, and the e'spuma is created using a classic cream whipper – a stainless steel vessel fitted with a screw top and a non-return valve which you charge with nitrogen dioxide (which constitutes 78% of the air we breathe); this has minimum water solubility therefore it will not affect the product that is being charged. The principle role of this gas, then, is to force the liquid out of the canister under pressure through two nozzles, making the cream more voluminous due to mechanical agitation of the fats. Although this statement may seem quite convoluted it is necessary to explain the mechanics of this machine for the purists among us. However, the simple version is: this canister, once charged, will whip cream the same as a whisk – it is as simple as that! Below are listed the key factors that are essential to a successful preparation.

Cold fat based

- In a litre canister: 750 g is the maximum product to be placed in the canister. Depending on the viscosity, 1 or 2 charges can be used: low viscosity (thin mixtures) – 2 charges; high viscosity (thicker mixtures) – 1 charge.
- Once the product has been charged, it will need to be treated like any fat-based product likely to be aerated, and not stored at room temperature because the aeration will be reduced dramatically.

Warm fat based

- In a litre canister: 600 g is the maximum product to be placed in the canister.
- Warm products tend to need 2 charges to ensure good aeration.

- 50–55°C is the optimum temperature to hold the canister charged and ready for use. Any hotter and the expansion in the canister will be too great and uncontrollable when the trigger is pressed. Too cold and the fat molecules will tend to coat the tongue and not give optimum flavour.

Gelatine based

- In a litre canister: 750 g is the maximum product to be placed in the canister.
- Obviously the product will be liquid when it is poured into the canister. It will need to be charged immediately, placed in the fridge and agitated every 10–15 minutes to prevent total setting.
- This preparation will give you a purer flavour as there is little or no fat involved, hence the use of gelatine – as fat coats the tongue, this absence of fat will increase flavour.

Why use e'spumas?

The 'holy grail' boundaries of gastronomy have changed somewhat over the last 20 to 30 years and will no doubt continue to do so for the next 20 to 30, but the current approach is 'less volume, more flavour'. By offering more flavours, the dining experience will be heightened; by reducing the volume that is taken, more flavour combinations than previously can be offered – e'spumas are excellent vehicles to achieve such a result.

However, this is a marvel that should be used in slight moderation as too much on one menu will become repetitive to the palate and what was initially your motivation for using them will extinguish advantage from the outset.

Pâte à bombe

	Makes 350 ml
caster sugar	150 g
water	100 ml
glucose	10 g
egg yolks, large	5
flavouring	

1. Boil the sugar, water and glucose together in a heavy-based pan. Continue to gently boil. Wash down the sides of the pan to prevent crystallisation.

2. Meanwhile put the egg yolks in a Kitchen Aid mixer and start mixing, while watching the sugar.
3. When the sugar reaches 121°C, pour onto the eggs in a steady stream. Add flavouring.
4. Carry on whisking to a sabayon until the mixture has increased in volume and is cold.
5. Use as required.

 This is used as a base for parfaits or soufflés.

French meringue

energy	kcal	fat	sat fat	carb	sugar	protein	fibre
3491 KJ	831 cal	0.0 g	0.0 g	210.0 g	210.0 g	10.8 g	0.0 g

	4 portions	10 portions
egg whites, pasteurised	4	10
caster sugar	200 g	500 g

1. Whip the egg whites stiffly.
2. Sprinkle on the sugar and carefully mix in.
3. Place in a piping bag with a large plain tube and pipe the desired shapes onto silicone paper on a baking sheet.
4. Bake in the slowest oven possible or in a hot plate (110°C). The aim is to dry out the meringues without any colour whatsoever.

Use as required.

Whipping egg whites

The reason egg whites increase in volume when whipped is because they contain so much protein (11%). The protein forms tiny filaments, which stretch on beating, incorporate air in minute bubbles then set to form a fairly stable puffed-up structure expanding to seven times its bulk. To gain maximum efficiency when whipping egg whites, the following points should be observed.

- Because of possible weakness in the egg white protein it is advisable to strengthen it by adding a pinch of cream of tartar and a pinch of dried egg white powder. If all dried egg white powder is used no additions are necessary.
- Eggs should be fresh.
- When separating yolks from whites *no* speck of egg yolk must be allowed to remain in the white; egg yolk contains fat, the presence of which can prevent the white being correctly whipped.
- The bowl and whisk must be scrupulously clean, dry and free from any grease.
- When egg whites are whipped the addition of a little sugar (15 g to 4 egg whites) will assist the efficient beating and reduce the chances of over-beating.

Italian meringue

	Makes 300 g
granulated or cube sugar	200 g
water	60 ml
cream of tartar	pinch
egg whites	4

1. Boil the sugar, water and cream of tartar to hard ball stage (121°C).
2. Beat the egg whites to full peak and, while stiff, beating slowly, pour on the boiling sugar. Use as required.

 It is important that the whites are reaching full peak at the same time that the sugar reaches 121°C.

4 Swiss meringue

	Makes 420 g
egg whites	4
icing sugar	300 g

1. Combine the egg whites and half of the icing sugar in the mixing bowl.
2. Stand the bottom of the bowl in a bain-marie set over direct heat.
3. Beat the mixture continuously until it reaches a temperature of about 40°C.
4. Remove the bowl from the bain-marie. Add the remaining sugar and continue to beat until the mixture is completely cold.
5. Preheat the oven to 120°C.
6. Spoon the mixture onto baking parchment or greaseproof paper using 2 soup spoons, or use a piping bag fitted with different nozzles to pipe it into various shapes and sizes.
7. Lower the oven temperature to 100°C and cook the meringues for 1 hour 45 minutes.
8. They are ready when both the top and bottom are dry.

5 Vanilla soufflé

energy	kcal	fat	sat fat	carb	sugar	protein	fibre
757 KJ	180 cal	9.1 g	3.5 g	16.6 g	14.6 g	9.1 g	0.1 g

	4 portions	10 portions
butter	10 g	25 g
caster sugar, for soufflé case	50 g	125 g
milk	125 ml	300 ml
natural vanilla or pod		
eggs, separated	4	10
flour	10 g	25 g
caster sugar	50 g	125 g
icing sugar, to serve		

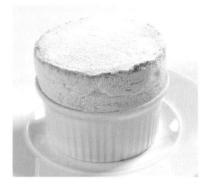

1. Lightly coat the inside of a soufflé case/dish with fresh butter.
2. Coat the butter in the soufflé case with caster sugar as needed, tap out surplus.
3. Boil the milk and vanilla in a thick-bottomed pan.
4. Mix half the egg yolks, the flour and sugar to a smooth consistency in a bowl.
5. Add the boiling milk to the mixture, stir vigorously until completely mixed.
6. Return this mixture to a clean thick-bottomed pan and stir continuously with a wooden spoon over a gentle heat until the mixture thickens, then remove from heat.
7. Allow to cool slightly. Add the remaining egg yolks and mix thoroughly.
8. Stiffly whip the egg whites and carefully fold into the mixture, which should be just warm. (An extra egg white can be added for extra lightness.)
9. Place the mixture into the prepared case(s) and level it off with a palette knife – do not allow it to come above the level of the soufflé case.
10. Place on a baking sheet and cook in a moderately hot oven (approximately 200–230°C) until the soufflé is well risen and firm to the touch – this will take approximately 15–20 minutes. (For individual soufflés, reduce time by 5 minutes.)
11. Remove carefully from oven, dredge with icing sugar and serve at once. A hot soufflé must not be allowed to stand or it may sink.

Add a pinch of egg white powder (meri-white) when whisking the whites, to strengthen them and assist in the aeration process.

Grand Marnier soufflé

	4 portions
egg yolk	1
whole egg	1
sugar	100 g
strong flour	75 g
milk	250 ml
vanilla pod, split	¼
egg yolks	5
egg whites	7
biscuit à la cuillère	4
Grand Marnier	100 ml

1. Whisk the single egg yolk and the egg together, add the flour and the sugar.
2. Boil the milk with the vanilla pod.
3. Add the boiled milk to the mixture and return to the heat. Cook until it thickens.
4. Place in a mixer, whisk the lumps out, then add the five egg yolks.
5. Take four soufflé moulds and 'chemise' by brushing with melted butter and lining with sugar.
6. Whisk the egg whites with a touch of salt until stiff.
7. Soak the chopped biscuit à la cuillère in Grand Marnier.
8. Add a small amount of egg white into the basic mixture, incorporate well, then gently fold the rest of the egg into the mixture.
9. Pour a spoonful of the mixture into the mould, then add the soaked biscuit and then the rest of the mixture up to the rim.
10. Cook for about 14 minutes at 200°C in the oven.

This soufflé could be accompanied with a sauceboat of whipped cream with chocolate chips folded into it.

This recipe was contributed by René Pauvert.

Crêpe soufflé

	4 portions	10 portions
soufflé mix		
Crêpes		
flour, white or wholemeal	100 g	250 g
salt	pinch	large pinch
egg	1	2–3
milk, whole or skimmed	250 ml	625 ml
melted butter, margarine or oil	10 g	25 g
oil for frying		
caster sugar to serve		

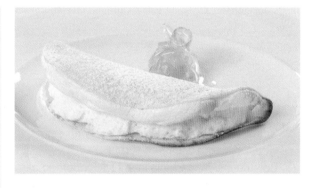

1. Make a batch of under-cooked crêpes by combining the ingredients and shallow frying one at a time.
2. Place the crêpes on a non-stick mat or silicone paper and pipe the soufflé mix (see recipe 5) across half of each crêpe.
3. Fold the remaining half of the crêpe over the soufflé mix and bake at 200°C for 5–6 minutes.
4. Lift carefully onto warmed plates using a palette knife or spatula and dust with icing sugar.
5. Serve with a suitable sauce, e.g. crème anglaise, cream, ice cream or syrup.

8   # Apple strudel

	4–5 portions	8–10 portions
Paste		
strong flour	100 g	200 g
salt	pinch	pinch
egg	1	1
butter, margarine or oil	12 g	25 g
hot water	40 ml	85 ml
icing sugar, for dusting		
Filling		
cooking apples	500 g	1 kg
breadcrumbs (white or brown)	25 g	50 g
butter, margarine or oil	12 g	25 g
brown sugar	50 g	100 g
sultanas	50 g	100 g
raisins	50 g	100 g
ground almonds	25 g	50 g
nibbed almonds	25 g	50 g
lemon, zest and juice of	1	2½
mixed spice	1½ g	3 g
ground cinnamon	1½ g	3 g

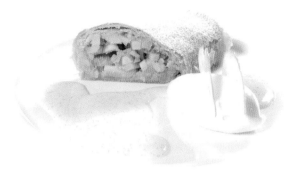

1. First, make the paste: sieve together the flour and salt and make a well in the middle. Place the egg, fat and water in the centre and work until a smooth dough forms.
2. Cover the dough with a damp cloth and relax for 20 minutes.
3. Peel and core the apples. Cut into thin, small slices and place in a basin.
4. Fry the breadcrumbs in the fat. Add to the apples. Add the other filling ingredients and mix well.
5. Roll out the dough in a square ¼ cm thick. Place on a cloth and brush with melted fat or oil.
6. Stretch the dough on the backs of your hands until it is very thin.
7. Spread the filling on the paste to within 1 cm from the edge.
8. With the aid of a cloth, roll up the paste tightly and seal the ends.
9. Place on a lightly greased baking sheet and brush with melted fat or oil.
10. Bake at approx. 190°C for 35–40 minutes.
11. When baked, dust with icing sugar.

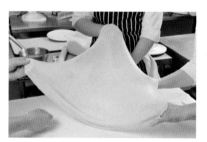
Pulling the dough

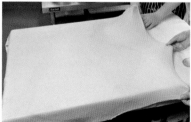
Fully stretched pastry

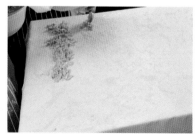
After dusting, adding the filling

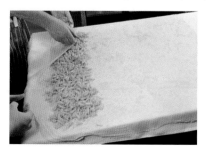
Folding the side in

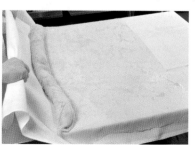
Rolling up in a cloth

9 Brioche pudding

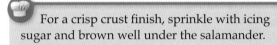

energy	kcal	fat	sat fat	carb	sugar	protein	fibre
1093 KJ	260 cal	11.6 g	5.9 g	30.4 g	23.4 g	10.6 g	1.0 g

	4 portions	10 portions
sultanas	50 g	100 g
slices of brioche	2	5
eggs	3	7
sugar, caster or unrefined	50 g	125 g
vanilla essence or a vanilla pod	2–3 drops	5 drops
milk, whole or skimmed	500 ml	1 ¼ litres

1. Wash the sultanas and place in a pie dish or individual dishes.
2. Remove the crusts from the brioche and cut each slice into four triangles; neatly arrange the triangles so that they are overlapping in the pie dish.
3. Prepare an egg custard: whisk the eggs, sugar and vanilla essence together. Warm the milk and pour it on to the eggs, whisking continuously.
4. Pass through a fine strainer on to the brioche. Dust lightly with sugar.
5. Stand in a roasting tray half full of water and cook slowly in a moderate oven at 160°C for 45 minutes to 1 hour.
6. Clean the edges of the pie dish and serve.

For a crisp crust finish, sprinkle with icing sugar and brown well under the salamander.

For a modern presentation, make individual puddings. Use small moulds instead of a pie dish, and cut discs from a cylindrical brioche mousseline (see page 298).

10 Chocolate fondant

energy	kcal	fat	sat fat	carb	sugar	protein	fibre
2830 KJ	675 cal	46.8 g	29.6 g	55.9 g	40.9 g	11 g	0.6 g

	4 portions	10 portions
chocolate couverture	150 g	375 g
unsalted butter	125 g	312 g
eggs	3	7
egg yolks	2	5
caster sugar	75 g	182 g
flour	75 g	182 g
white chocolate pieces (optional)		

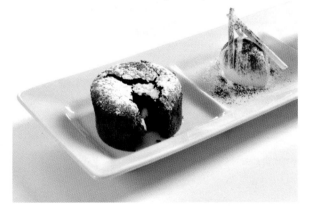

1. Lightly grease and flour individual dariole moulds or a ring mould.
2. Carefully melt the chocolate and butter in a suitable bowl, either in a microwave or over a pan of hot water (bain-marie).
3. In a separate bowl, whisk the eggs, egg yolks and caster sugar until aerated to ribbon stage. Pour into the chocolate and butter mix, then whisk together.
4. Add the flour, then mix until smooth.
5. Pour into the moulds. Place white chocolate pieces at the centre to give a two-tone effect. Bake in the oven at 200°C for 15 minutes.
6. Remove from the oven, leave for 5 minutes before turning out onto suitable plates.
7. Serve with a suitable ice cream (e.g. vanilla, pistachio, almond or Baileys).

11   Griottines (cherries) clafoutis

	Makes 1750 g, 15 portions
griottines (cherries)	105 (approx.)
neige-decor	
Batter 1	
eggs	4
caster sugar	80 g
milk	360 ml
kirsch, from the griottines	4 tsp
flour	80 g
Batter 2	
plain chocolate	400 g
butter	200 g
eggs	4
flour	20 g
cornflour	20 g
caster sugar	70 g

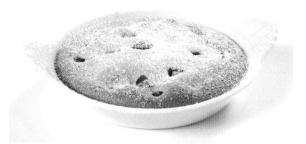

For batter 1

1. In a large bowl, beat the eggs and sugar together until well dissolved, add the milk and kirsch.
2. Sieve in the flour, mix well, then strain the batter through a sieve and set aside.

For batter 2

1. Melt the chocolate and butter in a bowl placed over a pan of simmering water on a low heat.

Meanwhile, place the eggs in a mixing bowl or a mixer with a whisk attachment and whisk to a thick white foam.

2. Switch the machine to the slowest speed, add both flours and mix for 30–60 seconds. Stir the chocolate and butter together, then use a hand whisk to fold this mixture into the whisked egg mixture, ensuring total incorporation.

To make the clafoutis

1. Place the griottines liberally into flat dishes (sur le plat dishes, approx. 10 cm). Cover with the batter.
2. Bake at 200°C for approx. 15 minutes until the batter has risen and set.
3. Serve warm, dusted with neige-decor.

12   Chocolate mousse

	12 portions
stock syrup at 30° baumé	125 ml
egg yolks, pasteurised	80 ml
bitter couverture	250 g
leaf gelatine	2
whipping cream, whipped	500 ml

1. If using leaf gelatine, soak in cold water.
2. Boil the syrup (see page 374).
3. Place the yolks into the bowl of a food processor. Pour over the boiling syrup and whisk until thick. Remove from the machine.
4. Drain the gelatine, melt it and fold it into the chocolate sabayon mixture.
5. Add all the couverture at once, and fold it in quickly.
6. Add all the whipped cream at once, and fold it in carefully.
7. Place the mixture into prepared moulds. Refrigerate or freeze immediately.

The gelatine makes sure the mousse will keep its shape when unmoulded. If serving the mousse in the mould, omit the gelatine.

13 Raspberry or strawberry mousse (bavarois)

energy	kcal	fat	sat fat	carb	sugar	protein	fibre
1102 KJ	265 cal	17.7 g	10.0 g	19.0 g	19.0 g	8.5 g	0.6 g	*

	4 portions	10 portions
gelatine	10 g	25 g
egg yolks	2	5
sugar, caster or unrefined	50 g	125 g
milk, whole, semi-skimmed or skimmed	180 ml	500 ml
raspberries or strawberries (picked, washed and sieved)	200 g	500 g
whipping or double cream or non-dairy cream	125 ml	300 ml

1. If using leaf gelatine, soak in cold water.
2. Cream the egg yolks and sugar in a bowl until almost white.
3. Bring the milk to the boil in a thick-based saucepan. Whisk the milk into the egg yolks and sugar mixture; mix well.
4. Clean the milk saucepan and return the mixture to it.
5. Return to a low heat and stir continuously with a wooden spoon until the mixture coats the back of the spoon. The mixture must not boil.
6. Remove from the heat; add the (drained) gelatine and stir until dissolved.
7. Pass through a fine strainer into a clean bowl, leave in a cool place, stirring occasionally until almost at setting point.
8. When the custard is almost cool, add the fruit purée.
9. Fold in the lightly beaten cream.
10. Pour the mixture into a mould or individual moulds (which may be very lightly greased with almond oil).
11. Allow to set in the refrigerator.
12. Shake and turn out on to a flat dish or plates.
13. Decorate with whole fruit and whipped cream.

Using whole milk and whipping cream.

14 Orange mousse with biscuit jaconde

	6 portions
Chocolate paste	
butter, soft	40 g
icing sugar	40 g
egg whites	40 g
flour	30 g
cocoa powder	15 g
Sponge	
soft flour	50 g
ground almonds	125 g
eggs	5 (250 g)
icing sugar	190 g
orange zest, grated	1
egg whites	190 g
caster sugar	25 g
butter, melted	35 g
cocoa butter	
Orange mousse	
orange juice	200 g
egg whites, pasteurised	30 g

caster sugar	30 g
gelatine, soaked in ice water	2 leaves
lemon juice	few drops
whipping cream	225 g
orange segments, to garnish	
Glaze (jelly)	
stock syrup (see page 374)	50 ml
gelatine, pre-soaked and drained	1 leaf
orange juice	100 ml

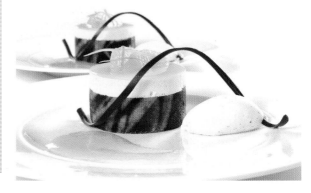

To make the biscuit jaconde

1. Make up the chocolate paste by combining the ingredients. Spread over a silicone mat and mark with a pattern. Freeze.
2. Sieve the flour and ground almonds onto paper.
3. Warm the whole eggs, icing sugar and orange zest. Whisk them to the ribbon stage.
4. Whisk the egg whites and sugar to stiff peaks.
5. Fold both the egg mixtures into the flour and almonds, then fold in the melted butter.
6. Spread over the frozen chocolate paste. Bake immediately at 230°C.
7. Allow to cool, then remove the silicone mat. Spray with cocoa butter.
8. Line individual rings with the sponge to ¾ height. Place a disc of sponge in the base of each ring.

To make the orange mousse

1. Reduce the orange juice by half.
2. Whisk the egg whites and half of the sugar over a bain-marie until firm peaks form (this is Swiss meringue). Remove from the heat and whisk in the rest of the sugar.
3. Drain the gelatine and dissolve it in the reduced orange juice. Add a few drops of lemon juice.
4. Fold the meringue into the juice, then fold in the cream.
5. Fill the lined moulds to the top and level off.
6. Chill to set.
7. To make the glaze, heat the stock syrup. Add the gelatine and stir until it dissolves. Add the orange juice and pass through a muslin.
8. When the mousses are cold, spoon the glaze over the top. Return to the fridge to set.
9. Unmould and decorate with orange segments.

15 Vanilla bavarois

energy	kcal	fat	sat fat	carb	sugar	protein	fibre	
970 KJ	231 cal	18.2 g	10.9 g	11.8 g	11.8 g	5.8 g	0.0 g	*

	6–8 portions
gelatine	10 g
egg yolks	2
caster sugar	50 g
milk, whole or skimmed	250 ml
vanilla pod or vanilla essence	
whipping or double cream or non-dairy cream	125 ml

1. If using leaf gelatine, soak in cold water.
2. Cream the yolks and sugar in a bowl until almost white.
3. Whisk in the milk, which has been brought to the boil with the vanilla pod or a few drops of vanilla essence; mix well.
4. Clean the milk saucepan, which should be a thick-based one, and return the mixture to it.
5. Return to a low heat and stir continuously with a wooden spoon until the mixture coats the back of the spoon. The mixture must not boil.
6. Remove from the heat; add the (drained) gelatine and stir until dissolved.
7. Pass through a fine strainer into a clean bowl, leave in a cool place, stirring occasionally until almost at setting point.
8. Fold in the lightly beaten cream.
9. Pour the mixture into a mould or individual moulds (which may be very lightly greased with almond oil).
10. Allow to set in the refrigerator.
11. Shake and turn out onto a flat dish or plates.
12. Decorate with vanilla-flavoured, sweetened cream.

* Using whole milk and whipping cream.

16 Rice bavarois (Empress rice)

	12 portions
Topping	
gelatine, soaked in ice water	3 leaves
stock syrup (see page 374)	200 ml
raspberry purée	200 ml
Bavarois	
milk	750 ml
vanilla pod (or use essence)	½
Carolina rice, washed	85 g
gelatine, soaked in ice water until limp	5½ leaves
caster sugar	165 g
salpicon (small dice) of glacé fruits	75 g
whipping cream, ¾ whipped	340 ml
To decorate	
raspberries	12
Chantilly cream	
moulded chocolate	

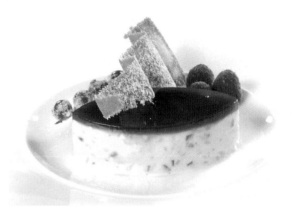

1. To make the topping, drain the gelatine. Boil the stock syrup and add the gelatine and raspberry purée. Stir over ice.
2. Pour the topping into the bottom of individual (7 cm) rings, to a depth of 3 mm. Set in the fridge.
3. Boil the milk with the vanilla. Rain in the washed rice. Cover and simmer until the rice is tender.
4. Drain the gelatine and mix with the caster sugar.
5. Remove the rice from the heat and add the sugar and gelatine. Mix well.
6. Place in a large bowl and stir over ice. When the mixture begins to gel, fold in the salpicon of glacé fruits, then the whipped cream.
7. Pour into the moulds and allow to set in the fridge overnight.
8. Unmould onto plates and decorate.

Variation: Maltaise rice

Follow the recipe above with the following changes:
- Use orange juice instead of raspberry purée for the topping.
- Instead of vanilla, boil two cubes of orange sugar with the juice of 1 orange and 30 ml of Grand Marnier – use this to flavour the milk.
- Use glacé orange instead of mixed fruits.
- Decorate with orange segments.

17 Banana, coffee and rum gratin

	12–16 portions
dark rum	100 ml
bananas	500 g
caster sugar	75–100 g
Genoese sponge, 1 cm thick	1 sheet
pastry cream, beaten	500 g
coffee essence	
double cream, whipped	500 g
dark muscavado sugar	30 g

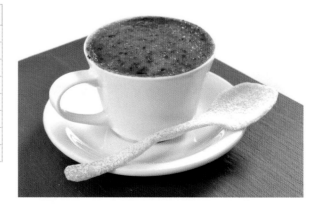

1. Macerate (soak) the rum, bananas and caster sugar together for 1 hour.
2. Place the sponge into the base of the dish or individual cups or moulds (cut to fit).
3. Spoon in the banana mixture.
4. Carefully blend the pastry cream, coffee essence and whipped double cream to form a *crème*

diplomat. Completely cover the banana mixture with this, and fill the dish to the top.
5. Sprinkle with muscavado sugar.
6. Place in the oven at 230°C for 2 minutes, then finish under the salamander to glaze.
7. Serve with an edible spoon made from tuile mixture.

18 Strawberry Charlotte

	6 portions
sponge	
biscuit à la cuillère	
kirsch syrup (½ kirsch, ½ syrup)	200 ml
strawberry mousse	
strawberries, diced	100 g
whipping cream, half whipped	200 ml
small strawberries, halved, to garnish	12

Make up the strawberry mousse using the instructions for orange mousse in recipe 14. Use strawberry purée instead of orange juice and do not reduce it.

1. Line the inside of a cake hoop with a strip of biscuit à la cuillère to three-quarters of the height of the hoop.
2. Place a disc of sponge inside the hoop to form a base. Moisten the sponge with kirsch syrup.
3. Fold the diced strawberries into the strawberry mousse.
4. Half fill the ring with mousse. Place a second disc of sponge on top.
5. Fill ring to the top with mousse and level off.
6. Allow to set in the fridge for at least 12 hours.
7. Spread the top with cream. Make a pattern using a serrated knife.
8. Remove the cake hoop. Garnish with strawberry halves.

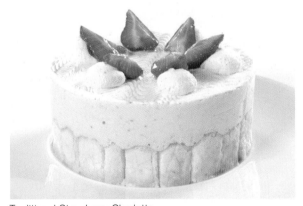
Traditional Strawberry Charlotte

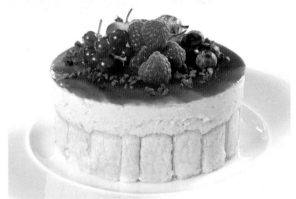
Modern Strawberry Charlotte

19 Blackcurrant delice (*miroir au cassis*)

	24 portions
vanilla sponge discs	4
cassis syrup	250 ml
gelatine, soaked in ice water	10 leaves
cassis liqueur	66 g
blackcurrant purée	666 g
Italian meringue	340 g
whipping cream, ¾ whipped	666 g
Glaze	
stock syrup at 30° baumé (density 1.2624)	150 ml
gelatine, soaked in ice water	3 leaves
blackcurrant purée	150 ml

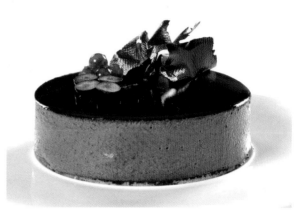

1. Place two stainless steel torten rings on a board. Place a sponge disc inside each to form a base.
2. Moisten the sponge with cassis syrup.
3. Drain the gelatine. Warm it with the cassis liqueur and one quarter of the blackcurrant purée until the gelatine has dissolved.
4. Add the rest of the blackcurrant purée. Fold this mixture into the Italian meringue (see recipe 3).
5. Fold in the whipped cream.
6. Half fill each ring with the mousse mixture. Place a smaller sponge disc on top of the filling and moisten it with syrup.
7. Fill to the top with more mousse. Level the top.
8. Allow to set in the fridge.
9. To make the glaze, warm the syrup. Add the gelatine and stir until it dissolves.
10. Add the blackcurrant purée. Pass through a fine chinois.
11. Carefully mask the top of each delice with the glaze. Allow to set in the fridge.
12. Carefully remove the rings. Garnish with blackcurrants *en branche*.

20 Tiramisu torte

	Makes 2 (12 portions)
biscuit or sponge bases	4
egg yolks, pasteurised	60 g
sugar	150 g
gelatine	3 leaves
mascarpone cheese	600 g
double cream	200 g
coffee syrup	100 ml
rum	40 ml
cocoa powder	

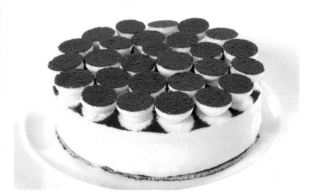

1. Cut the biscuit or sponge bases into shape: cut two to the size of the flan ring, and two to the same shape, but slightly smaller.
2. Mix the egg yolks and sugar. Cook over a bain-marie to 75°C, to form a sabayon.
3. Soak the gelatine in iced water. Drain and add it to the sabayon.
4. Beat the cheese well. Add the sabayon.

5. Lightly whip the cream and fold it into the mixture.

6. Place a large biscuit or sponge base into each flan ring, on a board. Soak the base with a mixture of coffee syrup and rum.

7. Half fill each ring with the cheese mixture.

8. Place the smaller circles of biscuit or sponge on top of the filling. Again, soak with syrup and rum.

9. Fill the rest of the ring with the cheese mixture, to a level top.

10. Chill in the fridge until set.

11. Decorate with small meringues and dust with cocoa powder.

21 Raspberry and chocolate truffle cake

	Makes 3 (36 portions)
chocolate Génoise	1 sheet
Mousse	
dark chocolate, melted	600 g
caster sugar	300 g
water	100 ml
glucose (boiled to 118°C)	1 'blob' the size of a large marble
eggs	4
egg yolks	6
gelatine, soaked in cold water	10 leaves
raspberry purée	750 ml
double cream, whipped	900 ml
Glaze	
stock syrup	250 ml
raspberry purée	250 ml
gelatine, soaked in ice-cold water	5 leaves

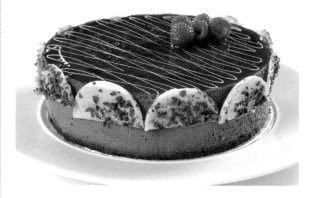

1. To make the mousse, melt the chocolate over a bain-marie. Boil the sugar, water and glucose until they reach 118°C.

2. Meanwhile, put the eggs and yolks in a food processor and start mixing. When the sugar reaches the required temperature, pour it over the eggs and whisk until thick and cold. Melt the gelatine in 100 ml of the raspberry purée, strain; add to the egg mixture and take out of the machine.

3. Fold in the chocolate followed by the rest of the raspberry purée and the whipped cream.

4. Line the ring with the sponge, soak with some stock syrup, and fill up with the mousse, level off and freeze.

5. To make the glaze, bring half the syrup to the boil and pour into a bowl. Squeeze the water from the soaked gelatine and dissolve in the heated syrup. Add the remaining syrup and the raspberry purée, and allow to cool.

6. To serve, pour the glaze over the top and leave to set. Turn out with a blow torch. Decorate with chocolate and raspberries.

22 Baked apple cheesecake

	16 portions		cream cheese, full fat	800 g
Base			caster sugar	230 g
biscuit crumbs	225 g		cornflour	75 g
butter, melted	110 g		eggs	2 (120 g)
caster sugar	30 g		vanilla arome or essence	
Filling			double cream	290 ml
apples, cooked, halved	approx. 8			

1. Combine the ingredients for the base. Press the mixture into the bottom of two lined cake tins.
2. Place the cooked apple halves into the tins.
3. Cream the cheese and sugar together. Stir in the cornflour, eggs, vanilla and double cream.
4. Divide the filling between the two tins.
5. Bake at 160°C for approximately 40 minutes.
6. Allow to cool slightly, then remove from the mould and dust with icing sugar. Decorate with apple crisps.

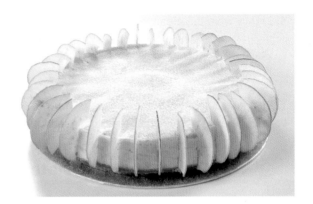

23 Strawberry floating island (*iles flottantes*)

	12 portions
Compote	
strawberries	500 g
caster sugar	50 g
champagne	250 ml
Anglaise	
vanilla pods, split	3
double cream	750 ml
egg yolks	240 ml
caster sugar	160 g
Poached meringue	
egg whites	250 ml
caster sugar	500 g
lemon juice	2 drops

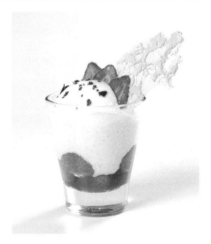

To make the compote

1. Cut any large strawberries in half.
2. Place all the fruit in a clean pan and sprinkle with caster sugar.
3. Stir over heat until hot and starting to produce liquid.
4. Douse with champagne and chill over ice.

To make the anglaise

1. To make the anglaise, add the split vanilla pods to the cream. Bring to the boil slowly.
2. Whisk the egg yolks and sugar together.
3. Pour half the boiling cream over the egg yolk mixture.
4. Return this to the pan of cream. Cook to 84°C.
5. Pass and chill over ice.

To make the poached meringue

1. Whisk the egg whites and 125 g of the sugar at a medium speed until soft peaks form.
2. Increase the speed and rain in 250 g of the sugar.
3. Fold in the remaining sugar by hand.
4. Pipe or spoon into prepared spherical moulds, or form into quenelles using spoons. Poach in a bain-marie until firm.

To serve

1. Fill glasses with a layer of compote followed by a layer of anglaise.
2. Top each glass with a meringue.
3. Garnish with pink bubble sugar.

24   Unmoulded *crème brûlée* with spiced fruit compote

	16 portions
Crème brûlée	
whipping cream	750 g
milk	250 g
vanilla pods	2
egg yolks, fresh	300 g
caster sugar	150 g
demerara sugar for sprinkling	
Spiced fruit compote	
plums	500 g
peaches	500 g
star anise	2
vanilla pods	2
cinnamon sticks	2
cloves	2
caster sugar	
red wine	
stock syrup	

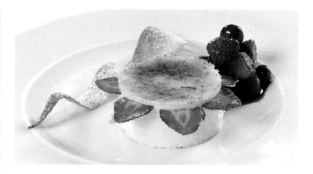

To make the *crème brûlée*

1. Prepare individual stainless steel rings: cover the bases with 2 layers of cling film and bake them to seal.
2. Boil the cream, milk and vanilla pods.
3. Whisk the egg yolks and sugar together.
4. Pour the boiling liquid onto the egg mixture. Pass, then stir well.
5. Using a dropper, pour into the prepared rings. Bake in a fan oven at 100°C for 30 minutes.
6. Thoroughly chill. Unmould onto plates.
7. Sprinkle demerara sugar on top and caramelise.
8. Serve with chilled fruit compote.

To make the compote

1. Butter a deep roasting tray.
2. Cut up the fruit and break up the spices.
3. Spread the fruit and spices over the tray. Sprinkle with caster sugar and wine.
4. Roast in a moderate oven until the fruit starts to soften.
5. Carefully remove the fruit. Deglaze the pan with more wine and a little stock syrup (see page 374).
6. Pass the sauce back onto the fruit. Chill.

25   Chocolate ice cream

Ice cream base

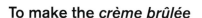

	Makes 760 g
cream	250 ml
milk	250 ml
egg yolks	100 g
glucose	20 g
trimoline	40 g
sugar	100 g

1. Bring the cream and milk to the boil together.
2. Mix the egg yolks, glucose, trimoline and sugar together until smooth.
3. Pour the cream over the egg mixture while whisking.
4. Return to the stove and cook until it coats the back of a spoon.
5. Pass. Mix in flavouring at this point (see below for chocolate) and chill in an ice bain-marie.
6. When cooled, churn, then freeze.

Chocolate ice cream

	12 portions
ice cream base (see above)	550 ml
plain chocolate, in pieces	125 g
chocolate chips (optional)	

1. Make the ice cream base as described above. While it is still hot, add the chocolate pieces. Mix until combined.
2. Chill, then churn.
3. Fold in chocolate chips if required. Store in a freezer at −18°C.

26 Malt ice cream and caramel sauce

	12 portions
milk	400 ml
inverted sugar, e.g. trimoline, staboline	100 g
Horlicks	150 g
egg yolks, pasteurised	120 g
caster sugar	100 g
Jersey or double cream	400 ml
Caramel sauce	
Carnation condensed milk	200 ml

1. Bring the milk and inverted sugar to the boil together. Whisk in the Horlicks until dissolved.
2. Whisk the egg yolks and sugar together until white.
3. Add half the boiling milk to the eggs, then return all to the saucepan. Cook well without allowing the mixture to boil.
4. Add the cream and cool over ice. Churn until frozen and set.
5. To make the sauce, place the condensed milk in a double boiler with a lid. Bring the water to the boil and cook gently for 40 to 50 minutes, stirring occasionally.
6. When the sauce is thick, with a light caramel colour, remove from the heat. Beat until smooth.

i Horlicks is a commercial powdered drink, widely available.

27 American orange ice cream

	8–10 portions
milk	300 ml
caster sugar	250 g
stabiliser	200 g
orange rind	
lemon rind	
orange juice	250 ml
lemon juice	10 ml
single cream	250 ml

1. Slowly bring the milk, sugar, stabiliser and rinds to the boil.
2. Remove from the heat and leave to cool. When cold, add the juice and cream.
3. Pass, then churn in an ice cream machine.
4. Place into a frozen container, seal and freeze.

28 Grapefruit water ice

	8–10 portions
water	250 ml
sugar	100 g
grapefruit juice	250 ml
orange juice	100 ml
white wine	25 ml
lemon (juice of)	1
stabiliser	50 g

1. Bring the water and sugar to the boil.
2. Add the rest of the ingredients, mix well and cool.
3. Churn and place into a frozen container.
4. Freeze until required.

Vanilla sorbet

	4 portions
water	255 ml
caster sugar	110 g
glucose	25 g
vanilla pod, scraped	1

1. Mix all the ingredients together and bring to the boil. Allow to cool fully.
2. Pass and then churn.

Lemon sorbet

	12 portions
lemon juice	250 ml
water	250 ml
milk	250 ml
caster sugar	300 g

1. Bring all the ingredients together and heat to dissolve the sugar.
2. Pass, cool and churn.

Bombe (individual)

	16 portions
egg yolks, pasteurised	120 g
water	100 ml
sugar	150 g
glucose	10 g
fruit purée (e.g. strawberry, raspberry, mango)	230 g
liqueur	10 ml
whipped cream	800 ml

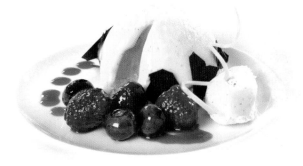

1. Line the outside of a frozen bombe mould (semi-spherical mould) with ice cream or sorbet. Fill the centre with *pâté à bombe*, as follows (steps 2 to 5).
2. Whisk the egg yolks.
3. Boil the water, sugar and glucose to 120°C.
4. Pour over the yolks and continue whisking until cold.
5. Fold in the fruit purée, liqueur and whipped cream.
6. Pour into lined bombe mould. Cover and freeze.

Examples

Ice cream/ sorbet lining	*Pâté à bombe* filling	Classical name
Apricot	Vanilla	Andalouse
Pineapple	Strawberry	Creole
Strawberry	Kirsch	Aida
Orange	Praline	Fedora
Vanilla	Rum/glacé fruits	Frou-Frou

32 Raspberry parfait

	6–8 portions
egg yolks, pasteurised	80 g
caster sugar	60 g
gelatine, soaked	1½ leaves
raspberry liqueur	10 ml
lemon juice	10 ml
raspberry purée	120 g
whipped cream	150 ml
Italian meringue	
egg whites	200 g
water	80 ml
glucose	20 g
caster sugar	150 g

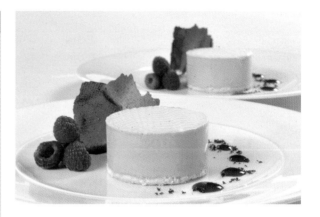

1. Make up the Italian meringue (see recipe 3 for instructions).
2. Combine the egg yolks and caster sugar in a stainless steel bowl. Whisk over a bain-marie to make a sabayon.
3. Drain the gelatine and dissolve it in the liqueur and lemon juice.
4. Fold the gelatine mixture into the sabayon, then fold in the raspberry purée.
5. Fold in half the Italian meringue, then fold in the whipped cream.
6. Place into prepared moulds and freeze.

33 Orange and Cointreau iced soufflé

	8 portions
oranges (juice and zest)	3
whipping cream, half whipped	800 ml
egg yolks	100 g
caster sugar	75 g
gelatine, soaked in cold water	2 leaves
Cointreau	20 ml
oranges (juice only)	8 (400 ml)
Italian meringue	
caster sugar	100 g
glucose	10 g
water	80 ml
egg whites	100 g

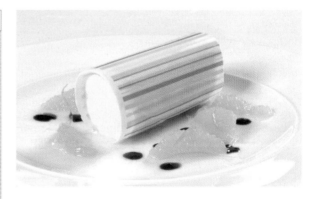

1. Use a microplane grater or similar to zest three oranges. Bring a small pan of water to the boil, add the zest and simmer for 5 minutes. Refresh the zest in cold water and reserve.
2. Juice all the oranges (11 in total). Measure the juice; pass and reduce until you have 200 ml. Leave to cool.
3. Whip the cream to soft peaks and chill.
4. Make a sabayon by whisking the egg yolks and sugar over a bain-marie until the mixture reaches 75°C. Mix the sabayon until it goes cold.
5. Make the Italian meringue by carefully boiling the sugar, glucose and water in a clean stainless steel pan until it reaches 120°C. Whisk the egg whites until they form soft peaks. Pour the sugar mixture onto the whites gradually and keep mixing until the meringue is tepid.
6. Drain and melt the gelatine. Heat it in the Cointreau with the orange zest and reduced juice until it becomes a liquid. Pass.
7. Fold the gelatine into the sabayon.

8. Fold the Italian meringue into the sabayon mixture, then fold in the cream.
9. Line the mould and fill it with the mixture. Freeze overnight.

The chocolate wrap

The iced soufflé shown in the photo is wrapped in white chocolate.
1. Spread tempered white chocolate very thinly onto a patterned acetate.

2. Cut to shape, curl and fasten with a paper clip.
3. Once set, remove the clip and peel away the acetate. The chocolate will retain the curled shape and the coloured pattern.

> *i* A microplane grater is a very efficient, hand-held grater, especially useful for zesting citrus fruit.
>
> Patterned acetate sheets for chocolate work are available in many colours and designs.

34 Chocolate sauce

	Makes ½ litre
Method 1	
double cream	175 g
butter	40 g
milk or plain chocolate pieces	225 g
Method 2	
caster sugar	40 g
water	120 ml
dark chocolate (75% cocoa solids)	160 g
unsalted butter	25 g
single cream	80 ml

Method 1

1. Place the cream and butter in a saucepan and gently bring to a simmer.
2. Add the chocolate and stir well until the chocolate has melted and the sauce is smooth.

Method 2

1. Dissolve the sugar in the water over a low heat.
2. Remove from the heat. Stir in the chocolate and butter.
3. When everything has melted, stir in the cream and gently bring to the boil.

35 Fruit coulis (boiled sugar)

	Makes 1500 ml
fruit purée	1 litre
caster sugar	500 g
water	200 ml
glucose	50 g

1. Warm the purée.
2. Boil the sugar with the water and glucose to soft ball stage (121°C).

3. Pour the soft ball sugar into the warm fruit purée while whisking vigorously.
4. Bring back to the boil, then cool. This will then be ready to store.

> *i* The reason the soft ball is achieved and mixed with the purée is that this stabilises the fruit and prevents separation once the coulis has been put onto the plate.

36 Fruit coulis (pectin)

	Makes 1.3 litres
orange juice	1 litre
sugar	300 g
pectin	10 g

1. Bring the orange juice to the boil with 200 g of sugar.
2. Mix the remaining sugar and pectin together.
3. When the orange juice is boiled, add the sugar and pectin mixture.
4. Re-boil, chill and use as required.

37 Butterscotch sauce

	Makes 500 ml
butter	125 g
soft brown sugar	125 g
golden syrup	125 g
vanilla pod, split	2
lemon juice	1 lemon
double cream	175 ml

1. Place the butter, brown sugar, golden syrup and vanilla pod in a small saucepan. Bring to a gentle simmer.
2. Remove from the heat and add the lemon juice to taste.
3. Stir in the double cream.
4. Remove the vanilla pod and serve hot.

38 Caramel e'spuma

	Makes approx. 600 ml
yoghurt	250 g
cream	50 g
milk	100 g
caramel sauce	166 g
icing sugar	104 g

1. Mix all ingredients together.
2. Pour into an e'spuma gun and charge with two gas cartridges.

i An e'spuma is usually dispensed from the gun into individual glasses. The e'spuma gun is also known as a siphon.

39 Hot chocolate e'spuma

	Makes 650 g
milk chocolate	300 g
dark chocolate	50 g
white chocolate	100 g
hot water	200 g

1. Melt the three types of chocolate over a bain-marie until at 45°C.
2. Add the hot water and whisk until smooth.
3. Pour mix into an e'spuma gun and charge with two cartridges.
4. Place in a bain-marie to keep warm.

40 Pernod foam

	Makes 800 ml
skimmed milk	450 ml
sugar	170 g
leaf gelatine, pre-soaked	3 leaves
Pernod	160 g

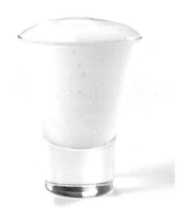

1. Boil the milk and sugar. Add the pre-soaked gelatine leaves and allow them to dissolve.
2. Allow the mixture to cool.
3. Add the Pernod.
4. Pour into an e'spuma siphon and charge with 2 cartridges. Refrigerate.
5. Once chilled, shake well before using.

41 Coconut foam

	Makes 400 ml
coconut purée, e.g. boiron	250 g
sugar	50 g
double cream	100 g

1. Blitz the ingredients together.
2. Place in an e'spuma gun and chill.

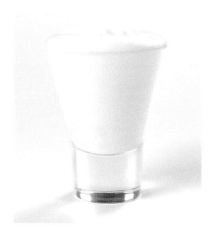

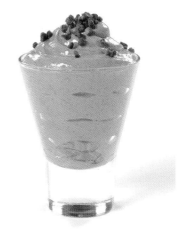

Example of a fruit foam: raspberry

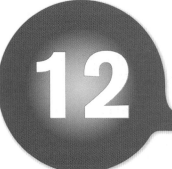

Biscuits, cakes and sponges

This chapter covers Unit 312: Produce Biscuits, Cakes and Sponges.

In this unit, you will learn:

1. how to produce biscuits, cakes and sponges
2. how to finish and evaluate biscuits, cakes and sponges.

For information about the key commodities used in many of these dishes, refer to Chapter 8.

Batters and whisked sponges

Batters and sponges allow us to make a large assortment of desserts and cakes. Basically, they are a mix of eggs, sugar, flour, and sometimes butter, and the air incorporated when these are beaten. Certain other raw materials can be combined – for example, almonds, hazelnuts, walnuts, chocolate, fruit, ginger, anise, coffee and vanilla.

Sponge cakes

When preparing light batters, specifically for sponge cakes, the aim is to achieve a spongy, honeycombed effect. This goal is reached when the eggs are beaten with sugar, which causes small air bubbles to form. These are held in place by the fat in the eggs while other ingredients are added.

Once in the oven, these bubbles expand and increase the volume of the batter. Then, after some time in the oven, the egg congeals because of the heat, giving the batter the desired consistency.

There are two methods for making sponge cakes: whole egg mixes and separated egg mixes. In the direct process, whole eggs are beaten. In the indirect one, yolks and whites are beaten separately; this yields a lighter sponge cake but makes it less dense and elastic.

What you need to know about sponge cakes

- You should never add flour or ground dry ingredients to a batter until the end because they impede the air absorption in the first beating stage.
- When making sponge cakes, we must always sift the dry ingredients (flour, cocoa powder, ground nuts, etc.) to avoid clumping.

- Fold in the flour as quickly and delicately as possible, because a rough addition of dry ingredients acts like a weight on the primary batter and can remove part of the air already absorbed.
- Flours used in sponge cakes are low in gluten content. In certain sponge cakes, a portion of the flour can be left out and substituted with cornstarch. This yields a softer and more aerated batter.
- The eggs used in sponge cake batters should be fresh and at room temperature so that they take in air faster.
- Adding separately beaten egg whites produces a lighter and fluffier sponge cake.
- Once sponge cake batters are beaten and poured into moulds or baking trays, they should be baked as soon as possible. Otherwise, the batter loses volume.

Marzipan

Most marzipan that is used today for culinary purposes is produced by large manufacturers. Much of this is of high quality, made from sweet and bitter almonds.

There are two distinct types of almond: hard- or soft-shelled. The hard-shelled types are grown in Italy, Sicily, Spain, Majorca and other European countries. Their kernels are sweeter and more tender than those of the soft-shelled type, which are grown in California.

Sugar and water is added to the almonds and this is refined to a smooth paste through granite rollers and then roasted. The paste is then cooled before packing ready for use. Almond pastes are made from this marzipan by the addition of sugar and glucose.

Hard granulated sugar and egg white is added to the almond paste to produce commercial macaroon paste.

1   Spiced hazelnut shortbread

	Makes 50 pieces (2.3 kg)
butter	500 g
icing sugar	375 g
pulp from split vanilla pod	1
eggs	2
soft flour	750 g
clove powder	5 g
hazelnuts, whole	250 g
hazelnuts, chopped	250 g
For dusting	
caster sugar	25 g
clove powder	5 g
ground cinnamon	5 g

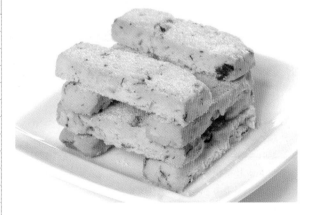

1. Cream the butter and icing sugar together, with the vanilla pulp. Work very lightly and do not over-mix.
2. Add the eggs to the mixture, one at a time.
3. Sieve the flour and clove powder. Add to the butter mixture. Add the whole and chopped hazelnuts. Mix together.

4. Press into a plastic tray covered with cling film. The layer should be about ½ cm thick. Refrigerate overnight.
5. Cut into batons 5 × 1.5 cm.
6. Bake at 180°C.
7. While still hot, dust the shortbread with a mixture of caster sugar, clove powder and ground cinnamon.

Chocolate Genoese

	Makes 2 × 16 cm
eggs	8
caster sugar	225 g
dark chocolate	50 g
flour	175 g
cocoa powder	50 g
melted butter	65 g

1. Whisk the eggs and sugar together to form a sabayon, then incorporate the melted chocolate.
2. Slowly fold in the flour and cocoa powder, followed by the melted butter.
3. Place in a lined mould and bake at 180°C for 15–20 minutes.

Make sure you have prepared all the equipment before you start.

Flourless chocolate sponge

	Makes 2 × 16 cm cake tins or 1 large silicone sheet
egg yolks	11
caster sugar	125 g
cocoa powder	90 g
egg whites	11
sugar	175 g

1. Whisk the yolks and caster sugar until it becomes a sabayon.
2. Fold in the sieved cocoa powder.
3. Make cold meringue with the egg whites and sugar. Fold in.
4. Bake at 180–200°C in a deck oven.

This sponge is used for gâteaux, pastries and lining sweets. It may be useful to cater for someone on a wheat-free diet.

Roulade sponge

whole eggs	900 ml
egg yolks	5
caster sugar	510 g
soft flour	340 g

1. Whisk the eggs, yolks and sugar by hand over boiling water until warm.
2. Whisk in a planetary mixer until the ribbon stage.
3. Sieve the flour onto paper.
4. Preheat the oven to 230°C.

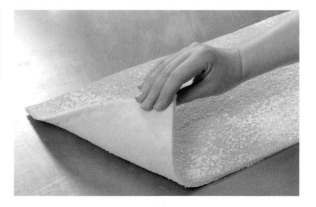

5. Fold the flour into the egg mixture as quickly and lightly as possible (ask someone else to help).
6. Divide the mixture between two prepared baking sheets, as quickly as possible. Spread evenly.
7. Bake for 5–7 minutes.
8. Cool completely.
9. Cut the sheets in halves.
10. To store, wrap individually in cling film and freeze, making sure they are not bent or squashed.

5   Patterned jaconde sponge

	Makes 2 sheets
Decorating paste (nature)	
butter, soft	200 g
icing sugar	200 g
colouring (optional)	
egg whites	105 g
soft flour	100 g
Decorating paste (chocolate)	
butter, soft	80 g
icing sugar	80 g
egg whites	80 g
soft flour	60 g
cocoa powder	30 g
Jaconde sponge	
ground almonds	250 g
soft flour	100 g
egg whites	375 ml
caster sugar	50 g
eggs	500 ml
icing sugar	375 g
butter, melted	75 g

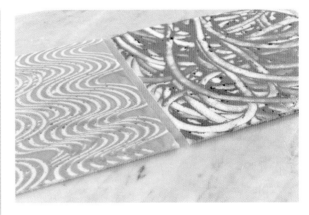

1. Make up a decorating paste (nature, coloured or chocolate) by creaming the butter and sugar until light and white (with colouring if required). Add the egg whites gradually while beating. Stir in the flour (and cocoa powder for chocolate paste).
2. Spread the paste evenly and thinly (1 to 2 mm) on a silicone mat. Mark with a pattern. Set in a freezer or fridge: the mat must be flat.
3. To make the jaconde sponge, sieve the almonds and flour onto paper.
4. Whisk the egg whites and sugar into a meringue.
5. Whisk the eggs and icing sugar together to the ribbon stage.
6. Fold the flour, meringue and egg mixture together. Finally, fold in the melted butter.
7. Spread over the patterned paste – it must have set first, so make sure it will be ready when needed.
8. Bake at 230°C for 6 minutes.

This sponge is used as a base for desserts and petits fours, a wrap for desserts, and for layering gâteaux and pastries.

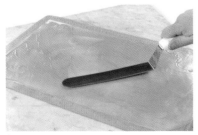
Spreading the cigarette mixture

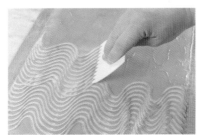
Making the pattern

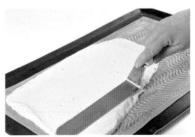
Spreading the layer of sponge over the pattern

6 | Dobos torte

	Makes 1 × 20 cm (12 portions)
Biscuit paste	
butter	120 g
icing sugar	120 g
vanilla arome or essence	a few drops
eggs	2
soft flour	120 g
Chocolate buttercream	
eggs, pasteurised	3
granulated sugar	175 g
water	150 ml
unsalted butter, small cubes	340 g
dark chocolate couverture, to taste	
Caramel	
water	100 ml
granulated sugar	250 g
glucose	25 g

1. Make up the biscuit paste by creaming the butter and sugar together with the vanilla. Beat in the eggs, then fold in the flour.
2. Spread the paste on a silicone mat and bake at 180°C until lightly coloured.
3. Cut out 7 evenly sized discs of paste.
4. To make the buttercream, whisk the eggs. Boil the sugar and water together to 118°C. Pour onto the eggs and whisk until just warm.
5. Add the cubes of butter gradually. Add couverture to taste.
6. To make the caramel, boil the ingredients together to 160°C. Leave to stand.
7. Take 6 discs of paste and layer them with buttercream between each layer.
8. Coat the top and sides with buttercream. Smooth the top and comb scrape the sides. Mask the bottom edge with grated chocolate.
9. Coat the remaining disc of paste with caramel and allow to set. Cut into segments. Pipe bulbs of buttercream on top of the torte and place a segment on each bulb.

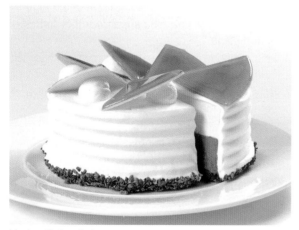

Modern Dobos torte

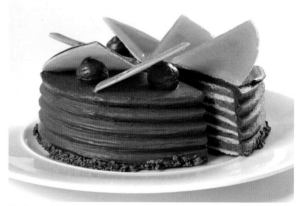

Traditional Dobos torte

7 Sachertorte

	Makes 2
butter, cut into pieces	280 g
vanilla essence	
caster sugar	310 g
egg yolks	12
dark chocolate couverture, melted	350 g
egg whites	16
plain flour	210 g
cocoa powder	70 g
apricot jam	100 g
chocolate glaze (recipe 21)	

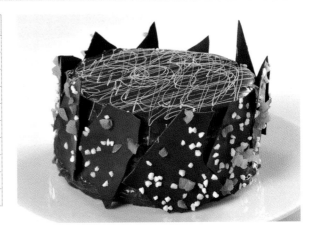

1. Prepare 2 sponge tins (16 cm diameter) by buttering them twice and then flouring them.
2. Cream the butter and vanilla with 225 g of caster sugar until white (warm slightly if necessary).
3. Beat in the egg yolks one by one, then stir in the melted couverture.
4. Whisk the egg whites and the remaining caster sugar until creamy, to make a meringue.
5. Sieve the flour and cocoa powder onto paper together.
6. Fold the flour and the meringue alternately into the butter mixture.
7. Divide the mixture between the 2 sponge tins and bake with steam at 180°C for 40–50 minutes. Turn and check at least twice during baking.
8. Unmould and allow to cool.
9. When cold, split each sponge in half. Spread apricot jam over each layer and sandwich the two halves together. Spread jam thinly on the sides and top.
10. Place the tortes on wire racks with trays underneath. Nap with the glaze and then allow to set. Finally, write 'SACHER' on top for a traditional presentation, or present in a modern style as shown here.

8 Opera

	16–18 portions
buttercream	800 g
coffee compound	
jaconde	3 small sheets
stock syrup	250 ml
rum	100 ml
ganache	800 g
chocolate glaze (recipe 21)	400 g

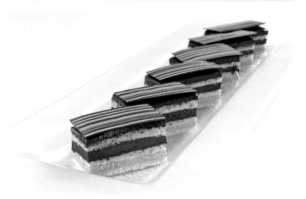

1. Mix the buttercream (see recipe 17) and coffee compound together.
2. Place down a layer of jaconde. Moisten it with a mixture of syrup (see recipe 16) and rum.
3. Cover with a layer of the coffee buttercream.
4. Place down another layer of jaconde and moisten it.
5. Spread ganache over this layer (see recipe 20). Top with another layer of jaconde and moisten it.
6. Coat the top with chocolate glaze.
7. Cut into slices approximately 8 × 3 cm. For a traditional presentation, pipe 'Opera' on each slice; for a modern presentation, top with chocolate patterened with an acetate, as shown here.

9 Himmel cheese torte

	Makes 2 × 20 cm
butter, cut into pieces	675 g
caster sugar	340 g
vanilla essence	
egg yolks	9
soft flour, sieved	675 g
jam	100 g
icing sugar	50 g
soft fruit (strawberries or raspberries)	400 g
Filling	
soft cheese	900 g
caster sugar	225 g
double cream	570 ml

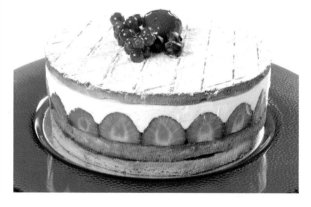

1. Place the butter in a mixing bowl and warm it slightly. Add the sugar and vanilla and cream until white.
2. Add the egg yolks one by one. Fold in the flour.
3. Spread the mixture inside six buttered rings (approx. 20 cm). Bake for 15–20 minutes at 180°C.
4. Allow to cool. Sandwich together two of the pieces with jam to form the base of one torte. (Repeat with two more for the second torte.)
5. To make the filling, cream the soft cheese and caster sugar together. Fold in the double cream.
6. Pipe filling on top of the base in concentric circles to 2½ cm thick. Fill in gaps with soft fruit, then smooth over.
7. Invert a third piece of sponge and place it on top of the filling. Press gently.
8. Allow to set in the chiller for at least 1 hour.
9. Dust with icing sugar.

10   Red wine cake

	Makes 3
butter	500 g
caster sugar	500 g
vanilla arome	
eggs, large	7
self-raising flour	500 g
cocoa powder	1 tbsp
ground cinnamon	1 tbsp
clove powder	½ tbsp
red wine	312 ml
dark chocolate chips or grated couverture	250 g
To finish	
water	100 ml
sugar	60 g
red wine	250 ml
redcurrant glaze	
water icing or white chocolate	

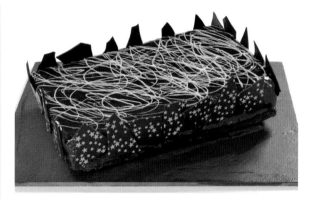

1. Prepare savarin rings or rectangular cake tins (approx. 16 cm) by buttering each tin twice, then flouring it.
2. Cut the butter into small pieces, place in a mixing bowl and warm it until soft.
3. Add the sugar and vanilla and beat until white – at least 5 minutes on a fast speed.
4. Whisk the eggs and add them gradually while beating.
5. Sieve the flour. Add the cocoa powder and spices to it, and sieve again.
6. Fold the flour into the egg mixture.
7. Stir in the red wine and chocolate.
8. Pipe the mixture into the rings or tins so that they are three-quarters full. Place on a baking sheet and bake at 160°C for 35–45 minutes (50–60 minutes for rectangular tins).
9. Unmould immediately, then allow to cool.
10. Boil the water, sugar and red wine together. Pour this into the cleaned cake tin, and invert the cake back in, to soak.
11. Turn out the soaked cake. Brush with hot redcurrant glaze. To decorate, mask with water icing or spin with white chocolate.

11   Chocolate and pecan nut brownies

	20–24 portions
sugar	450 g
eggs	6
butter	330 g
dark chocolate coverture	330 g
soft flour	150 g
cocoa powder	50 g
vanilla extract	
roasted and chopped pecans	100 g
Glaze	
whipping cream	250 ml
glucose	25 g
dark chocolate	250 g

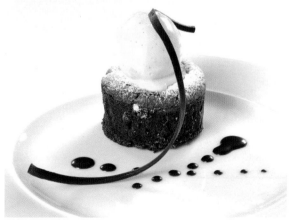

A brownie served as a dessert

1. Whisk the sugar and eggs together until they have reached ribbon stage, making a sabayon.
2. Mix together the butter and chocolate.
3. Mix together the flour, cocoa and vanilla.
4. Fold the chocolate and butter mix into the sabayon, then the pecans and finally the flour mixture followed by the nuts.
5. Prepare the tins and cook at 165°C for 30 minutes.
6. The brownies should be soft in the middle.
7. For the glaze, boil the cream and glucose together, whisk in the chocolate.
8. To finish the brownies, melt the glaze and pour it over the brownies. Allow to set. Comb scrape, pipe over fine lines of dark and white chocolate.

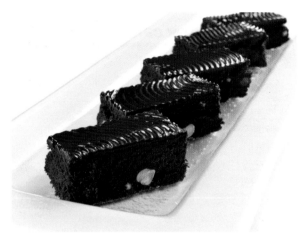

Brownies prepared as pastries

12 Muffins

	Makes 16–20
eggs	2
milk	230 ml
butter – melted	115 g
caster sugar	90 g
salt	pinch
soft flour	290 g
baking powder	5 g

1. Mix the eggs, milk, butter, sugar and salt together.
2. Sift the flour and baking powder onto the wet mix and bring together gently.
3. Allow to rest in the refrigerator before adding flavours (see below).
4. Pipe into muffin trays or paper muffin cases and bake at 210°C for 25 minutes.
5. Turn out onto wire racks to cool.

Variations

A variety of flavours can be incorporated into this recipe; the following are only examples. The additions should be incorporated once the mix has rested in the fridge.

● Apricot and cinnamon: 50 g dried apricots, chopped; 5 g cinnamon.
● Banana and coconut: 100 g mashed banana; 40 g dried coconut.
● Blueberry and pecan: 50 g blueberries; 50 g pecans, chopped.
● Choc-chip and orange: 80 g chocolate chips; zest of 3 oranges.

13   Financiers

	Makes 50–60 petits fours
butter	250 g
caster sugar	350 g
ground almonds	250 g
plain flour	50 g
egg whites	6 (180 ml)

1. Place the butter in a saucepan. Heat to make a beurre noisette.
2. Leave to stand for 2 minutes. Pour off and retain the fat. Discard the sediment. Cool the fat to room temperature.
3. Mix the sugar, almonds and flour together.
4. Whisk the egg whites.
5. Beat the butter into the sugar mixture. Fold in the egg whites.
6. Allow to rest, preferably overnight.
7. Three-quarters fill small muffin trays or suitable cake moulds with the mixture.
8. Bake at 200°C for 8–10 minutes, until peaked and coloured.

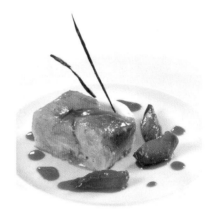
Financier with rhubarb

i   Fruit (e.g. rhubarb or apple) may be added to this recipe. The financiers may be glazed with apricot glaze.

14   Madeleines

	45 portions (585 g)
caster sugar	125 g
eggs	3
vanilla pod, seeds from	1
flour	150 g
baking powder	1 tsp
beurre noisette	125 g

1. Whisk the sugar, eggs and vanilla seeds to a hot sabayon.
2. Fold in the flour and the baking powder.
3. Fold in the beurre noisette and chill for up to 2 hours.
4. Pipe into well buttered madeleine moulds and bake in a moderate oven.
5. Turn out and allow to cool.

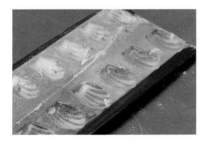
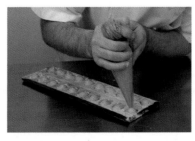
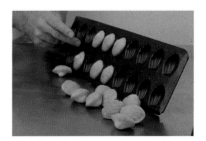

15 Success (dacquoise)

	Makes 2 sheets
hazelnuts, skinned	200 g
egg whites	160 g
caster sugar	80 g
icing sugar	150 g

1. Toast the hazelnuts until they are golden brown.
2. Make a cold meringue from the egg whites and caster sugar.
3. While the nuts are still hot, blitz them with the icing sugar in a food processor, then fold this mixture into the meringue.
4. Spread onto a silicone mat, ½ cm thick. (Alternatively, it may be piped.)
5. Bake at 170°C for 10 minutes, until half cooked.
6. Cut out and return to the oven at 150°C to dry out.

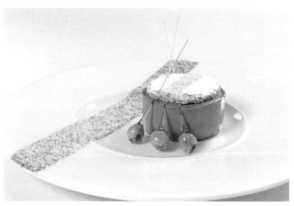

A dessert decorated with dacquoise

Prepare all the equipment and preheat the oven to 170°C before you start making this recipe.

16 Stock syrup

	500 ml	1 litre
water	500 ml	1 litre
granulated sugar	500 g	1 kg
glucose	100 g	200 g

1. Boil the water, sugar and glucose together for approx. 5 mins.
2. Strain and cool.

17 Boiled buttercream

	Makes 900 g
eggs	2
icing sugar	50 g
granulated sugar or cube sugar	300 g
water	100 g
glucose	50 g
unsalted butter	400 g

1. Beat the eggs and icing sugar until at ribbon stage sabayon (sponge).
2. Boil the granulated or cube sugar with water and glucose to 118°C.
3. Gradually add the sugar at 118°C to the eggs and icing sugar at ribbon stage, whisk continuously and allow to cool to 26°C.
4. Gradually add the unsalted butter while continuing to whisk until a smooth cream is obtained.

18 Chantilly cream (*crème Chantilly*)

	Makes 500 ml
whipping cream	500 ml
caster sugar	100 g
vanilla arome	a few drops

1. Place all ingredients in a bowl. Whisk over ice until the mixture forms soft peaks. If using a mechanical mixer, stand and watch until the mixture is ready – do not leave it unattended.
2. Cover and place in the fridge immediately.

19 Chantilly-style whipped ganache

	Makes 1.8 kg
cream, 35 per cent fat	450 g
inverted sugar, e.g. staboline, or similar stabiliser	55 g
glucose	55 g
dark chocolate couverture, 72 per cent cocoa solids, broken into pieces	380 g
whipping cream	

1. Boil 450 g of cream with the inverted sugar and glucose.
2. Pour the boiling cream over the chocolate pieces and emulsify.
3. Weigh the chocolate mixture. Measure out the same weight of whipping cream, and add it to the mixture. Chill overnight.
4. Whip the mixture at a moderate speed until a piping consistency is achieved.

20 Ganache

Version 1	
double cream	300 ml
couverture, cut into small pieces	350 g
unsalted butter	85 g
spirit or liqueur	20 ml
Version 2	
double cream	300 ml
vanilla pod, seeds from	½
couverture, cut into small pieces	600 g
unsalted butter	120 g

1. Bring the cream (and the vanilla for version 2) to the boil in a heavy saucepan.
2. Pour the cream over the couverture. Whisk with a fine whisk until the chocolate has melted.
3. Whisk in the butter (and the liqueur for version 1).
4. Stir over ice until the mixture has the required consistency.

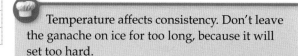

Temperature affects consistency. Don't leave the ganache on ice for too long, because it will set too hard.

21 Chocolate glaze

	Makes 600 ml
double cream	188 g
water	175 g
caster sugar	225 g
cocoa powder	75 g
gelatine, soaked in cold water	4½ leaves (10 g)

1. Bring the cream, water, sugar and cocoa to the boil slowly in a heavy-bottomed saucepan.
2. Simmer for 2–3 minutes, then remove from the heat.
3. Drain the gelatine and add it to the mixture. Stir until dissolved.
4. Pass, then cool by stirring over ice.
5. Store in a plastic container with cling film pressed directly onto the surface.

22 Lemon curd

	Makes 450 ml	1½ litres
granulated sugar	450 g	1 kg 125 g
zest of lemon, grated	2	5
freshly squeezed lemon juice	240 ml	600 ml
eggs, large	8	20
egg yolks, large	2	5
unsalted butter, cut into pieces	350 g	875 g

1. Place the sugar into a bowl. Grate the lemon zest into it and rub together.
2. Strain the lemon juice into a non-reactive pan. Add the eggs, egg yolks, butter and zested sugar. Whisk to combine.
3. Place over a medium heat and whisk continuously for 3–5 minutes, until the mixture begins to thicken.
4. At the first sign of boiling, remove from the heat and strain into a bowl and cool.

13 Food product development

This chapter covers Unit 314: Food Product Development. You will learn how to research, design, develop and produce food products.

Factors to consider when developing new recipes and menus

Why produce new recipes and new menus?

In order to create or to develop customer or consumer satisfaction it is essential to prevent menu apathy and to produce interest, and thus enable the discovery of new flavours and combinations. Producing new menus and dishes with the selection of foodstuffs available from all over the world is a stimulating and exciting task. So much so that it is easy to overlook or dismiss traditional and classical dishes as being old-fashioned and out of date.

There are, however, customers who welcome the opportunity of being able to choose a traditional or classical dish occasionally. You should consider, therefore, including a small number of such dishes on almost any type of menu. While the creator of new recipes may enjoy the experience, it must be clear that the exercise is twofold: to satisfy (a) the customer and (b) management. For this reason, the prime considerations are the cost of the development and the selling price. It is also essential to consider the style or type of establishment and the kind of clientele for whom the changes are intended, as well as regional variations and food fashions.

The reasons for change could include:
- Menu fatigue
- Changes in clientele
- Food fashion changes
- Availability of supplies
- Seasonal demands
- Need to stimulate business
- New chef and staff
- The opening of a similar local establishment.

Whatever the cause, it is necessary to introduce new recipes and menus in accordance with the organisation's objectives. It follows that, in every sphere of catering, recipe and menu changes may need to occur – whether this involves school meals, hospital food, speciality outlets, exclusive restaurants, or wherever. If new developments are intended, it is essential to evaluate:
- The cost of development
- The effect the change or changes will have on the existing situation
- The ability of the staff to cope
- Whether adequate equipment is present and suitable suppliers are available
- The presentation of the dishes
- The format of the menu.

Depending on the quality and expertise of staff it can be an interesting and possibly useful exercise to offer them the opportunity of contributing to recipe development and/or suggesting new dishes or variations to existing ones. If successful, this can boost staff morale and assist in developing team spirit.

Recipe development: preparation

Before beginning to prepare for the practical aspect of producing new recipes, you will need to construct a method of recording that includes accurate details of ingredients; their cost, quality and availability (for example, by drawing up a chart). You must also record how much time is needed for preparation and production and the yield. Space should be available on the chart to specify several attempts so that comparisons can be made, and there should be adequate space for making notes.

An evaluation sheet is required so that a record can be made of the opinions of the tasting panel or persons consulted. This sheet will, as appropriate, be constructed so as to include space for details of flavours, colour, texture, presentation, and so on.

Research

Before deciding to develop new products, recipes and menus it is important to research the market and ask the questions: Who are our customers? What are their needs and wants? Talk to your existing customers to find out what they want and would like to see changed.

Carrying out consumer research does not have to be costly. Simple questionnaires can be devised and distributed in your restaurant and local businesses.

You may find it useful to conduct brainstorming exercises with the staff and small groups of potential customer groups.

Always consider seasonality and the availability of local produce when developing new products. Locally sourced food is a significant selling point. Explore both new and traditional ingredients.

Part of the research activity is to assess what is the best way to package the new recipe, dish or product. Consider plate service or silver service. Consider the production system to be used: cook/chill; cook/freeze; or conventional.

If cook/chill or cook/freeze systems are to be used, the recipes will require moderation and much more careful development using modified starches and other specialist ingredients.

You will need to cost all new recipes and products carefully and calculate the desired gross and net profits.

Developing new ideas

Before proceeding to develop new ideas it is essential to have a basic foundation on which to build.

Developing new recipes is challenging, stimulating and creates new interest, but where do original ideas come from? Many are triggered by the creations of others. It is particularly worthwhile to keep abreast of what is happening in the industry, perhaps by some of the means listed below.

- Publications:
  - trade magazines such as *Caterer and Hotelkeeper*
  - books produced by leading chefs
  - consumer magazines, food journals
  - newspaper articles
  - visit the library
  - use the internet, e.g. chef blogs, social media.

- TV and radio:
  - *Masterchef*
  - *Great British Menu*
  - *Ready Steady Cook*
  - *Saturday Kitchen*
- Contacts:
  - visiting other establishments
  - visiting catering exhibitions
  - attending lectures, demonstrations
  - visiting competitors
  - catering organisations, etc.

Extra care needs to be taken when introducing new recipes to patients in hospitals and nursing homes, and in the provision of meals in schools and residential establishments, so as to ensure the nutritional content is suitable. Dietitians can provide advice on the dietary requirements of these persons.

Communication and information

Information sources for recipes are available everywhere to the open and enquiring mind. Every kind of establishment, from the local Chinese restaurant to the five-star hotel, can present innovative ideas. You may find particular value in sourcing ideas when travelling abroad, if it is possible, as well as being alert to new dishes in the UK. Visits to department stores, exhibition centres, outdoor events and the like may well stimulate ideas. The range of ingredients available from catering suppliers is immense, but you should not ignore local markets and supermarkets as sources of supply.

If you have new developments in mind, you will need to pass on your proposals to both senior management (who will be responsible for their implementation) and fellow members of the kitchen brigade, for their constructive comments. If possible, put your ideas to the test with respected members of the catering profession with whom you are acquainted. Your proposals should include estimated food costings, time taken to produce, labour costs, equipment and facilities needed, and details of staff training if required. Knowledge of the establishment's organisation is important so that the right person or persons are involved.

Quality of materials

The highest possible standards of ingredients should be used so that a true and valid result is available for assessment of the recipe.

Staff abilities

Before implementing new recipes and menus, the standard of staff members' craft skills should be appraised in order to assess their capacity to cope with innovation. Failure to do so could jeopardise the whole project. Not only should you assess their craft skills but also seek their cooperation and suggestions in putting new ideas into practice, and give encouragement if the outcome is successful.

Equipment and facilities

You may find that new recipes could affect the utilisation of existing equipment by overloading at peak times. The capacity of items such as pastry ovens, deep-fat fryers, salamanders, and so on, may already be fully used. It is important that you bear in mind the fact that new items can affect the production of the current menu so that service is not impaired.

Implementation

Having tested and arrived at the finished recipe, staff may need to practise production and presentation of the dish. This may include making both small and large quantities, depending on the establishment. In all cases, careful recording of all aspects of the operation can help in the smooth running of the exercise; in particular, basic work study should be observed. Seek constructive comments from staff and discuss any problems that may arise.

The results of such trial runs should be conveyed to senior personnel and any problems that have been identified should be resolved.

Having validated the recipe, checked on a reliable supplier and ensured the capability of the staff, it is important that all concerned know when the dishes will be included on the menu. Storekeepers, kitchen staff and serving staff need to be briefed, as do any other departments involved, as to the time and date of implementation.

Presentation of dishes

When a dish is received by a customer it needs to appeal to the senses of sight and smell even before taste. For this reason, you need to consider presentation early in the development of the idea: what dish will be used, what will accompany it, are any particular skills needed to serve it? Foods in some establishments are prepared and cooked in front of the customer; some require the dish to be cooked fresh while the customer waits; therefore details of presentation must be recorded and, where possible, a test carried out in the actual situation.

Should the new recipe be for a food service operation that involves preparation, cooking and presentation before the customer, so that all or part of the process is seen by the potential consumer, then attention needs to be paid to the skills of the chef. Extra training – not only culinary skills, but customer-handling skills – may be needed, and particular attention should be paid to hygiene. These factors need to be observed at the development stage so that customer satisfaction is guaranteed as soon as the new recipe is implemented.

Organisation

Adequate time needs to be allowed to test and develop any new recipe, to train staff, to appraise comments and modify the recipe if necessary. Staff (particularly serving staff) must be briefed on the composition of the dish, as well as being told when it will be included on the menu. They need to be asked if there are any problems; if required, this could be in a written form. Senior personnel need to be apprised orally or in writing of the implementation of the new items.

Should the new dish or dishes require skills that are unfamiliar to some staff, then the workload of individuals may need to be changed while the relevant staff are trained in the appropriate skill. In estimating how long it will take to implement the new dish factors to take account of are:

- The skills of the staff
- That suitable equipment is available
- That suppliers can produce the required ingredients in the right quantity, at the desired quality and at a suitable price.

Clear written instructions may need to be provided; this means the sequence in which the ingredients are to be used, with the appropriate amount (for example, for 10 portions or 50 portions). This should be followed by the instructions in the order that the recipe is to be followed, so that it is logical.

The introduction of new dishes will perhaps affect the existing style of operations. If dishes are prepared in front of the customer – for example, in a department store – the new dish may require more time in preparation than others on the menu, which may cause a bottleneck. The introduction of a salad bar or sweet trolley to include new dishes can affect the service of the usual dishes. If the clientele require, say, vegetarian dishes, or people of certain cultural or religious groups have special needs, then adaptations may be necessary to accommodate this in the existing set-up.

In addition to obtaining feedback (that is to say information) from staff, it is just as important, if not more so, to obtain comments from the customer or consumer.

Finally, consider the following points:

- The elimination of waste
- The control of materials and ingredients
- The careful use of energy
- The wise use of time.

Ensure that a record is kept so that no resources are misused. Failure to control and monitor resources can be expensive in terms of time, materials and effort, and can be very wasteful.

Menu design

The function of a menu is to inform potential customers what dishes are available and, as appropriate, the number of courses, the choice on the courses and the price. The wording should make clear to the kind of customer using the establishment what to expect. The menu may be used to promote specific items, such as when an ingredient is in season, children's menus, reductions for senior citizens, what is served at particular times, and so on.

If printed, the type should clear and of readable size; if handwritten, the script should be of good quality so as to create a good impression; the spelling must be correct. Menus are expensive to produce but when they are attractive and fulfil the function of informing the customer, they may enhance the reputation of the establishment and increase custom.

Specific considerations

When considering any development, it is necessary to take into account any current problems and issues that may affect the outcome, and also those of historic origin based on culture and religion.

It is essential to keep up to date on factors such as, for example, BSE and the effect on consumers' choice or rejection of beef. The increasing use of 'organic' foods may increase customer demand for such foods to be used; all foods are organic, but the term has become restricted to mean those grown without the use of pesticides or processed without the use of additives. There is little difference nutritionally between organic and non-organic foods. The *Manual of Nutrition* published by HMSO is a useful reference book for those seeking information on nutrition.

Certain groups of people have restrictions on their eating habits (religious or cultural) that must be observed when producing new recipes for them. The following list offers some examples:

- *Hindus:* no beef, mainly vegetables, no alcohol.
- *Muslims:* no pork, no alcohol, no shellfish, halal meat (requires a Muslim to be present at the killing).
- *Sikhs:* no beef, no alcohol, only meat killed with one blow to the head.
- *Jews:* no pork, meat must be kosher, only fish with fins and scales, meat and dairy produce not to be eaten together.
- *Rastafarians:* no animal products except milk, no canned or processed foods, no salt added, foods should be organic.

Development of recipes and menus for special diets

A balanced diet is important for health, providing the right amount and type of nutrients required to maintain a healthy lifestyle. However, some customers require special diets for health reasons. Others choose special diets for ethical, cultural and/or religious reasons.

The chef may be required, on occasion, to provide menus for individuals on special diets, such as those described below.

Low-salt diet

A high-salt diet increases the risk of high blood pressure, which in turn increases the risk of stroke and heart attack.

Milk-free diet

Soya or rice milk can be used as an alternative to cows' milk for customers who have a milk allergy or lactose intolerance.

Low-cholesterol diet

People on a low-cholesterol diet avoid high-cholesterol foods such as liver, kidney, egg yolks, fatty meats, fried foods, full-cream milk, cream, cheeses, biscuits and cakes. The chef should use lean meat or fish (grilled or poached), and low-fat milk and cheeses.

Diabetic

When someone is suffering from diabetes, their body is unable to control the level of glucose in the blood. This can lead to comas, and long-term problems such as increased risk of blindness, and cardiovascular and kidney disease. Avoid serving high-sugar dishes, fatty meats, eggs, full-cream milk, cream cakes, biscuits, and so on.

Coeliac

Someone suffering from coeliac disease has an allergy to gluten, exposure to which results in severe inflammation of the gastrointestinal tract, pain and diarrhoea, and malnutrition due to the inability to absorb nutrients. Avoid serving all products made using wheat, barley or rye.

Vegetarianism

A vegetarian is someone who lives on a diet of grains, pulses, nuts, seeds, vegetables and fruits, with or without the use of dairy products and eggs (preferably free range). A vegetarian does not eat any meat, poultry, game, fish, shellfish or crustacea, or slaughter by-products such as gelatine or animal fats.

Strict vegetarians will not wish the utensils with which their food is prepared or served to be contaminated with any animal products. For this reason, chefs have to take special care in the preparation of vegetarian foods in a kitchen that also caters for meat and fish eaters.

Types of vegetarian

There are several types of vegetarian including:

- *Lacto-ovo-vegetarian:* eats both dairy products and eggs.
- *Lacto-vegetarian:* eats dairy products but not eggs.
- *Ovo-vegetarian:* will include eggs but not dairy products.
- *Vegan:* does not eat dairy products, eggs or any other animal product (e.g. honey).
- *Fruitarian:* a type of vegan who eats very few processed or cooked foods; the fruitarian's diet consists mainly of raw fruit grains and nuts; fruitarians believe that only plant foods that can be harvested without killing the plant should be eaten.
- *Macrobiotic:* requires a diet that follows spiritual and philosophical codes; it aims to maintain a balance between foods seen as yin (positive) and yang (negative); the diet progresses through ten levels, becoming increasingly restrictive – not all levels are vegetarian, although each level gradually eliminates animal products.
- *Demi-vegetarian:* eats little or no meat and may eat fish.
- Those who eat fish but not meat are sometimes called *pescetarians*.

Issues the chef has to consider

These issues include:

- Many ingredients are derived from the slaughter of animals (for example gelatine, which is used in confectionery, ice cream and other dairy products).
- The term 'animal fats' refers to carcass fats and may be present in a wide range of foods (for example biscuits and cakes); suet and lard are also types of animal fats.
- Cheese is made with rennet, which is a substance extracted from the stomach lining of slaughtered calves. Vegetarian cheese is made with rennet from a microbial source.
- Many vegetarians who eat eggs will eat only free-range eggs. This is usually due to moral objections to the battery farming of hens.

Vegetarian foods

The main vegetarian food groups are:

- Cereals and grains (for example wheat, and include bread and pasta, oats, maize, barley, rye and rice)
- Potatoes
- Pulses (beans, lentils, peas), nuts and seeds
- Fruit and vegetables
- Dairy products, or soya products (tofu, tempeh, soya protein)
- Vegetable oils and fats.

Exclusion of animal-derived products

The following products should be excluded from vegetarian diets, recipes and menus:

- Non-vegetarian alcohol: some wines or beers may be refined using isinglass (a fish product) or dried blood.
- Animal-fat ice cream: replace with vegetable-fat ice cream.
- Animal fats (suet, lard, dripping): replace with vegetable fats/oils.
- Oils containing fish oil: replace with 100 per cent vegetable oil.
- Gelatine: replace with agar-agar.
- Meat stock: replace with vegetable stock.
- Rennet or pepsin: replace with vegetarian cheeses (that is, made with vegetarian rennet) or non-rennet cheeses such as cottage and cream cheese (these should not be used for vegans, unless made with soya milk).

Guidelines on serving healthy food

It is recommended that everyone should follow a diet that is rich in fresh fruit and vegetables, fish, wholegrain breads, pulses, rice and pasta, and that is low in fats of all types, especially animal fats. Recommended cooking methods are grilling, poaching, steaming and *en papillote* (cooking in an envelope/parcel), and reducing the amount of shallow-fried and deep-fried food.

Some guidance on how to 'think healthy' when preparing food is given below.

Meat, fish and alternatives

Ensure that you:

- Always use lean cuts of meat, trim off any excess fat, and remove the skin from chicken or chicken portions.
- Bake, grill or roast meats and fish, and do not baste with additional fats. Fish may be steamed. If frying is unavoidable, ensure that the fat is at the correct temperature and drain the food well on absorbent paper before serving. As mentioned above, cooking *en papillote* is a healthy alternative as there is no need to use additional fats and all flavours (of the herbs, spices, vegetables used) are retained.
- Alternatives to meat, fish and eggs, are pulses, nuts, tofu, Quorn, and so on (see also the section on 'Vegetarianism', above). Dishes can also be prepared using a combination of meats and pulses, to cut down on the amount of meat used.

Fats and oils

Consider the following:

- If there is a need to use fat, consider which type and how much.
- Use olive oil for flavour, and rapeseed oil where any flavour will be masked.
- Low-fat margarines or spreads cannot be used for baking as they contain a large amount of water, which evaporates.
- Full-fat polyunsaturated margarines contain as many calories as butter.
- Margarines contain flavourings, colours and other additives to provide that 'buttery' taste.
- Thicken sauces and gravies with cornflour, arrowroot, fécule (potato starch/flour), rice flour or barley flour rather than a fatty 'roux'.
- Always offer polyunsaturated or low-fat spreads as an alternative to butter.
- Offer low-fat sauces, salad dressings and mayonnaises separately.

Sugar

You should:

- Avoid adding sugar to savoury dishes.
- Consider the possibility of reducing the amount of sugar in any dish.
- Consider lower-fat, lower-sugar, fruit-based desserts.

Salt

Ensure that you:

- Reduce salt in recipes and leave it to customers to add more if they wish. Many people have reduced their salt consumption so they may find highly salted foods unpalatable.
- Remember that most stock cubes and stock powders are high in salt.
- Explore the use of fresh herbs to add flavour to dishes.

Fibre

Where possible, increase the fibre content of dishes by using pulses, vegetables, fruit, wholemeal bread, wholemeal pasta, and so on.

Breads, cereals and potatoes

You should:

- Offer a wide variety of interesting bread products, including teabreads, and serve with a choice of spreads.
- Provide a wide range of breakfast cereals, particularly low-sugar, high-fibre products, and ensure that customers can choose low-fat milk, yoghurts, fresh and dried fruit, and artificial sweeteners if desired.
- Make pasta an inviting choice, offering good portions of fresh varieties and serving with low-fat sauces.
- Remember that providing generous portions of starchy foods incurs little additional cost.

Fruit and vegetables

Ensure that you:

- Offer a range of interesting salads. Dressings should be offered separately, including a low-fat alternative.
- Bake or steam vegetables to retain their colour, flavour and texture, and use only small quantities of fat when stir- or shallow-frying.
- Make vegetables appealing by exploring the range and variety available.
- Use a wide variety of fresh fruits, low-fat cream, ice cream, fromage frais and yoghurts.

Milk and dairy

It is good practice to:

- Reduce the amount of fresh cream used in recipes.
- Substitute cream with crème fraîche or fromage frais.
- Where possible, use skimmed milk.

- If possible, use low-fat cheeses such as Edam and Gouda.

Food allergies

Some customers have a very serious adverse reaction to certain foods. A reaction can occur within a few minutes of exposure to the allergen; typically the lips and tongue tingle and swell. There may be abdominal cramps and diarrhoea, and sometimes the person vomits. There may also be wheezing and shortness of breath followed, in rare cases, by cardiovascular failure and collapse, leading to death if very prompt action is not taken.

It is important to be aware that almost any substance can trigger an allergic reaction in someone. Although peanuts are the most common food to trigger such a reaction, other common potential 'problem foods' are:

- Beef and pork
- Cashew, pecan and brazil nuts, and walnuts
- Eggs
- Milk
- Mushrooms
- Sesame seeds
- Shellfish
- Wheat.

Other foods that, less commonly, may trigger an allergic reaction are:

- Chocolate
- Coffee
- Oranges
- Soya
- Strawberries
- Sugar
- Tomatoes
- Yeast.

It is important that chefs train their staff in product knowledge. They should know what ingredients are in the dishes. For details of foods containing sugar and foods containing yeast see Table 13.1.

While food allergies are mainly a medical issue, it is necessary for those concerned with providing meals to be aware of the situation. Therefore, in any catering establishment, should a customer enquire if a substance or food to which they are allergic is included in the recipe ingredients, it is important that staff give an accurate and clear answer. Failure to provide the correct information could have dire consequences; for example, a person who is allergic to nuts would need to know if there were walnuts in the Waldorf salad, almonds garnishing the trout, marzipan on the gâteau or nuts in the ice cream. If a person inadvertently consumes a food item to which they are allergic, medical assistance will be urgently needed.

A person who is intolerant to milk would need to know if cheese was included in a dish, and a person allergic to nuts must know if, say, peanut butter has been used. Therefore, persons *serving* the food, as well as those *preparing* it, must be knowledgeable regarding its composition so as to give accurate information to potential customers.

Tables 13.2 and 13.3 are examples of checklists that can be used to make staff aware of the breadth of restricted items.

Because a person is allergic to one item in a family of foods, there is a possibility of their being allergic to other items in the family (as in the checklists of plant and animal families below).

Unfortunately, some staff employed in the catering industry are themselves allergic to handling certain items of food. In the event of an employee becoming aware of this (for example, coming out in a rash), medical advice must be obtained. In certain cases, if the person cannot be cured, they may be advised to transfer to other work. Examples of foods that may cause this problem include flour, tomatoes and fish.

Specialised cookery books are available to assist those who have an allergy, or those who need to develop recipes for them. For further information on this topic see the resources listed at the end of this chapter.

Packaging and labelling

Packaging

If food is to be packaged it must protect the food against contamination. The packaging must also label the product based on what it contains:

- Name of product
- How to store the food
- Ingredients
- The average filled weight.

Packaging materials

Packaging technology is a specialised science. In hospitality a limited number of materials are used. These include:

- Paper and board
- Solid white board made from chemical wood pulp

Table 13.1 Foods containing sugar and food containing yeast

Foods containing sugar	Foods containing yeast
All types of sugar	Bread (not matzo or chapatis)
Honey	Buns
Golden syrup	Yeast extract (Marmite/Vegemite)
Treacle	Stock cubes
Molasses	Bovril, Oxo
Malt	Dried fruit
Jam	Unpeeled fruit
Marmalade	Yoghurt
Chutney	Synthetic cream
Cakes	Soy sauce
Maple syrup	Vinegar
Peanut butter	Quorn, mycoprotein (meat substitute)
Dried fruits	Edible fungi
Foods labelled dextrose, fructose, maltose or sucrose	Malt
Biscuits	Cheese – Brie and Camembert
Pudding	
Sweeteners	

Table 13.2 Checklist of plant families

Fungi or moulds	Grains or grasses	Onion or lily
Baker's yeast	Wheat	Onion
Brewer's yeast	Corn	Asparagus
Mushroom	Barley	Chive
Truffle	Oats	Leek
Chanterelle	Cane sugar	Garlic
Cheese	Bamboo shoots	Shallot
Vinegar	Rice	

Mustard	Rose	Pulses
Broccoli	Apple	Peas
Cabbage	Pears	Lentils
Cauliflower	Quince	Soya beans
Brussels sprouts	Apricot	Peanuts
Horseradish	Cherry	Haricot beans
Radish	Raspberry	Chickpeas
Swede	Strawberry	Runner beans
Turnip	Loganberry	Mangetout
Watercress	Blackberry	Kidney beans

Citrus	Grape	Parsley
Orange	Wine	Parsley
Lemon	Brandy	Carrot
Grapefruit	Sherry	Dill
Lime	Raisins	Celery
Tangerine	Currants	Fennel
Ugli fruit	Sultanas	Parsnip

Potato	Gourd	Mint
Potato	Melon	Mint
Tomato	Cucumber	Basil
Aubergine	Squashes	Marjoram
Chilli	Gherkin	Oregano
Paprika	Courgette	Sage
	Pumpkin	Rosemary
	Marrow	Thyme

Table 13.3 Checklist of animal food families

Bovines	Beef, dairy products, mutton, lamb, goat
Poultry	Chicken, eggs, duck, goose
Grouse	Grouse, guinea fowl
Pig	Pork, bacon, ham, sausage
Fish	All types of fish
Shellfish (crustaceans)	Lobster, prawns, shrimps, crab, crayfish
Molluscs	Snail, clam, mussel, oyster, scallop

- Chipboard made from recycled paper
- Plastics: flexible and rigid
- Low density polythene
- High density polythene which resists boiling temperatures
- Polythene: poor barrier to oxygen
- Nylon (polyamide): good oxygen barrier
- Aluminium foil: can be laminated with polythene
- Plastic bottles (polyethylene terephthalate): very light and strong
- Cellulose films or 'cellophane': wide range of types, denoted by letter codes, for example 'P' to indicate it is permeable and moisture proof
- Glass.

Packaging of individual foods

There is a need to know the nature of the food and the degree of protection required. For instance:
- Fresh fruit and vegetables require oxygen but must allow loss of some moisture
- Fresh meat requires oxygen to form bright red oxymyoglobin
- Cured meat needs protection against oxygen to prevent discolouration
- Dehydrated foods need protection against moisture, oxygen and mechanical damage
- Frozen foods need protection against moisture loss to prevent 'freezer burn' and require low oxygen permeability to minimise tainting problems.

Source: RK Proudlove (2010) *The Science and Technology of Food* (Forbes)

Labelling

Labels should include information about the durability of the food contained in the package. Durability is indicated by 'best before' followed by the date up to which the food remains in first-class condition if stored correctly. See Table 13.4

Table 13.4 Information shown on labels to indicate durability

Date to be declared	Period of durability
'Best before' – day, month	Within 3 months
'Best before end' – month/ year	3 – 18 months
'Best before end' – month/year or year	More than 18 months

The 'use by' date should be indicated by 'use by' followed by the date/day/month or for longer periods, day/month/year. Details of necessary storage conditions must be given.

Nutritional labelling

This must be in tubular form or in linear form on small labels. It should include the following information per serving and per 100 g:

Table 13.5 Information required in nutritional labelling

Nutrient	Units used
Energy	Kilojoules (KJ) and kilocalories (Kcal)
Protein	Grams (g)
Carbohydrate	Grams (g)
Of which sugars	Grams (g)
Polyols	Grams (g)
Starch	Grams (g)
Fats	Grams (g)
Of which saturated	Grams (g)
Monounsaturated	Grams (g)
Polyunsaturated	Grams (g)
Cholesterol	Grams (g)
Fibre	Grams (g)

Nutrient	Units used
Sodium	Grams (g)
Vitamins*	Units as appropriate
Minerals*	Units as appropriate
* Give name, e.g. vitamin C, folacin	

Assessing the taste and quality of dishes

It is important for chefs to assess the quality of dishes by tasting. In this way they learn about flavour and are able to become skilled in blending and mixing different flavour components.

Organoleptic assessment

This simply means using our sense to evaluate food. We detect the flavour of food through the sense of taste and smell. The overall taste of food is made up of one or more primary tastes, of which there are five. These are:

- Sweet
- Sour
- Salt
- Bitter
- Umami.

In the West salt, sweet, sour and bitter were the known basic tastes. In Japan, they talk of the fifth taste called 'umami', or 'xian' as it is known in China. Asian cuisine is based on umami-rich ingredients.

The Chinese have been referring to umami for more than 1200 years. In his book *The Physiology of Taste*, published in 1825, Brillat-Savarin makes reference to osmosone, generally considered a forerunner to the concept of umami.

Umami is found naturally in many foods, both animal and vegetable. It is a combination of proteins, amino acids and nucleotides, which include not only glutamates, but also inosinates and ganylates. When the proteins break down through cooking, fermenting, aging or ripening, the umami flavours intensify.

To find out more, visit the Umami Information Centre website at www.umaminfo.com.

The sensation of taste is detected by taste buds in the mouth, mostly on the upper surface of the tongue. Different parts of the tongue are particularly sensitive to different primary tastes. The notion that the tongue is mapped into four areas – sweet, sour, salt and bitter is wrong. It was a century old misunderstanding that no one challenged. Only in recent years have taste receptors been identified. The entire tongue can sense all of the five basic tastes more or less equally – salt, sweet, sour, bitter, umami.

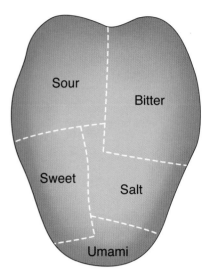

Tongue map

Our sensitivity to different primary tastes varies greatly.

Colour of food

The colour of food is extremely important to our enjoyment of it. People are sensitive to the colour of the food they eat and will reject food that is not considered to have the accepted colour. Colouring matter is sometimes added to food to enhance its attractiveness. There is a strong link between the colour and the flavour of food. Our ability to detect the flavour of food is very much connected with its colour, for if the colour is unusual our sense of taste is confused. For example, if a fruit jelly is red it is likely that the flavour detected will be that of a red-coloured fruit, such as raspberry or strawberry, even if the flavour is lemon or banana.

The depth of colour in food also affects our sense of taste. We associate strong colour with strong flavours. For example, if a series of jellies all contain the same amount of a given flavour, but are of different shades of the same colour, then those having a stronger colour will appear also to have a stronger flavour.

The flavour of food

Because the nose shares an airway, the pharynx, with the mouth, we smell and taste our food simultaneously, and what we call the flavour or the 'taste' of the food is really a combination of these two sensations. To quote Brillat-Savarin:

Smell and taste form a single sense, of which the mouth is the laboratory, the nose is the chimney, or to speak more exactly, of which one serves for the tasting of actual bodies and the other for the savouring of their gases.

With taste and smell, therefore, we first decide whether a particular food is edible and then go on to sample its chemistry simply to enjoy it.

Temperature of food

Foods are chemical mixtures, so that we seldom encounter any of the basic taste sensations in isolation. The temperature of food also affects our sensitivity to its taste. Low temperatures decrease the rate of detection. Maximum taste sensitivity ranges from 22–44°C. Sweet and sour are enhanced at the upper end, salt and bitter at the lower end. At any given temperature, however, we are much more sensitive to bitter substances than we are to sweet, sour or salty ones, by a factor of about 10,000. Synthetic sweeteners are effective at concentrations nearer to bitter substances than to table sugar.

Developing a discriminating palate

Our sensitivity to the flavour of food in our mouth is greatest when we breathe out with the mouth closed; air from the lungs passes along the back of the mouth on its way to the nose and brings some food vapours with it.

It is important when assessing food to remember that taste, smell and colour are closely linked and contribute to the overall assessment of the dish. Training and knowledge are therefore essential if one is to develop a discriminating palate and to acquire the ability to identify individual flavours.

Presentation of food

Food must be presented in such a way that it can be fully appreciated by the customer. This will vary according to the culture and customs of the various groups in society. It may vary in the different sectors of the industry. For example, airline catering will be different in presentation from a Michelin Star restaurant; school meals will differ from staff feeding. In all cases, the food should look appetising, colourful and easily identifiable. Particular attention must be paid to colour, presentation, size, nutritional balance, texture, flavour and consistency of the various components that make up the dish. The garnish must also be in harmony with the dish.

Tasting panels

Tasting panels are usually set up in controlled environments so that tasters are not influenced by outside factors or by each other. These panels are set up to obtain feedback on the quality, texture, flavour, and so on, of a product or dish.

Different tests are often agreed with either a pair of unknown food products or dishes, or three in a triangle in which two are identical and the third is separated. In ranking, a series of samples have to be put in order by the panel according to increasing sweetness, saltiness, flavour or any other characteristic.

A flavour profile is an elaborate evaluation of a flavour by a trained panel. The flavour is broken down into its components, which are described by any term that accurately describes it such as, for example, 'spicyness fragrant'. The individual flavour notes are considered; the order of their appearance in the mouth; their strength; and the presence of any aftertaste.

Taste panel

Set up a taste panel and prepare samples to be tasted by difference (two samples) or by triangle test (three samples, two being identical).

Vary one ingredient in the recipe; for example use a soup recipe for tomato soup. Vary the suet level, sugar level, amount of tomato puree or fresh tomato used. Pick out the one the panel prefers or the one that is different.

You could use and compare a manufactured tomato soup with a fresh tomato soup.

Healthy eating and menu development

A recap on nutrition

Foods contain nutrients, water and fibre. In the right quantities, all of these food components do some sort of job to help people live. The nuts and bolts of what you need to know about nutrition in order to make sense of the rest of this chapter are summarised in Table 13.6.

Nutrition and health

Over the decades our eating habits have changed. This dietary evolution, together with other shifts in lifestyle, has brought massive health problems. In particular, obesity is now hitting the headlines and the statistics for the UK are sobering:

- In 2008, almost a quarter of adults (24 per cent of men and 25 per cent of women aged 16 or over) in England were classified as obese
- A greater proportion of men than women (42 per cent compared with 32 per cent) in England were classified as overweight in 2008
- In 2008, 16.8 per cent of boys aged 2 to 15, and 15.2 per cent of girls were classed as obese, an

increase from 11.1 per cent and 12.2 per cent respectively in 1995.

Connected to this growing epidemic are the escalating rates of diabetes and our high rates of coronary heart disease. In addition, many cancers are related to the food we eat.

To tackle these health problems all of us need to change our patterns of eating. The messages are simple:

- Base meals on starchy foods such as rice, bread, pasta (ideally whole grain varieties) and potatoes
- Eat lots of fruit and vegetables (at least five portions a day)
- Eat moderate amounts of meat, fish and alternatives (including a portion of oily fish each week)
- Cut down on saturated fat, sugar and salt.

There are clear quantitative nutritional targets for the UK population and these have been translated into the daily guidance reproduced in Table 13.7.

Table 13 .6 Nutrition basics

Nutrient	Comment	Function
Carbohydrate	Two main types are starch and sugars	Energy provider (3.75 kcals/g)
Protein	Animal (e.g. meat, milk, eggs) or vegetable (e.g. beans) sources	Body builder (4 kcals/g)
Fat	Two main types are unsaturated (liquid, e.g. vegetable oils) or saturated (hard, e.g. butter)	Provide energy (9 kcals/g) – fat is twice as calorie dense as carbohydrate (e.g. small (30 g) cube cheese = 124 kcals compared to one (100 g) jacket potato = 136 kcals)
Vitamins and minerals	Needed in minute quantities	Regulate body processes (e.g. growth, immune and nervous functions); some act as antioxidants
Other food constituents		
Fluid	Need 1.2 litres fluid/day = 6–8 mugs of drinks daily	Essential for helping the body to function properly (e.g. kidneys, regulating body temperature, lubricant)
Fibre	Not digested/absorbed; found in wholegrain cereals, pulses, vegetables and fruit	Essential for gut health and prevents constipation

Table 13.7 Nutritional targets for the adult UK population

Nutritional targets for adults
● Reduce total fat intake (the target is to keep below 95 g/day for men and 70 g/day for women)
● Reduce saturated fat (the target is to keep below 30 g/day for men and 20 g/day for women)
● Reduce sugars not found naturally in foods or milk (around 60 g/day max)
● Reduce salt intake (no more than 6 g/day)
● Increase intakes of starchy carbohydrate (around 37 per cent of total energy intake should be starchy foods)
● Increase fibre intake (around 18 g/day)
● At least five portions of a variety of fruit and vegetables per day
● Two portions of fish per week (at least one should be oily fish like salmon)

Source: Department of Health (1991) *Dietary Reference Values for Food Energy and Nutrients for the United Kingdom.* London: HMSO; Scientific Advisory Committee on Nutrition (2003) *Salt and Health.* London: The Stationery Office.

The chef's expertise is vitally important to the translation of these nutritional targets into food on the plate. They have the skills and knowledge to make healthy eating a positive experience. Some of the best cuisines of the world are based on the sort of guidelines summarised above. Dishes and meals can be built around lots of starchy foods with generous helpings of a wide range of vegetables, salad and fruit, and including relatively small amounts of lower-fat meats plus an abundance of fish dishes, all made with unsaturated oils like sunflower, olive or sesame oil. Many recipes from Italy, the eastern Mediterranean, China, India and Thailand echo these principles.

The concept of balance

Healthy eating is about balance. Chefs can help people achieve this balance by threading the principles listed above through their practice. This section illustrates how chefs can do this.

Energy balance

One of the keys to healthy eating is balancing energy input (through food) with output (through physical activity). Put simply, too much energy consumed leads to obesity. Energy is measured in calories (or joules in metric). A 24-year-old male chef, for example, needs

about 2550 kcals/day to keep his body ticking over and fuel any additional physical activity such as preparing food, walking round the kitchen or going to the gym. Rates of calorie expenditure vary between activities. Table 13.8 below lists a range of activities together with their expenditure rates. As a rule, the harder the crème body works, the higher the rate of energy expenditure.

Table 13.8 Energy expenditure for selected activities

Activity	Expenditure rate (kcals/per minute)
Running	6–20
Swimming	5–15
Cycling	4–20
Cooking/preparing food	2–3
Fitness training	4–12
Walking	3–6

Chefs can make significant calorie reductions simply by making a few small changes that concentrate on driving down fat levels, which will help those customers who want to control their weight. For example, large calorie savings can be made by:

● Trimming the fat from meat
● Reducing the amount of cream, butter or oils in sauces
● Swapping whole milk for semi-skimmed in béchamel sauces
● Dry-frying meat to seal before braising.

Balancing recipes

There are countless small steps chefs can take to drive down levels of fat, salt and sugar and, at the same time, also bump up the starch, fibre, fruit and vegetable content of their recipes. This balancing process may involve:

● Changing ingredients (for example, swapping full-fat crème fraîche for the half-fat version)
● Manipulating proportions within recipes (such as using relatively larger quantities of rice and white fish to meat in paella, or serving more tortillas and vegetables in relation to meat in a fajita recipe)
● Switching cooking methods (for example, oven-baking samosas instead of deep-frying; oven-roasting aubergine slices for moussaka instead of frying them in olive oil).

The example shown in Table 13.9 below shows how

a traditional recipe for sole mornay can be modified to make it healthier. The modified version ends up much lower in fat (particularly saturated fat) and calories because the sauce is made with semi-skimmed milk and unsaturated margarine. The sauce is then finished with fromage frais and flavoured with smaller amounts of Parmesan instead of large quantities of high-fat Gruyère cheese.

Table 13.9 Modifying a traditional recipe for sole mornay to create a healthier version

Traditional sole mornay ♥	Modified sole mornay ♡
Béchamel sauce made with butter, flour, whole milk Egg yolks and cream used to finish sauce Large quantities of Gruyère cheese used to flavour dish	Béchamel sauce made with polyunsaturated margarine, flour and semi-skimmed milk Fromage frais and small quantities of Parmesan used to add flavour and texture
Per portion: 28.0 g fat 15.7 g saturated fat 420 kcals	*Per portion:* 11.8 g fat 3.5 g saturated fat 272 kcals

Balancing plates

The next level of balance comes within individual courses. The idea is to:

- Boost amounts of starchy foods, which can be done in lots of different ways (for example, adding bread rolls, increasing portion sizes of potatoes, rice or pasta, using thicker dough for pizza)
- Increasing the content of vegetables by, for example:
  - serving more vegetables (variety and amount) with the main course
  - adding side salads
  - garnishing dishes with bunches of watercress or rocket
  - serving cucumber or fresh tomato relishes with curries
  - offering more dishes where vegetables are integral (for example, moussaka, boeuf bourguignon)
- Maximising the fruit content of puddings (for example, using fruit coulis instead of cream; increasing the proportion of fruit in classic dishes like apple charlotte and tarte tatin; decorating classic cold desserts with combinations of fresh fruit).

The example shown in Table 13.10 below indicates how the balance of an individual course can change depend-

ing on the recipes used and accompaniments chosen from a menu.

Table 13.10 Comparison of fat content in a main course

Higher-fat main course ♥	Lower-fat main course ♡
Traditional sole mornay recipe using béchamel sauce made with whole milk and flavoured with cream and Gruyère cheese Sauté potatoes Grilled mushrooms	Modified sole mornay recipe using béchamel sauce made with semi-skimmed milk and flavoured with fromage frais and Parmesan New potatoes Broccoli and carrots
Per course: 45.3 g fat 18.0 g saturated fat 688 kcals	*Per course:* 12.3 g fat 3.5 g saturated fat 380 kcals

Balancing complete meals

Chefs can help customers to balance individual courses so meals consumed are healthier. For example, higher-fat first courses (like deep-fried Camembert, or avocado stuffed with cream cheese and walnuts) can be balanced with lower-fat main courses (for example, steamed sole with garlic, spring onion and ginger) and again with lower-fat desserts (for example, fruit sorbets or strawberry pavlova). The example given in Table 13.11 below shows how consistently lower-fat choices across a menu, together with small changes to a traditional recipe, can improve the 'health profile' of a complete meal.

Table 13.11 'Health profile' of a complete meal

Higher-fat meal	Lower-fat meal
Duck and chicken terrine Sole mornay (traditional recipe) with sauté potatoes and grilled mushrooms Sticky toffee pudding with butterscotch sauce	Terrine of chicken and vegetables Sole mornay (modified recipe) with new potatoes, broccoli and carrots Pears in red wine
Per meal: 128 g fat 64.2 g saturated fat 1995 kcals	*Per meal:* 29.8 g fat 12.9 g saturated fat 769 kcals

Balancing menus

In terms of healthy eating, chefs have a delicate pathway to tread. Some customers will want to indulge themselves and forget about fat and calories, while others will be consistently looking for healthier choices and ways to control calories. The demand for healthier choices will be particularly high in 'everyday eating environments' like workplace restaurants or venues that serve business lunches. In addition, the food culture in the UK has undergone a revolution over the last decade. There is now a much stronger emphasis on the highest-quality fresh ingredients put together to craft dishes that reflect many of the principles of healthy eating. Following these rules, creative chefs can help people understand that healthy eating does not necessarily have to be brown and boring.

Never before has the demand for healthier options been higher. For these reasons chefs need to consider including:

- A variety of fish dishes (white fish is lower in fat than meat, and oily fish like salmon, fresh tuna or trout contains beneficial omega-3 fats)
- A wide range of exciting vegetable dishes (if people are going to reach their five-a-day goal, they need to learn to love vegetables, and chefs can play a vital role in helping people try something different – for example, roasted butternut squash, steamed asparagus, mashed celeriac or stir-fried pak choi)
- Pasta dishes, which inherently contain proportionately more starch than other types of dishes, or adding bread to meals or using thicker dough in pizza dishes
- Desserts based on, or including, fruit (for example, pears in red wine, blackcurrant sorbet, apple crumble, vacherin with strawberries and half-fat crème fraîche).

In this way chefs can help people achieve the sort of dietary balance required over time, as depicted below. The eatwell plate shows the proportions of different food groups that make up a healthy eating pattern.

Fat facts

This chapter has talked a lot about fat. One of the key drivers in healthy catering is to reduce fat in recipes; the other is to change the type of fat used from saturated to unsaturated (including monounsaturated and polyunsaturated fats). Foods contain different types of fats in varying amounts. Generally, foods of animal origin contain predominantly saturated fats (which are solid at room temperature) and foods from vegetable sources tend to contain much more of the healthier unsaturated fats (which are liquid at room temperature). Many commercial spreads and margarines contain a mixture of saturated and unsaturated fats. Softer spreads tend to

contain more unsaturated fats (for example, sunflower spreads) and harder 'block' margarines are usually predominantly saturated. See Table 13.12 for more information about saturated and unsaturated fats.

Table 13.12 Foods containing saturated and unsaturated fat

Saturated fat	Unsaturated fat
Lard, suet, hard margarine Butter Fat in meat Dairy products like cheese Hidden in cakes, pastries, biscuits Egg yolk	**Monounsaturated** Olive, rapeseed, groundnut oils **Polyunsaturated** Sunflower spread and oil, corn and soya oils **Beneficial omega-3 fats** Oily fish like salmon, trout, fresh tuna

The concept of reducing fat in products, but at the same time moving towards unsaturated fats, is often difficult for people to translate into practice. An example of the direction of required change is given in the examples shown in Table 13.13 below.

Table 13.13 Sandwiches: traditional versus healthier options

Traditional sandwich ♥	Healthier sandwich ♡
Two slices of well-buttered white bread Filled with large portion of Cheddar cheese (60 g)	Two thick slices of wholegrain bread spread thinly with low-fat polyunsaturated spread Filling of cold chicken, teaspoon of low-calorie mayonnaise Salad vegetables additionally packed into sandwich
Per sandwich: 41.4 g fat 25.9 g saturated fat 558 kcals	*Per sandwich:* 7.6 g fat 1.9 g saturated fat 289 kcals

Reducing fat and cholesterol levels in the diet

For those wishing to reduce fat and cholesterol levels in the diet, the following suggestions may be useful.

Consider, where suitable, using:

- Oils and fats high in monosaturates and polyunsaturates in place of hard fats

The eatwell plate

Use the eatwell plate to help you get the balance right. It shows how much of what you eat should come from each food group.

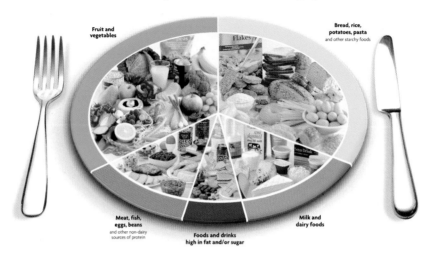

The eatwell plate

- The minimum of salt or low-sodium salt
- Wholemeal flour in place of, or partly in place of, white flour
- Natural yoghurt, quark or fromage frais (all lower in fat) in place of cream
- Skimmed milk, or semi-skimmed, instead of full-cream milk
- Minimum amounts of sugar or, in some cases, reduced-calorie sweeteners
- Low-fat cheese instead of full-fat cheese.

Many of the recipes in this book have been adjusted, incorporating some of these principles as alternatives to be used as and when required. Where we state oil, sunflower oil is recommended other than for fierce heat; in such instances pomace olive oil is more suitable. When yoghurt is stated, we mean natural yoghurt with a low fat content.

Table 13.14 offers an example of how traditional recipe ingredients may be replaced by healthier ones.

Table 13.14 Substituting healthier recipe ingredients

Instead of	Choose
Whole milk	Skimmed milk (or semi-skimmed)
Butter or hard margarine	Polyunsaturated margarine
Lard, hard vegetable fats	Pure vegetable oils, e.g. corn oil, sunflower oil
Full-fat cheeses, e.g. Cheddar	Low-fat cheeses, e.g. low-fat Cheddar has half the fat
Fatty meats	Lean meats (smaller portion), or chicken or fish
Cream	Plain yoghurt, quark, smetana, fromage frais

A number of non-dairy creamers are now available. Some are produced specifically for pastry work and, being sweetened, are unsuitable for savoury recipes. However, there are also various unsweetened products that may be used in place of fresh cream for soups, sauces, and so on. It is important to determine the heat stability of these products before use, that is, by testing whether they will withstand boiling without detriment to the product.

Table 13.15 indicates which cooking oils, fats and margarines are healthiest, that is, those with the smallest percentage of saturated fats.

Table 13.15 Comparison of cooking oils, fats and margarines showing levels of different types of fat

Oil/fat	Saturated %	Monounsaturated %	Polyunsaturated %
Coconut oil	85	7	2
Butter	60	32	3
Palm oil	45	42	8
Lard	43	42	8
Beef dripping	40	49	4
Margarine, hard (vegetable oil only)	37	47	12
Margarine, hard (mixed oils)	37	43	17
Margarine, soft	32	42	22
Margarine, soft (mixed oils)	30	45	19
Low-fat spread	27	38	30
Margarine, polyunsaturated	24	22	54
Ground nut oil	19	48	28
Maize oil	16	29	49
Wheatgerm oil	14	11	45
Soya bean oil	14	70	11
Sunflower seed oil	13	32	50
Safflower seed oil	10	13	72
Rapeseed oil	7	64	32

A word about salt

There is now strong evidence that points to the need for us to cut back on salt intake for our health. Currently, average daily intakes are around 9 g and we all need to ensure that we consume no more than 6 g/day (even less for children). Up to 80 per cent of this is hidden in everyday foods (like bread, breakfast cereals, baked beans and meat products) bought from the supermarket and some manufacturers are gradually reducing levels of salt in their products. It is important to check the label (see box). In addition, food eaten away from home can also contain significant amounts of salt.

Chefs can help customers drive down their salt intakes by being very careful about:

- The products they use in the kitchen: for example, many commercial bouillons, soups and sauce preparations have high levels of salt
- The amount of salt they add to recipes: a heaped teaspoon holds about 8 g salt, so adding one of these to a four-portion recipe will bump up someone's salt intake by around 2 g, which is a considerable part of the 6 g maximum daily allowance.

Salt or sodium? Checking the label

Most food labels show the amount of sodium per 100 g rather than salt per serving.
To convert sodium to salt you need to multiply the amount of sodium by 2.5 (1 g sodium = 2.5 g salt)
An adult should have less than 6 g salt/day = 2.4 g sodium.

A quick guide
A *lot of salt* in food is more than 0.5 g sodium/portion (or per 100 g for main meals).
A *little salt* in food is less than 0.1 g sodium/portion (or per 100 g for main meals).

Further resources

- *The Allergy Cookbook*, by Stephanie Lash Ford (Ashgrove Press, 1983)
- *The New Allergy Diet*, by J. Hunter, E. Workman and J. Woolner (Vermilion, 2000).
- *The Allergy Handbook*, by Keith Mumby (Thorsons, 1988)
- *Food Allergy and Intolerance*, by Jonathan Brostoff and Linda Gamlin (Bloomsbury, 1998)
- *HCIMA Technical Brief* No. 43
- *National Institute of Allergy and Infectious Diseases* www.niaid.nih.gov
- *Dietary Reference Values for Food Energy and Nutrients for the United Kingdom* (Department of Health, 1991)
  Sets the current main benchmarks for nutrient intakes in the UK. Available from the Stationery Office.
- *Catering For Health* (Department of Health/Food Standards Agency, 2001)
  Provides further detail on nutrition, plus practical advice on how to integrate healthy eating principles into catering practice. Available from the Stationery Office for £5.00.
- *Catering For Health: The Recipe File* (The Stationery Office, 1988)
  Provides healthier recipe ideas for caterers. Available from the Stationery Office.
- *Tipping The Balance* (1999)
  A 23-minute video on practical tips aimed at encouraging healthier catering practice in the workplace. Available from the Food Standards Agency.
- *The Balance of Good Health* (1996)
  A pictorial model for food selection. Available in A4 leaflet or A3 poster format. Available from the Food Standards Agency (see www.food.gov.uk). The FSA's website is a useful source of valuable information on healthy eating relevant to caterers.

Appendix 1: Food safety and business

A business with sound food safety practices in place will see many benefits as a result. These include the following:

- It is less likely that food safety problems will occur or that a food poisoning outbreak will be linked to the business
- The business is not breaking the law
- There will be greater customer confidence and fewer complaints
- There will be less food waste
- There will be less likelihood of problems with pests
- The business will be a pleasant workplace for staff, which should result in higher productivity
- Cleaning processes will be efficient and easier to complete
- The running costs of the business will be lower
- The future of the business will be more secure, and so will the employment of the staff.

Poor food safety practices will have negative effects on a business, including:

- Possible legal costs from civil action and legal action
- Loss of customer confidence, and poor reputation of the business and its products
- Production halted, causing loss of income and therefore loss of profit
- Reduced market share in the local area
- Loss of staff/difficulty in recruiting new staff
- Increased costs because of inefficiency and the cost of putting the business back on track
- Spoilage and wastage of food stocks.

Appendix 2: Reported cases of food poisoning

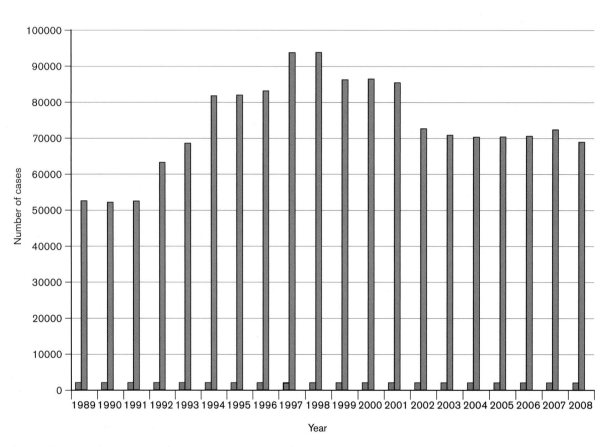

Cases of reported food poisoning (England and Wales figures)
Source: Health Protection Agency

Appendix 3: Food safety legislation and food premises

This appendix outlines the main food safety legislation affecting supervisors of food premises.

In 2006, there was an update of the existing food safety legislation for England. Most things stayed the same but were brought into line with EU legislation, and it became law for all food premises to have a **Food Safety Management System** based on the principles of **HACCP**, including all the relevant documentation that goes with that system.

Before the changes in 2006, the main acts covering food safety were the Food Safety Act 1990 and related regulations. These were concerned mainly with food standards.

Under the 1990 Act it is an offence:

- To render food injurious to health
- To sell food which fails to comply with food safety requirements
- To sell food which is unfit
- To sell food that is not reasonable to eat in the state it is offered
- To sell food that is not of the nature, substance or quality demanded by the customer:
  - 'Not of the nature demanded' means different to the food that was asked for
  - 'Not of the substance demanded' means not of the required composition
  - 'Not of the quality demanded' means, for example, that the food has deteriorated.

Food Hygiene (England) Regulations 2006

Part 1

Part 1 defines many of the key words used in the legislation, for example, the meaning of 'food', 'premises' and 'Enforcement Officer'. (These are also covered in the main text.)

Part 1 also states that it is presumed that any food found on premises was intended for human consumption.

Part 2 (Hygiene improvement notices)

If an authorised officer thinks there is a lack of compliance with the regulations, he or she may serve the business with one of the following:

- Hygiene improvement notice
- Hygiene prohibition order
- Hygiene emergency prohibition order/notice.

This is covered under regulations 6, 7 and 8. For more information about these notices and orders, see pages 37–8.

Part 3 Administration and enforcement

Regulations 12 and 13 state that an authorised officer may buy or take any food, substance or material that could be used for evidence. The samples may be examined or analysed if required.

Regulations 14 and 15 state that authorised officers have powers of entry to premises at any reasonable time and must be given access to relevant records. It is an offence to obstruct an officer or to give misleading information.

Regulations 17 and 18 are about offences and the resulting penalties. A person guilty of non-compliance would be liable to:

- Summary conviction in a magistrates' court (maximum fine £5,000)
- Conviction at a crown court (imprisonment for up to 2 years and/or an unlimited fine).

A corporate body can be guilty of the same offences.

Regulations 20, 21 and 22 make it possible to appeal against decisions. This could be in a magistrates' court or crown court. Regulation 22 is specifically about appeals against improvement notices and remedial action notices.

Part 4 Temperature control regulations

Chill holding

Chilled food that is likely to support the growth of microorganisms must be kept at or below 8°C, unless:

- It is a low risk food meant to be kept at ambient temperatures
- It has gone through a process to make it safe, e.g. canning
- It needs to be at ambient temperature to ripen
- It will go through a process to make it safe
- It is covered by other marketing standards, e.g. eggs
- The food producer/processor can prove there is another process in place to keep the food safe.

There is also a defence for keeping foods above 8°C if:

- It was on display or waiting for service on one occasion, for not more than 4 hours

- It was being taken to a vehicle or area where it would be kept below 8°C
- It was hot food
- Time needs to be allowed for processing and preparation of food
- Equipment is being defrosted/cleaned
- There has been a temporary breakdown of equipment
- There are measures in place compliant with food safety legislation.

Hot holding

Hot food should be kept at a temperature of 63°C or above to control the growth of pathogens/toxins. It is permitted to store it at a lower temperature if:

- It has been cooked/reheated
- It is displayed for service/sale (for a maximum of 2 hours).

There is also a defence for keeping foods below 63°C if:

- A scientific assessment has concluded that it is safe to do so
- The food has been out of temperature control for less than 2 hours on one occasion only.

Regulation (EC) No. 852/2004 – Hygiene of Foodstuffs

These new regulations came into force in January 2006, replacing the Food Safety (General Food Hygiene Regulations) 1990 and 1995 regulations.

Most of the requirements remained the same. The main changes were:

- All food businesses must be registered with the local authority (Article 6).
- All food businesses must have a suitable food safety management system based on the principles of HACCP. Relevant records related to this system must be kept and be available for inspection.

Annex ii

Chapter i – General requirements

This deals with food premises and their design, siting, layout, size, design, construction, etc.

The requirements apply particularly to:
- adequate refrigerated storage

- allowing maintenance and cleaning/disinfection to take place properly
- protection against pests
- adequate ventilation
- protection against all kinds of contamination
- allowing for good hygienic practices.

There must be adequate toilet facilities not opening onto the main kitchen, facilities for effective hand-washing, and changing facilities for staff.

Lighting must be sufficient for work carried out and to allow cleaning to take place; cleaning materials must be kept away from where food is handled; drainage must be suitable for the work being completed.

Chapter ii – Specific requirements

This deals with specific requirements for rooms where foodstuffs are prepared, processed or treated.

The design and layout of fittings and equipment must permit good hygiene practices and help prevent contamination.

Items discussed and considered are floors, walls, ceilings, windows, doors, surfaces and facilities for washing equipment and food. All of these items must be well maintained and in sound condition.

Generally surfaces must be impervious, non-toxic, prevent accumulation of dirt, be easy to clean and disinfect, avoid contamination of any kind, discourage pests.

Chapter iii

Chapter iii deals with temporary food premises, for example, marquees, market stalls, vehicles and vending machines.

These must all be designed, constructed, cleaned and maintained in good repair/condition to avoid any contamination.

- Appropriate personal hygiene facilities must be provided (toilet, hand wash, changing facilities).
- Surfaces used for food should be easy to clean and disinfect, and suitable for the task.
- There must be adequate provision for cleaning/disinfection to take place and hygienic food washing to take place.
- There must be adequate supplies of hot, cold and potable water.
- There must be adequate temperature control equipment.
- Suitable provision must be made for the removal of waste.
- Food must be protected from contamination.

Chapter iv – Transport

Vehicles for transporting foodstuffs must be clean and maintained in good repair to protect food from contamination and allow cleaning and disinfection. Where necessary, vehicles must be capable of maintaining the required temperature of food.

Chapter v – Equipment

Food equipment must be:

- Effectively cleaned/disinfected at a frequency to avoid contamination
- Made of materials that allow cleaning and disinfection and minimise risk of contamination
- Installed in a way that allows cleaning/disinfection of the equipment itself and the surrounding areas.

Chapter vi – Food waste

- Adequate provision must be made for waste.

- Waste must be removed from food rooms as quickly as possible to avoid accumulation.
- Waste should be stored in closable containers of sound construction that allow cleaning and disinfection.
- Refuse areas should be managed and cleaned to keep them free of pests.
- Waste must be dealt with in a hygienic, environmentally friendly way and avoid being a source of contamination.

Chapter vii – Water supply

- There must be an adequate supply of potable water to ensure that food is not contaminated.
- Ice must be made from potable water
- Ice must be properly stored to protect it from contamination.

Chapter viii

Everyone working in a food handling area must maintain a high degree of personal cleanliness, wear suitable clean clothing/overclothing.

No one who is suffering from or is a carrier of a disease that can be transmitted through food, or who has skin infections, sores, vomiting or diarrhoea, must handle food. They must not enter the food area if there is any possibility of contamination.

Any person affected by the above who is likely to come into contact with food must report the illness/symptoms to the owner/manager/supervisor.

Chapter x – Provisions applicable to food

- Raw foods/ingredients must not be accepted if they are suspected of being contaminated and would still be unfit to consume after processing.
- Storage of foods/ingredients must be in appropriate conditions to prevent harmful deterioration and contamination.
- Food must be protected from contamination that would make it unfit for consumption.
- Procedures must be in place to control pests and the entry of pests (including domestic animals) to areas where food is prepared.
- Raw materials and any foods likely to support the growth of pathogenic microorganisms or toxins must not be kept at temperatures that may result in a risk to health. For practical reasons some limited time out of temperature control is permissible (see above). When food is to be

served cold/chilled, it must be cooled as quickly as possible to chill temperatures.

- Frozen foods must be thawed in a way that minimises the risk of growth of pathogens and formation of toxins which could be a risk to health.
- Hazardous or inedible items must be labelled and stored in separate secure containers.

Chapter xi – Wrapping and packaging

- Materials for wrapping and packaging food must not cause contamination, and must not be stored where they are exposed to contamination.
- Wrapping and packaging must be carried out in a way that avoids contamination: cleanliness must be assured.

Chapter xii – Training

Food businesses must ensure that:

- Food handlers are supervised/instructed/trained as required for their work activity
- Those responsible for setting up and maintaining a HACCP system must have received suitable training in the principles of HACCP.

Appendix 4: Disinfectants

Disinfectants must be suitable for kitchens and food areas. Select a disinfectant that has a BS (British Standard) 2462, 5305 or 6424.

Normal hypochlorites (bleach) are very efficient in killing bacteria and are inexpensive, but they are corrosive to metals, irritate skin and can cause burns. They also have a strong smell that can taint food, utensils and equipment.

Disinfectants work best at room temperature (but follow individual manufacturer's instructions). Always dilute correctly, allow sufficient contact time and rinse off correctly, all according to manufacturer's instructions.

 ## Disinfectant types

Quaternary ammonium compounds

Quaternary ammonium compounds (QAC) are taint-free, odour-free and non-corrosive, so they are very useful for kitchen and other food areas. QACs can usually be left on a surface and do not need extra rinsing. Always carefully follow instructions for use.

QACs may be rendered less effective by hard water, organic soiling and some plastics. Manufacturers sometimes include additives to overcome this.

Biguanides

Biguanides are similar to QACs but are more efficient and perform better. They often form the 'disinfectant content' of sanitisers, and are included in specific glass-washing products.

Amphoterics

Amphoterics have very low toxicity, are non-corrosive and will not taint or leave an odour. They tend to be very efficient disinfectants but are expensive for general use.

Peroxy compounds

Peroxy compounds are strong disinfectants that can work well even at temperatures as low as 0°C. They tend to be used in agricultural settings such as dairies.

Alcohols

Alcohols are used when quick and efficient disinfection is needed without the use of water, and where the more usual methods cannot be used.

Alcohol hand rubs are provided throughout hospitals and increasingly at the entrances of other buildings. They are also available in gel and disposable wipes for small items such as food probes that may need to be quickly disinfected between uses. They are typically a mixture of a suitable alcohol and a QAC.

Normal hypochlorites (bleach)

Normal hypochlorites are efficient and inexpensive disinfectants that are widely available, but they are not suitable for use in kitchen areas.

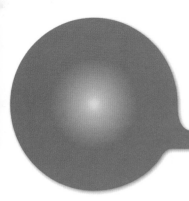

Appendix 5: Salmonella

There are over 2,000 known serotypes of salmonella, with new strains emerging frequently. However, not all salmonella causes illness in humans: the strains most associated with food poisoning are salmonella typhimurium and salmonella enteritidis.

Salmonella typhimurium

Salmonella typhimurium lives in the gastrointestinal tract of many animal species, where it usually causes no problems. However, if it multiplies in food it can cause salmonellosis (food poisoning), 6 to 48 hours after eating the contaminated food (usually poultry or beef).

Illness may begin with nausea and vomiting, often followed by diarrhoea. In healthy adults the disease is very unpleasant and uncomfortable, usually followed by a speedy full recovery. However, it is much more serious in the young, the old and those with other medical conditions. The fatality rate can be as high as 5 to 10 per cent in nurseries and nursing homes. The incidence of food poisoning from this organism has decreased in recent years in developed countries, primarily because of modern methods of animal husbandry, food preparation, and distribution.

Salmonella enteritidis

Salmonella enteritidis is mostly associated with eggs, though occasionally with meat. The organism may be inside eggs and on the shells, and so eggs are a potential cause of illness, especially if they are raw or undercooked. Thorough cooking of eggs is recommended, especially for those in the high risk groups. Handling eggs may lead to cross-contamination, so take care and use good hygiene practices when handling them.

A person infected with the salmonella enteritidis bacterium usually has fever, abdominal cramps and diarrhoea beginning 12 to 72 hours after consuming the contaminated food. The illness usually lasts 4 to 7 days, and most persons recover quickly. However, the diarrhoea can be severe, and occasionally the person may be ill enough to require hospital treatment.

The elderly, babies and those with impaired immune systems may have a more severe illness. In these cases, the infection may spread from the intestines to the blood stream, and then to other body sites; it can cause severe illness and even death unless the person is treated promptly.

Typhoid fever (salmonella typhi)

Typhoid fever is an acute illness caused by the salmonella typhi bacteria. Salmonella paratyphi is a related bacterium that usually causes a less severe illness. The bacteria are deposited in water or food by a human carrier and are then spread to other people.

Symptoms of typhoid include fever, exhaustion, slow pulse rates, red spots on the abdomen, constipation and/or diarrhoea.

The incidence of typhoid fever in the UK has decreased rapidly since the early 1900s. Today, most cases occur in people who have recently have travelled to areas where the disease is still a problem. India, Pakistan and Egypt are known high-risk areas for developing this disease.

Worldwide, typhoid fever affects more than 13 million people annually, with over 500,000 dying of the disease.

Those suffering or who have recently suffered from this disease must not handle food and must not return to food handling until they have had six negative faecal samples confirmed by their doctor.

Appendix 6: Scores on the Doors

The Scores on the Doors scheme is fully supported by the Food Standards Agency.

Star ratings are allocated by Environmental Health Officers when they inspect food premises. Currently it is not a mandatory requirement to display the scores, although it is very much encouraged. All the scores of all premises visited can be seen on the internet.

The scoring system is based on the following three criteria taken from the Food Standards Agency's statutory risk rating system:

- The current level of compliance of food hygiene practices and procedures
- The current level of compliance relating to structure and cleanliness of premises
- Confidence in management of the business and food safety controls.

The star ratings have the following meanings:

***** Excellent: very high standards of food safety management; fully compliant with all food safety legislation.

**** Very good: good food safety management; high standards of compliance with food safety legislation.

*** Good: good level of legal compliance; some more effort is required.

** Broadly compliant: broadly compliant with food safety legislation but more effort is needed to meet legal requirements.

* Poor: poor level of compliance with food safety legislation; much more effort needed.

No stars Very poor: a general failure to comply with legal requirements; little or no appreciation of food safety; major effort for improvement needed.

Table A1 The risk rating system

Risk rating categories	Excellent					Poor
Food hygiene and safety	0	5	10	15	20	25
Structure and cleaning	0	5	10	15	20	25
Management/control	0	5	10	15	20	25

Index